Study Guide for
Leadership
and
Nursing Care
Management

THIRD EDITION

D1254638

Study Guide for
Leadership
and
Nursing Care Management

THIRD EDITION

Jean Nagelkerk, PhD, APRN, BC

Assistant Vice-President for Academic Affairs and
Professor of Nursing
Grand Valley State University
Grand Rapids, Michigan

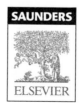
SAUNDERS

ELSEVIER

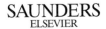

11830 Westline Industrial Drive
St. Louis, Missouri 63146

STUDY GUIDE FOR LEADERSHIP AND NURSING CARE MANAGEMENT
Copyright © 2006, Elsevier Inc.

ISBN-13: 978-1-4160-3161-1
ISBN-10: 1-4160-3161-8

NOTICE

Previous editions copyrighted 2000, 1996

ISBN-13: 978-1-4160-3161-1
ISBN-10: 1-4160-3161-8

Senior Editor: Yvonne Alexopoulos
Developmental Editor: Kristin Hebberd
Editorial Assistant: Sarah Vales
Publishing Services Manager: John Rogers
Project Manager: Helen Hudlin
Designer: Amy Buxton

Printed in the United States of America

Last digit is print number: 9 8 7 6 5 4 3 2

Contents

Answers to Text Study Questions revised by:
Lori Houghton-Rahrig, MSN, APRN, BC
Affiliate Instructor of Nursing
Kirkhof College of Nursing
Grand Valley State University
Grand Rapids, Michigan

Study Guide for
Leadership
and
Nursing Care
Management

THIRD EDITION

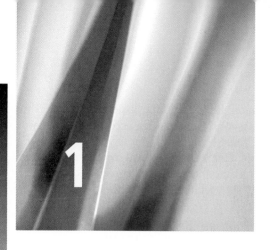

Leadership Principles

STUDY FOCUS

Nursing is a service profession with nurses filling two basic roles: (1) care provider and (2) care manager. In these roles, leadership is important to build teams, spark innovation, create positive communication, and accomplish goals. Leadership is crucial in health care because relentless change is affecting the organization, delivery, and financing of services. Leadership is the process of influencing people to accomplish goals by inspiring confidence and support among followers. Skill at interpersonal relationships and applying the problem-solving process is fundamental to leadership. Strong leadership empowers individuals and instills in them a belief and confidence in their ability to achieve and succeed. In contrast, *management* is the process of influencing employees to work toward the goals of the organization by integrating resources through planning, organizing, coordinating, directing, and controlling. Managers obtain power to accomplish objectives from their position and title.

The role of the leader is to facilitate the development of effective support systems to generate efficiencies directed to improving processes. *Leadership styles* are combinations of task and relationship behaviors used to influence others to accomplish goals. *Followership* is an interpersonal process of participating by following. *Empowerment* is the giving of authority, responsibility, and freedom to act. Empowerment instills in a person a belief and confidence in his or her ability to achieve. There are three levels of leadership. The individual level of leadership involves activities such as mentoring, coaching, and motivating others. The group level of leadership involves building teams and resolving conflict. The organizational level of leadership involves building culture.

The *five interwoven aspects of leadership* are (1) the leader, (2) the follower, (3) the situation, (4) the communication process, and (5) the goals (Kison, 1989). Leaders' values, experiences, skills, and expertise are important ingredients in their ability to lead effectively. *Transactional leaders* function in a caretaker role focusing on day-to-day operations. *Transformational leaders* motivate followers to perform to their full potential and provide a sense of direction. *Followers* reject or accept the leader and determine their own level of participation and the leader's power within the group. Followers may exhibit the *Pygmalion effect;* that is, acting according to what the leader expects. The situation includes the work to be done, control systems, available resources, the amount of time, the level of interaction, and the external forces affecting the type of decision task. The communication process is the vital means for leaders and followers to send and receive clear messages, verbal and nonverbal, through formal and informal channels. The goals include the organizational, personal, and professional goals of the leader and followers.

Leadership characteristics include taking risks, communicating a vision, empowering the followership, mastering change, and motivating groups to achieve goals. Effective leaders know that a leader is someone who has followers, leaders are visible and set examples, and leadership is not rank, but responsibility. Leadership is not popularity; leadership is results. Many leadership theories may be categorized as trait, attitudinal, or situational. *Trait theories* emphasize the characteristics of the leader; *attitudinal theories* measure attitudes toward leader behavior, and *situational theories* focus on leader behaviors and how leadership style can be matched to the situation. Examples of different leadership theories include attitudinal leadership, situational leadership, Fiedler's contingency, and Hersey and Blanchard's tri-dimensional leader effectiveness model. Kouzes and Posner (1987) identify five behaviors correlated with leadership excellence. These behaviors are challenging the process, inspiring shared vision, enabling others to act, modeling the way, and encouraging the heart. Leadership style often is discussed in terms of task and relational behavior. *Task behavior* is the extent to which leaders organize roles, explain activities, and manage work, whereas *relationship behavior* is maintaining personal relationships through supportive behaviors.

Three styles of leadership are authoritarian, democratic, and laissez-faire. *Authoritarian leadership* refers to directive and controlling behaviors by which the leader in isolation determines policies and makes decisions and then orders subordinates to carry out the tasks or work. This style is helpful in crisis situations. *Democratic leadership* is a team approach whereby the leader facilitates and coordinates material and human resources and shares responsibility for decision making and quality improvement. All members of the group are encouraged to participate actively in a cohesive fashion to accomplish team objectives. The democratic leadership style is useful when professional staff work together to establish and meet goals. A *laissez-faire leader* is one who does not interfere in decision making or policy setting through preference or incompetence. This style may be useful with highly qualified professionals who work well in teams to accomplish established goals.

Contemporary leadership research shows that a new view of leadership is emerging in which connectedness and relationships facilitate organizational work. *Quantum leadership* is one way to facilitate work by fostering an environment of curiosity, questioning, and exploration. *Servant leadership* is also a method of facilitating work by leaders who focus on serving others and nurturing autonomy and personal growth. The *feminist perspective* complements quantum and servant leadership by leader's building connections, empowering others, and supporting personal growth to promote team work and to accomplish work goals.

Nurse leaders are challenged in today's rapidly changing practice environment. They need to exert effective leadership in order to effect positive organizational and individual productivity. At a national level, nurses, representing the largest health care profession in the United States, need to band together to provide leadership and direction in health care delivery. Nurses also must provide leadership in advocating positive health care practices for clients and communities. The nursing leadership challenge is to develop strategies that help followers cope with change and develop the ability to adapt in a positive and productive way.

LEARNING TOOLS

Task Orientation and People Orientation Leadership Questionnaire: An Assessment of Style*

Purpose

To assess your leadership style in the areas of task and people orientation and to assess your leadership style profile in relation to autocratic, shared (democratic), and laissez-faire leadership.

---

*The T-P Leadership Questionnaire was adapted from Sergiovanni, Metzcus, and Burden's (1969) revision of the Leadership Behavior Description Questionnaire, American Educational Research Journal 6, *62-79.*

Directions

The following items describe aspects of leadership behavior. Respond to each item according to the way you would most likely act if you were the leader of a work group. Circle whether you would most likely behave in the described way: always (A), frequently (F), occasionally (O), seldom (S), or never (N).

A F O S N   1. I would most likely act as the spokesman of the group.

A F O S N   2. I would encourage overtime work.

A F O S N   3. I would allow members complete freedom in their work.

A F O S N   4. I would encourage the use of uniform procedures.

A F O S N   5. I would permit the members to use their own judgment in solving problems.

A F O S N   6. I would stress being ahead of competing groups.

A F O S N   7. I would speak as a representative of the group.

A F O S N   8. I would needle members for greater effort.

A F O S N   9. I would try out my ideas in the group.

A F O S N   10. I would let the members do their work the way they think best.

A F O S N   11. I would be working hard for a promotion.

A F O S N   12. I would tolerate postponement and uncertainty.

A F O S N   13. I would speak for the group if there were visitors present.

A F O S N   14. I would keep the work moving at a rapid pace.

A F O S N   15. I would turn the members loose on a job and let them go to it.

A F O S N   16. I would settle conflicts when they occur in the group.

A F O S N   17. I would get swamped by details.

A F O S N   18. I would represent the group at outside meetings.

A F O S N   19. I would be reluctant to allow the members any freedom of action.

A F O S N   20. I would decide what should be done and how it should be done.

A F O S N   21. I would push for increased production.

A F O S N   22. I would let some members have authority which I could keep.

A F O S N   23. Things would usually turn out as I had predicted.

A F O S N   24. I would allow the group a high degree of initiative.

A F O S N   25. I would assign group members to particular tasks.

A F O S N   26. I would be willing to make changes.

A F O S N   27. I would ask the members to work harder.

A F O S N   28. I would trust the group members to exercise good judgment.

A F O S N   29. I would schedule the work to be done.

A F O S N   30. I would refuse to explain my actions.

A F O S N   31. I would persuade others that my ideas are to their advantage.

A F O S N   32. I would permit the group to set its own pace.

A F O S N   33. I would urge the group to beat its previous record.

A F O S N   34. I would act without consulting the group.

A F O S N   35. I would ask that group members follow standard rules and regulations.

T _____   P _____

Scoring

1. Circle the item number for items 8, 12, 17, 18, 19, 30, 34, and 35. Write the number 1 in front of a circled item number if you responded S (seldom) or N (never) to that item.

2. Write a number 1 in front of item numbers not circled if you responded A (always) or F (frequently). Circle the number 1s which you have written in front of the following items: 3, 5, 8, 10, 15, 18, 19, 22, 24, 26, 28, 30, 32, 34, and 35.

3. Count the circled number 1s. This is your score for concern for people. Record the score in the blank following the letter P at the end of the questionnaire.

4. Count the uncircled number 1s. This is your score for concern for task. Record this number in the blank following the letter T.

Awareness of your leadership style will help you to tailor your responses in personal or work situations. You will be able to compare your perception of how people and task oriented you are with a score of how you respond in specific situations. The next step is to determine if your score matches your desired response and determine whether to continue your present leadership style or to make changes to become more participatory (if you score high on autocratic leadership style) or more directive (if you score high on laissez-faire leadership style).

Task-Orientation and People-Orientation Leadership Style Profile Sheet

Directions

To determine your style of leadership, see the diagram on p. 4 and mark your score on the concern for task dimension (T) on the left-hand arrow. Next, move to the right-hand arrow and mark your score on the concern for people dimension (P). Draw a straight line that intersects the P and T scores. The point at which the line crosses the shared leadership arrow indicates your score on that dimension.

Shared Leadership Results from Balancing Concern for Task and Concern for People

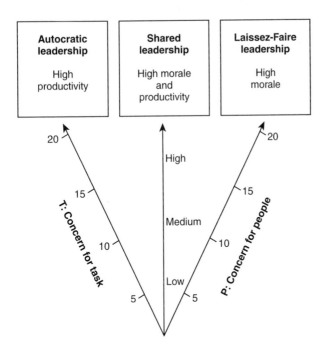

From Pfeiffer, J. W., & Jones, J. E. (1974). *A handbook of structured experiences for human relations training* (Vol. 1). San Diego, CA: Pfeiffer & Company.

CASE STUDY

Jennifer Yaur is the nurse manager of a 68-bed respiratory unit with 95 employees. Nurse Yaur tailors her leadership style according to the employees' needs, experience, and situation. She is helping a graduate nurse who is in orientation to learn how to use the documentation forms. Nurse Yaur provides detailed instructions to the new nurse, explaining step-by-step the process for documentation. In another situation, Nurse Yaur asks a seasoned clinical nurse to take responsibility for the total quality improvement process. She provides the nurse with information and offers to assist any time the clinical nurse needs consultation. Nurse Yaur promotes Susan Young, a clinical nurse, to a 3-11 charge position. Because this is Nurse Young's first management experience, Nurse Yaur is providing a structured orientation but is giving Nurse Young the opportunity to seek out the information she needs and to design learning objectives to meet her needs.

Case Study Questions

1. What type of leadership theory is Nurse Yaur using?
2. What are the benefits of changing the leadership style based on the employee's experience, knowledge, and situation?

3. What is the relationship between followership and leadership?
4. What levels of leadership is Nurse Yaur engaging in the work environment? Provide examples for each level.

LEARNING RESOURCES

Discussion Questions

1. Is a clinical nurse a leader?
2. What are the characteristics of effective leaders? Identify an effective leader.
3. What is situational leadership? Are the three styles of leadership—authoritarian, democratic, and laissez-faire—interchangeable? What are the differences?
4. How can nursing as a profession exhibit leadership in defining policy for health care delivery?
5. According to Kouzes and Posner (1987), what are the five practices common to exceptional leadership achievements?

Study Questions

Fill-in-the-Blank: Identify the appropriate leadership style for the following situations.
1. A code has been called. Which leadership style is most effective in this situation? _____
2. The nursing record is being revised. Which leadership style is most appropriate? _____
3. Nurses, physicians, dietitians, and social workers are working together to increase client services in a hospital. Which leadership style is useful? _____

True or False: Circle the correct answer.

T   F   4. Two critical skills in leadership are interpersonal and problem-solving skills.

T   F   5. Followership is a process whereby leaders participate in group decisions.

T   F   6. Empowerment is the ability to lead a group successfully.

T   F   7. Important skills for leading include diagnosing, adapting, and communicating.

T   F   8. Situational leaders tailor their leadership style based on the employee, experience, and situation.

T   F   9. Laissez-faire leadership entails minimal participation and directing by the leader, resulting in high productivity.

T   F   10. A transactional leader is one who motivates employees to their full potential.

T　F　11. The new role of leader/manager is to facilitate the development of effective support systems to generate efficiencies directed to improving processes.

T　F　12. Popularity is leadership.

T　F　13. Leadership is not rank, but responsibility.

Matching: Write the letter of the correct response in front of each term.

_____ 14. Leadership

_____ 15. Management

_____ 16. Followership

_____ 17. Empowerment

_____ 18. Pygmalion effect

_____ 19. Authoritarian

_____ 20. Democratic

_____ 21. Laissez-faire

A. Decisions are made by the leader, and followers are told what to do

B. Process of influencing people to accomplish goals

C. Instilling in people belief and confidence in their own ability to achieve

D. Coordinating and facilitating teamwork and group decision making

E. Complete freedom of individuals to make choices without direction or interference

F. Interpersonal process of participation

G. A process whereby individuals act according to expectations

H. Coordination of resources by planning, organizing, coordinating, directing, and controlling

REFERENCES

Kison, C. (1989). Leadership: How, who and what? *Nursing Management, 20*(11), 72-74.

Kouzes, J., & Posner, B. (1987). *The leadership challenge.* San Francisco: Jossey-Bass.

SUPPLEMENTAL READINGS

Epitropaki, O. (2004). Implicit leadership theories in applied settings: Factor structure, generalizability, and stability over time. *Journal of Applied Psychology, 89*(2), 293-310.

Fuimano, J. (2004). Add coaching to your leadership repertoire. *Nursing Management, 35*(1), 16-17.

Kleinman, C. S. (2004). Leadership: A key strategy in staff nurse retention. *The Journal of Continuing Education in Nursing, 35*(3), 128-132.

Rogers, A. (2003). Leadership styles and situations. *Nursing Management, 9*(10), 27-30.

Thompson, P. A. (2004). Leadership from an international perspective. *Nursing Administration Quarterly, 28*(3), 191-198.

Chapter 1: Leadership Principles (pp. 1-32)

1. How would you describe a leader? Identify one person who personifies leadership.

Leadership entails influencing others to accomplish goals. Leadership is an interactional process that involves the building and empowerment of teams, the ability to instill motivation, use of positive communication, and innovation to influence and engage individuals in goal attainment. In other words, managers are concerned with systems and structures, as well as the management of organizational resources. A leader is seen as one who is innovative, whereas the manager administers.

Florence Nightingale was a leader in nursing. Her visionary leadership, combined with her willingness to take risks and actively engage the environment, helped shape the profession of nursing. Who do you know that personifies leadership?

2. What are the important qualities of leadership?

Effective leaders are dynamic, visionary individuals. They are productive, responsible, flexible, and visible to their followers. Leaders demonstrate strong interpersonal skills to influence, motivate, empower, and guide groups of individuals toward goal achievement. The ability to be a change agent, take calculated risks, build team relationships, to lead by example, and to develop new cultures are important qualities of a leader. When these qualities are evident in leaders, followers perceive them as courageous, honest, and trustworthy.

3. What tools are available to assess leadership skills?

The best way to learn leadership skills is through education and practice. Nurses can become more effective leaders by analyzing their interactions with others, diagnosing areas for improvement, and practicing the skills needed to enhance their leadership ability. Diagnosing a problematic situation, adapting one's behavior to match the situation, and communicating clearly can improve leadership effectiveness.

Self-assessment tools such as LEAD instruments by Hersey and colleagues (2001), or leaders Behaviour Description Questionnaire-LBDQ-12, Leadership Practices Inventory, the Multifactor Leadership Questionnaire-MLQ, the Self-Assessment Leadership Instrument are available to assist the leader in evaluating leadership and followership behaviors.

4. Who are the leaders in nursing?

Two types of leaders in nursing include transactional and transformational leaders. Transactional nursing leaders work with the existing organizational culture. They maintain the status quo by coordinating and managing the environment and by focusing on the day-to-day operations. In contrast, transformational leaders influence and change the culture of the organization. They use innovation, charisma, individual consideration, and intellectual stimulation to effect change. Effective leaders are those who can change their leadership style to meet the needs of the situation when necessary.

5. Can you be a leader in nursing?

Many leaders are needed in the profession of nursing. Nurses can learn and practice leadership skills that will enable them to be effective leaders. According to Kouzes and Posner (1990), exceptional leadership practices include challenging the process, inspiring a vision, enabling others, modeling the way, and encouraging the heart.

6. What are some examples of leadership opportunities or challenges that you have faced? How did you handle them?

Leaders must assess the group with which they are working, match leadership behaviors to the environment, and adapt their style to accommodate the needs of the group. Groups take on a personality, and a skilled leader will be able to ascertain the maturity and the readiness level of the group. The selected leadership style will be different depending on the composition of the group. A more knowledgeable, experienced, and mature group will present different opportunities and challenges than a less experienced group. What opportunities and challenges have you encountered as a leader and as a group member?

7. What is a good follower?

Followers are essential because they accept or reject the leader and determine the scope of the leader's power. Although there are varying degrees of followership engagement, effective followers demonstrate initiative and independent thinking. In addition, effective followers are responsible, competent, and committed individuals who should be nurtured, developed, and valued as assets to the organization.

8. **What is your favored leadership style? Followership style?**

Leadership styles are a combination of task and relationship behaviors used to influence others to accomplish goals. A leader may select behaviors among three distinct leadership styles: authoritarian, democratic, and laissez-faire. If you primarily demonstrate directive behaviors, then authoritarian is your leadership style. Behaviors reflecting a relationship and person orientation indicate a democratic style, whereas behaviors that promote independence and freedom reflect a laissez-faire leadership style. One must recognize that one leadership style is not better than any other; each has its own advantages and disadvantages, depending on the situation. Followership styles include the "sheep" who lack initiative, a sense of responsibility, and critical thinking; "yes-people" who lack enterprise and yield to the opinions of others; and "alienated" followers who are independent and critical thinkers but passively resist open opposition.

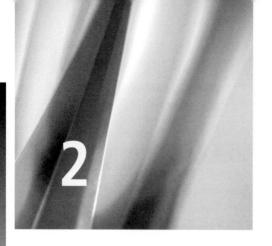

2

Management Principles

STUDY FOCUS

Management is the coordination and integration of resources through planning, organizing, directing, and controlling to accomplish specific organizational goals and objectives. *Nursing management* is coordinating and integrating nursing resources by applying the management process to organize and deliver high-quality client care to individuals, groups, and communities. The *management process* is composed of four steps: planning, organizing, directing, and controlling. A major task of management is to link the staff at the bottom of the organization with those at the top. Nurse managers continuously must balance two important—and at times competing—needs: those of the staff for growth and those of the organization for viability.

Planning for the needs of individuals and the organization is complex and requires time and skill. *Strategic planning* is a long-term process that provides direction and purpose for the organization. *Tactical planning* is typically a short-term process that focuses on the specific details of activities necessary to accomplish the broad organizational goals. To accomplish goals, the manager must organize the integration and coordination of resources. *Organization* is the mobilization of the human, financial, and material resources of the agency to achieve established goals. *Directing* employees by motivating and providing leadership is essential to goal accomplishment. Nurse managers must know the scope of nursing practice to assign and delegate tasks to appropriate personnel. After the nurse manager has assigned work to staff and goals have been accomplished, evaluation of the outcomes is necessary. *Controlling* refers to examining the results of activities (outcomes) in light of a predetermined standard for the purpose of quality control and then taking corrective actions when necessary.

A *nurse manager* is a registered nurse who holds 24-hour accountability for management of the health care unit(s). The nurse manager's role is complex and varied, encompassing multiple diverse tasks, many of which require immediate action. The components of the nurse manager role include managing care delivery, managing resources, developing personnel, complying with regulatory and professional standards, and fostering interdisciplinary and collaborative relationships. Mintzberg (1975) identifies 10 important role behaviors for managers that he categorizes into three role sets. The role sets are interpersonal (figurehead, leader, and liaison), informational (monitor, disseminator, and spokesperson), and decisional (entrepreneur, disturbance handler, resource allocator, and negotiator).

Managing difficult individuals is a challenging task for any manager. Difficult individuals may exhibit negative attitudes or behaviors. Lewis-Ford (1993) describes the following categories of difficult people: Sherman tanks, snipers, exploders, bulldozers, balloons, clams, negative nabobs, complainers, and stallers. Tactics to use with these individuals include trying to understand their behavior, preparing yourself psychologically to interact with them, and selecting disciplinary measures, if necessary.

Nurse managers who are skilled in coordination and integration are valuable resources in the changing health care environment. They are able to adopt new flexible strategies and structures to enhance productivity and quality client care while meeting community health care needs. Nurse managers who successfully manage large numbers of employees and balance complex job demands are developing creative strategies to manage proactively an increasingly complex, turbulent health care environment. Nurse managers are adapting systems, developing strategic plans, fostering interdisciplinary collaboration, and partnering with community members while integrating and reconfiguring health care services.

9

LEARNING TOOLS

Self-Assessment

Purpose

To explore your strengths and areas for improvement in leadership and management behaviors.

Directions

Circle the option that reflects how often you engage in the leadership or management behavior listed.

Management Self-Assessment Study Guide

A = Always; M = Most of the time; S = Some of the time; O = Occasionally; N = Never

A M S O N   1. Enjoys being visible and inter-acting at work

A M S O N   2. Communicates vision to others effectively

A M S O N   3. Is able to motivate others to accomplish goals

A M S O N   4. Seeks out new resources to resolve problems

A M S O N   5. Consistently evaluates outcomes

A M S O N   6. Coordinates client care

A M S O N   7. Plans daily activities and accomplishes them

A M S O N   8. Makes assignments

A M S O N   9. Sets goals for self

A M S O N   10. Negotiates with others to accomplish tasks

A M S O N   11. Is comfortable with change

A M S O N   12. Initiates change

A M S O N   13. Communicates effectively with others

A M S O N   14. Develops strong peer relationships

A M S O N   15. Is able to resolve conflicts

A M S O N   16. Establishes information networks

A M S O N   17. Feels comfortable making decisions in conditions of extreme ambiguity

A M S O N   18. Guards own perspective and avoids taking the behavior personally

A M S O N   18. Enjoys building teams and working cooperatively

A M S O N   19. Consistently meets deadlines

A M S O N   20. Is able to manage multiple priorities

Scoring

Identify the items that you marked *Always* or *Most of the time*. These are the leadership and management behaviors in which you are strong and excel. Now, identify the items that you marked *Some of the time, Occasionally,* or *Never*. These are the leadership and management behaviors that are areas for improvement or growth. By working on these areas, you can improve your leadership skills.

CASE STUDY

Ruth Anne Smith is a nurse manager of an oncology unit for Middle View Hospital in North Dakota. Nurse Smith has been a manager for 15 years and enjoys the role. She is proud of the fact that she has never once been over budget at year end, has maintained a high productivity level, and has a stable core staff. Nurse Smith is detail-oriented and organized. She conscientiously follows policies and procedures and implements new programs according to protocol. She meets monthly with the director of the medical/surgical areas and keeps her abreast of any changes in the unit. Nurse Smith is open to innovations that the director asks her to initiate. She treats all employees equitably and follows the personnel handbook for any human resource issue.

Case Study Questions

1. Does Nurse Smith exhibit managerial or leadership behaviors?

2. What management behaviors does she exhibit?

3. With the changing health care environment, what types of leadership and management behaviors will be important for Nurse Smith to use to improve performance and efficiencies on the oncology unit?

LEARNING RESOURCES

Discussion Questions

1. What are the legal aspects of management in the nurse manager's role?

2. What are some categories of difficult people? What are some effective methods to manage difficult people?

3. What is the management process? What is involved in each of the four steps?

4. What is the role of a nurse manager? What is the nature of managerial work?

5. How do management and leadership differ? Are there similarities between leadership and management?

Study Questions

True or False: Circle the correct answer.

T   F   1. Leadership is more important than management in a turbulent health care environment.

T   F   2. Transformational leaders focus on the maintenance of quality and quantity of performance.

T   F   3. Transformational leadership is necessary in periods of growth, change, and crisis.

T   F   4. Management is focused on tasks and accomplishing organizational goals.

T   F   5. Nursing management is the coordination and integration of resources using a political and computer science process.

T   F   6. The traditional management functions include planning, organizing, controlling, and coordinating.

T   F   7. Tactical planning is a broad-range process of establishing the purpose and direction of the organization.

T   F   8. Management is a discipline that uses a set of tools to achieve desired outcomes.

T   F   9. Organizing is determining the long- and short-term objectives and the corresponding actions to take to achieve objectives.

T   F   10. Nurse managers usually have 24-hour accountability for the coordination and delivery of care.

REFERENCES

Lewis-Ford, B. (1993). Management techniques: Coping with difficult people. *Nursing Management, 24*(3), 36-38.

Mintzberg, H. (1975). The manager's job: Folklore and fact. In M. Matteson & J. Ivancevich (Eds.), *Management classics* (3rd ed., pp. 63-85). Plano, TX: Business Publications.

SUPPLEMENTAL READINGS

Campbell, S. L. (2003). Cultivating empowerment in nursing today for a strong profession tomorrow. *Journal of Nursing Education, 42*(9), 423-426.

Cunning, S. M. (2004). Avoid common management pitfalls. *Nursing Management, 35*(2), 18.

Gokenbach, V. (2004). Infuse management with leadership. *Nursing Management, 34*(1), 8, 10.

Guo, K. L. (2002). Roles of managers in academic health centers: Strategies for the managed care environment. *The Health Care Manager, 20*(3), 43-58.

Chapter 2: Management Principles (pp. 33-58)

1. Discuss which concept is more important: leadership or management? Why?

One must recognize that leadership and management are equally vital processes. The focus of each process is different, though their outcomes may be interrelated. How important one process is over the other depends on what is needed at the time and the context in which it occurs.

2. Why is management important to a nurse?

As managers of care, management is an important concept to nurses. Nurses coordinate and deliver health services to clients. Nursing management is the coordination and integration of nursing resources to accomplish care provision through application of the management process.

3. Describe a scenario in which middle managers become obsolete?

According to the American Organization of Nurse Executives (1992), nurse managers are individuals who have 24-hour accountability for the management of client care unit(s) or area(s) within a health care institution. Essential components of the nurse manager's role are the management of human, fiscal, and other resources needed for nursing practice and care delivery. The complexity of the nurse management role and the skills necessary to manage multiskilled, cross-functional work groups will continue to intensify as organizations reconfigure, restructure, and integrate.

4. How do Mintzberg's 10 roles differ for nurses at different positions in a hierarchical bureaucracy?

Mintzberg (1975) identified 10 roles that describe a manager's role. The three interpersonal roles— (1) figurehead, (2) leader, and (3) liaison—evolve from the formal authority and status of the management position. Informational roles include monitor, disseminator, and spokesperson, and the decision-making roles include entrepreneur, disturbance handler, resource allocator, and negotiator. Engagement in these three roles, including the amount of time involved and the type of individuals with which they interact, depends on whether one is a care manager, nurse manager, or nurse executive in the hierarchical bureaucracy. Care managers provide direct care to clients and make clinical decisions through interactions with clients, physicians, and colleagues. The nurse manager focuses on the coordination of care delivery and manages interactions with employees and administrators, as well as with clients and families. The focus of the nurse executive is on strategic management, policy formation, and service delivery analysis and trending. Nurse executives interact most frequently with other administrators, managers, and board members.

5. Why is it easier for nurses to change to a new managerial role than it is for other types of health care workers?

Nurses are positioned well to move easily and naturally into the management realm because of their clinical expertise, ability to facilitate interdisciplinary coordination, and knowledge of human and resource management. Nurses blend these skills to produce positive outcomes such as quality client care, workforce stability, organizational productivity, and effective cost control.

6. In what way is case management a managerial role? How can the clinical focus be described as management?

Case management involves the four elements of the management process: planning, organizing, coordinating or directing, and controlling. Case management is a care delivery approach designed to plan, organize, and coordinate care to control costs, increase quality outcomes, and enhance accessibility to appropriate and needed health care services.

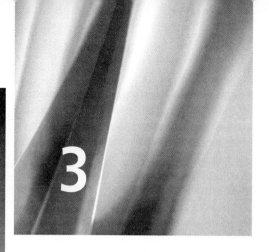

Professional Practice and Career Development

3

STUDY FOCUS

Individuals choose nursing as a profession for many different reasons. For some, nursing is their chosen field because of a desire to help people, for others the variety of jobs and job security affected their career choice. *Career commitment* is the nurse's attitude toward nursing as a profession and the nurse's motivation to work in his or her chosen career role. *Contemporary nursing* is a complex practice profession that in some part is shaped by knowledge, economics, society, and population demographics.

The practice of nursing is broad, and the scope and function of nursing practice continues to evolve. The profession of nursing is defined by licensure laws and practice regulations in each state. The four approaches to regulation are (1) designation/recognition, (2) registration, (3) certification, and (4) licensure. *Designation/recognition* is the least restrictive approach to regulation and provides the public with information about special credentials. *Registration* involves having the person's name on an official roster maintained by a particular agency that can provide services. Individuals who are registered and meet certain requirements are permitted to use specific titles. *Certification* imposes a more stringent form of regulation and is given when requirements are met. Individuals meeting certification requirements are able to use the title that recognizes their professional competence. *Specialty certification* implies that a standard has been met that usually is assessed by passing of a certifying examination. *Licensure* is the granting of permission by the state to engage in a given profession. Licensure indicates that an individual has attained a minimal degree of competence to perform within the scope of practice. *State Boards of Nursing* are regulatory agencies that are given the authority to enact the licensure laws that define the legal boundaries and scope of professional nursing practice that is passed by state legislation. The many

influences on professional nursing practice include laws, professional organizational activities, and workplace rules and standards.

The American Nurses Association (ANA) provides leadership in defining nursing by publishing the definition of nursing, an ethical code, and standards of practice. The ANA represents nursing in the health policy arena as the collective voice of nursing. The ANA was established in 1896 as the Nurses Associated Alumnae of the United States. Currently, only 5% of U.S. nurses belong to the ANA. Nurses have a responsibility to belong to their professional organization in order to have a strong collective voice to influence health care delivery and policy. *Magnet recognition* is an award of achievement confirmed by the ANA credentialing body, the American Nurses Credentialing Center, to recognize agencies that provide quality care and create positive work environments that reward and promote professional nursing and positive client outcomes. Characteristics of Magnet work environments include autonomous nursing practice, collaborative relationships among health care professionals, and control over practice.

Is nursing a profession or an occupation? A *profession* is comprised of a system of roles that is socially defined. An occupation is defined as on-the-job training, not having specialized training, and typically without lasting commitment (Larisey, 1996). Professions hold contracts with society to provide services for the public good. In return for these essential services, society affords professionals (one who is engaged in a profession and meeting standards and recognition requirements) higher prestige, income, and autonomy in their work. *Professionalism* is the extent to which an individual identifies with a profession and adheres to its standards. Members of society expect that professionals will uphold society's trust by possessing characteristics of expertise, engaging in rigorous academic preparation, and demonstrating commitment and responsible behavior.

13

Professionalization is the process by which occupations set standards to move from nonprofessional to professional status. Nurses perform many roles. *Role* is defined as the expected and associated behaviors of a specific job position (Hardy & Hardy, 1988). Nurses often perform the roles of clinician, educator, administrator, researcher, and consultant. One view of nurse's roles is twofold, that of a caregiver and integrator (McClure, 1991). The caregiver role is enacted in direct client care, whereas the integrator role is a coordinating function to ensure a seamless integration of client care.

The three most common criteria for a profession as identified by authors are service, knowledge, and autonomy. *Service* is providing society with essential activities. A service orientation includes committing to the standards of practice and lifelong learning, committing to the community of nurses that share common goals, and committing to civility despite individual differences (Logan et al., 2004). *Knowledge* is the strong base of specialized education from which a profession practices. Nursing knowledge has focused around the four main concepts of nursing, person, environment, and health (Fitzpatrick & Whall, 2005). *Professional autonomy* is having authority over and accountability for one's decisions and activities. All professions have a code of ethics that guides practice. Six principles of ethical decision making are justice (fairness), autonomy (freedom to decide and act), fidelity (accountability), beneficience (to do good), nonmalfeasance (to avoid harm), and veracity (truthfulness). Professionalization of an occupation can be viewed on a continuum. An occupational group can move along the continuum from nonprofessional to semiprofessional to professional.

Nursing requires a high level of expertise, sophisticated decision making, and a sense of service, which are characteristics of professional groups. Problematic areas for nursing have been a lack of differentiated practice (multiple educational levels equated with one job assignment), the absence of a unified voice, and the fact that nursing is a profession in which most workers are women. The three major educational paths to registered nursing are (1) a bachelor's degree in nursing, (2) an associate's degree in nursing, and (3) a diploma. The flexibility of multiple entry paths into nursing practice has been attractive to many individuals but also can be problematic for a unified voice for nursing practice. Nursing leaders must support autonomous nursing practice (job autonomy), continue to develop a strong nursing knowledge base, and use and contribute to nursing research while being role models of professional behaviors. Using positive media images, educating the public about the role of nursing in health care, supporting the National Institute for Nursing Research, acting altruistically in policy making, and dressing and acting in a professional manner also will enhance the status and profession of nursing.

Nurses enter the profession of nursing for many reasons. Some enter to help people, others enter for job security, and still others are influenced by strong nursing role models. Nurses may view their work as a job or a career. A *job* is a specific position that one fills for a specific amount of pay, whereas a *career* is a personal and professional plan comprised of a series of positions to meet a long-term goal. Career commitment is an individual's motivation and attitude to work in a professional role. Nurses assess their personal and professional goals in relation to their work, their personal goals, and their family obligations when determining a career trajectory or professional path. Examining adult life stages when assessing an individual's career trajectory assists the nurse in understanding choices throughout the life span in relation to developmental growth and task accomplishment. Early in an individual's career, between the ages of 18 and 22, one experiences an exploration phase; between 46 and 53 one balances one's life, and after the age of 70 one does what one is able to do. An individual's career choice is influenced by the work, personal and family needs, and roles in one's life.

Individuals who view nursing as a profession need to plan their career and then follow it up with periodic self-analysis to assess progress on personal needs and career goals. Self-assessments are important at annual intervals to evaluate progress toward personal and professional goals and again at times of decision points when one must make choices about changing positions, returning for advanced education, taking a certification examination, or moving to a new organization or geographic location.

Career anchors are personal needs and skills that help to explain individual values in career choices. Friss (1989) identified eight career anchors: (1) service, (2) managerial competence, (3) autonomy, (4) technical-functional competence, (5) security, (6) identity, (7) variety, and (8) creativity. Nurses tend especially to value the three primary anchors of technical-functional competence, security, and identity. An advantage for individuals pursuing a nursing career is the variety of roles available and the multiple part-time opportunities for employment. Many nurses are keenly aware of the social, political, and economic environment that has an impact on opportunities within the profession of nursing, as well as the timing of personal and family goals and demands.

Career planning is essential to meeting professional goals. Career planning is most effective when started early in an individual's career. Self-assessment is the cornerstone of career planning, and finding a supportive mentor is useful to advance your career. Vogel (1990) identified career planning as a lifelong process linked to each person's values, lifestyles, goals, and work style. Vogel identified six stages of career development: (1) self-analysis, (2) career analysis, (3) integrating, (4) planning, (5) implementing, and (6) evaluating. A written plan is beneficial in formulating personal and professional goals, and the nurse should reevaluate the plan annually. To meet professional goals, one must be aware of environmental changes, set goals, plan activities to enhance one's career, and anticipate future trends to attain additional education or certification in a specialty area. By keeping abreast of health care and community needs and changes, the nurse can capitalize on the changing health care environment by securing a coveted position or by starting a business venture. The nurse also may experience transition points in the career trajectory. *Transition points* are choices one makes that change the direction of one's career. Careful evaluation and reaffirmation of goals and aspirations at these junctures is essential. Methods for staying informed of health care changes include reading professional journals, reading about current events in the national news, joining the American Nurses Association, networking, and helping with political campaigns.

Benner's (1982) work describes *five levels of proficiency* through which a nurse progresses to mastery of content and skill. The five levels are novice, advanced beginner, competent, proficient, and expert. Experience and competence are gained over time and require practice and education. Individuals adjust to the work environment and personal and professional demands while gaining expertise. New graduates are commonly in the novice stage of proficiency, and during the transition from school to work, frequently experience reality shock. *Reality shock* is when a new nurse faces the challenge of implementing the ideal within a constrained work environment. During this period the nurse may become disenchanted. Kramer (1974) identifies the honeymoon, shock, recovery, and resolution of conflict as *phases of reality shock*.

Socialization is a process in which information, values, and ideals are transmitted (van Maanen & Schein, 1979). *Professional socialization* is how students learn through an educational process in which content and role modeling by faculty, preceptors, and mentors for professional nursing practice occurs. *Organizational socialization* is learning the culture of the environment by learning policies and procedures and becoming aware of acceptable behaviors and practices. A *mentor* is an experienced nurse who is a strong force in facilitating the professional development of new nurses or nurses who desire guidance and role modeling from a seasoned nurse. Characteristics of mentors include a caring approach to work, effective communication and listening, trustworthiness in communications and activities, experience and respect, and service as a professional role model. They have a long-term commitment to their protégé. In contrast, a *preceptor* is an experienced nurse assigned to a new nurse during orientation to facilitate acclimation to a practice environment. Seyboldt (1983) described *five phases of tenure* in an organization. Phase 1 is entry, and the time frame is less than 6 months. In this period employees are transitioning through orientation; feedback is essential. Phase 2 is early, spanning 6 months to 1 year. This phase is characterized by learning the basics of the job; strong mentoring is needed. Phase 3 is middle, comprising 1 to 3 years. This period is relatively stable, and autonomy and validation are important. Phase 4 is advanced, consisting of 3 to 6 years. It is important to employees that their work is validated and that contributions are meaningful. Phase 5 is the later period, which is the period of 6 years or more. These employees are informal leaders and pillars of the organization.

The health care environment is turbulent and constantly changing. We are in the midst of a nursing shortage, with the average age of a nurse being 45.2 years. Nursing leaders will be faced with restructuring outdated hierarchical and bureaucratic structures that are antithetical to autonomy. Learning organizations will be the wave of the future. The new models will foster teamwork, coaching, and advocacy. Leaders will need to work with the Baby Boomers who are loyal, reliable, and customer oriented and with the Gen Xers who seek autonomy, desire constant feedback, balance work with other priorities, and prefer flexible schedules. *Swift trust,* in which professionals work in a fluid, flexible environment quickly establishing trust-based work relationships, will be essential for efficient and effective care delivery. Nurses who strive for a competitive advantage in career advancement may look to future trends to position themselves to capitalize on opportunities. To conceptualize the future direction for nursing, the ANA convened a committee comprised of representatives from 19 professional organizations to describe what nursing should look like in 2010. The following 10 key areas were identified:

1. Having a unified voice and plan for nursing

2. Using integrated models of care

3. Implementing an unified standard of nursing education

4. Being equal partners in practice

5. Facilitating recruitment and retention efforts that result in adequate numbers of novice and experienced nurses

6. Gaining reasonable compensation

7. Sharing governance in practice

8. Maintaining a positive public image

9. Practicing in dynamic learning environments

10. Having a diverse workplace

Nurses who choose a career trajectory must be their own advocate for advancement and identify learning opportunities essential for their chosen career path. Marketing yourself is important. Finding a mentor, networking, developing and then assessing your career trajectory, and embarking on advanced preparation, certifications, or specialized training may be necessary to accomplish your goals. Opportunities in health care continually change, and keeping abreast of the trends will assist you with career planning. Labor projections and media report that nursing is one of the top 10 occupations for job growth. Opportunities are emerging in the areas of primary care and advanced nursing practice. Certification in advanced practice provides recognition by the public of a nurse's specialized area of practice. Advanced education and certification are two methods for nurses to demonstrate competence and quality.

LEARNING TOOLS

Self-Assessment Activity 1

*Valiga Concept of Nursing Scale**

Directions

The following statements attempt to ascertain the ideas that you currently hold about nursing as a profession, the role of the nurse, and the relationship of the nurse to the client and to the physician and other health team colleagues. Read each of the following statements carefully. Then for each statement, indicate whether you strongly agree (SA), agree (A), are undecided or do not know (U), disagree (D), or strongly disagree (SD) with the statement. Circle the one response that best expresses your opinion, and please be certain your response to each statement is marked clearly. There are no right or wrong answers, so please respond openly and honestly.

1. Nurses must be willing to work with clients on those health-related situations that they cannot face alone.   SA A U D SD

2. Nursing is concerned with helping people maximize their health potential in their particular life situation.   SA A U D SD

3. Overt action, directed by logical thought, toward meeting the client's need for help constitutes the practice of clinical nursing.   SA A U D SD

4. Nurses must assume responsibility for diagnosing and treating human responses to actual or potential illnesses.   SA A U D SD

5. The independent functions of nurses include supervising the care of clients, observing and recording, supervising nonprofessional personnel, and health teaching.   SA A U D SD

6. Nursing must be concerned equally with the prevention of disease and the conservation of health.   SA A U D SD

7. Nursing is an expression of one's commitment to others.   SA A U D SD

8. Nurses must be involved actively in professional organizations.   SA A U D SD

9. There is definitely a right and a wrong way to do things and approach nursing situations.   SA A U D SD

10. Nurses should make written or verbal contacts with all appropriate persons to ensure continuity of nursing care for clients.   SA A U D SD

11. The uniqueness of nursing lies in the reasons for what nurses do in society, rather than in the specific tasks they perform.   SA A U D SD

*_ Courtesy Theresa M. Valiga, RN, EdD, Dean and Professor, School of Nursing, Fairfield University, Fairfield, CT._

12. Nurses should be concerned primarily with giving physical care to clients as directed by the physician.　　SA　A　U　D　SD

13. There should be only one nursing theory.　　SA　A　U　D　SD

14. Evaluation of the work of their peers and other nursing personnel should be a responsibility of nurses.　　SA　A　U　D　SD

15. Nurses must follow doctors' orders without question.　　SA　A　U　D　SD

16. Nurses should be free to practice nursing as they define it within the scope of professional autonomy.　　SA　A　U　D　SD

17. Nurses should assume responsibility for the total nursing care of a caseload of clients.　　SA　A　U　D　SD

18. Nurses should update their knowledge through lifelong continuing education.　　SA　A　U　D　SD

19. Nurses must control and direct their own practice.　　SA　A　U　D　SD

20. Nurses should be responsible for conducting nursing care conferences routinely.　　SA　A　U　D　SD

21. Nurses must be aware that people who require their assistance are helpless and dependent and usually need to be told what to do.　　SA　A　U　D　SD

22. Nurses have a responsibility for discussing the proposed medical plan of care with the physician so it can be adjusted, if possible, to be more acceptable to the client.　　SA　A　U　D　SD

23. Nurses must assume responsibility for reviewing and evaluating care provided by nursing peers.　　SA　A　U　D　SD

24. Nurses must take deliberate action to attain independence in nursing situations.　　SA　A　U　D　SD

25. Nurses must not hesitate to assume the role of leader of the health care team when the client's problems are best met by nurses.　　SA　A　U　D　SD

Scoring

Each individual receives a score of +2 for each item with which they strongly agree, +1 for each item with which they agree, 0 for each item about which they were unsure, −1 for each item with which they disagreed, and −2 for each item with which he or she strongly disagreed. The minimum score is −50, and the maximum score is +50. The higher the positive score, the stronger the professional view.

Self-Assessment Activity 2

Purpose

To assist you in developing a career trajectory and to develop a cover letter and resume to market your special skills and abilities.

Career Trajectory

Introduction

To successfully plan a career, you need to take time to assess your personal and professional goals in order to develop a meaningful, efficient, and rewarding career trajectory. Once you identify your specific goals, you will be able to determine which resources, education, and experience are essential for you to meet your career goals.

Directions

Conduct a self-assessment of your personal and professional goals. Determine timelines for when you would like certain goals met. You may choose to look at early, middle, and late career and lifetime goal intervals. This will assist you in identifying activities and experiences that are necessary to progress to your ultimate career objective. The following categories are listed for you to identify goals for personal and professional areas. List those goals that you would like to complete in each time period. Form your goals, and then fill in the resource category with what you must do to attain your desired goal. For example, if your goal is to be a nurse practitioner, you must pursue advanced education, so put this activity into the resource column.

	GOAL INTERVAL			
Type of Goal	Early	Middle	Late	Resources
Career				
Lifestyle				
Personal/family				
Financial				
Living and retirement				

Summary

Complete a self-assessment annually to determine the goals that have been met and what activities you need to engage in to accomplish the remaining goals. Update your personal and professional goals and do not forget to celebrate your accomplishments.

Cover Letter

Directions

It is important to write a professional cover letter when applying for a position. Even if you choose to deliver the letter and resume in person, it provides a snapshot of how you present yourself and leaves a strong impression with the recruiter and interview committee. The letter should be written clearly, should be typed on bond paper, and should be grammatically correct. A sample cover letter is provided for your review (see below). Take the time to develop your own cover letter based on the position(s) you are interested in obtaining. Make sure you get the correct title and spelling of the recruiter's name.

3195 Hanna Ave.
Detroit, MI 68941

January 21, 2006

Phyllis Jones, RN, MSN
Nurse Recruiter
Cedarville Hospital
719 South Haven
Detroit, MI 68941

Dear Mrs. Jones:

I would like to apply for a position in the six-month graduate nursing internship program for new graduates at Cedarville Hospital that Miss Jason discussed during her visit to Mercy University. Upon graduation with a baccalaureate nursing degree on April 14, 2006, I will be available to begin employment immediately.

Miss Jason's description of Cedarville Hospital as a comprehensive medical center serving the southwestern Detroit community convinced me that the graduate nursing internship is an ideal learning opportunity. I have completed two clinical internships on the medical and surgical units at Cedarville Hospital and have been impressed by the high-quality care provided by the professional nursing staff. I am interested in joining your professional nursing team.

I am available on Tuesdays and Fridays for an interview. Please let me know if it is convenient for you to meet with me on these days. My telephone number is (313) 687-1519.

I am looking forward to meeting with you and discussing the graduate internship program.

Sincerely,

Sharon Smith

Resume

Directions

It is important to develop a clear, concise, accurate resume to convey your work experience, education, and achievements. It is important to devise a simple but clear format for your resume. Your resume should be typed, free from spelling and grammatical errors, and printed on high-quality bond paper. You need to explain gaps between employment dates. A brief description of your employment experience is helpful to highlight key performance areas. A sample resume follows for your review. Take the time to create a resume for yourself. This document highlights and markets your abilities. Take the time to make a sharp, professional, accurate resume. It is important that your resume stands out among the others and captures the recruiter's attention.

CASE STUDIES

Case Study 1

Kay Klements is a staff nurse on the oncology unit at Zimmer Hospital in Austin, Texas. She has been a registered nurse for 3 years. Nurse Klements graduated with a baccalaureate degree in nursing and has continued to enroll in one course per term toward her master's degree. She is active in the Texas Nurses Association, and she is the secretary for the local Oncology Nurses Association. Nurse Klements subscribes to two nursing

Meghan Sjots
220 South Appleville Drive
Hudsonville, MI 49604
(616) 245-7894

Objective	To work as a staff nurse on a medical-surgical unit.
Education	BSN, Grand Valley State University, Allendale, Michigan, December 2005
Experience May 1995–Present	Intern, Spectrum Health, Grand Rapids, Michigan Assisted registered nurses in providing direct client care. Assisted with feeding clients, bathing, taking vital signs, calculating intake and output, positioning, and reporting. Certified in CPR.
May 1997–May 1998	Volunteer, Spectrum Health, Grand Rapids, Michigan Coordinated recreation activities for the medical-surgical unit. Transported clients for testing and discharge.
Licensure	Scheduled to sit for the NCLEX in Grand Rapids, Michigan on January 20, 2006
Professional Organizations	Michigan Association of Nursing Students
Honors	Dean's Honor Roll 2001-2005 Kappa Epsilon, Chapter of Sigma Theta Tau Spectrum Health Volunteer Award
References	Available upon request

The following references are only provided as a guide of what to submit when you are asked for them.

Julie Brown, RN, BSN
Nurse Manager Medical-Surgical
Spectrum Health
1 Spillwood Avenue
Grand Rapids, MI 49580
(616) 791-3456

Mrs. Welch
Volunteer Manager
Spectrum Health
1 Spillwood Avenue
Grand Rapids, MI 49580
(616) 791-3467

Keverin James, RN, PhD
Professor of Nursing
Grand Valley State University
1 Campus Drive
Allendale, MI 49401
(616) 331-3558

journals and attends continuing educational programs at the hospital. She enjoys her work and volunteers for clinical projects.

Case Study 1 Questions

1. Does Nurse Klements demonstrate behaviors that indicate she is career- or occupation-oriented?

2. What characteristics of a professional nurse does Nurse Klements demonstrate?

3. What types of master's degree programs in nursing may Nurse Klements elect to pursue?

Case Study 2

Janice Day will be graduating from Grand Valley State University with her baccalaureate degree in December 2005. She will be interviewing for her first professional nursing position. Student Nurse Day has taken the time to develop a professional quality cover letter and resume. She has researched the available nursing positions in her community and in the surrounding areas. Ms. Day has applied for several positions to explore the organizational philosophy and work environment. She is offered two positions: a community health nursing position where she will be a case manager making home visits and helping to coordinate care for a group of families, and a clinical nurse position on a 45-bed medical-surgical unit.

Case Study 2 Questions

1. How should Student Nurse Day determine which is the best position for her?

2. How does Ms. Day's career trajectory help her make the best decision for her personal and professional goals?

3. Ms. Day has decided that her long-term goal is to become an advanced practice nurse. What is an advanced practice nurse, and how does this plan fit into her present dilemma of which job she should accept?

LEARNING RESOURCES

Discussion Questions

1. What is nursing's scope of practice? What are some examples of nursing roles that illustrate that nursing has a broad and evolving scope of practice?

2. What are the twofold roles of nursing that McClure identifies? Give examples of each role.

3. Does nursing fit the major three categories of a profession (service, knowledge, and autonomy)?

4. What is advanced practice nursing, and how does it relate to nursing careers and career planning?

5. How does advanced nursing practice fit into professional nursing practice?

6. How has the fact that the majority of nurses are women influenced the profession of nursing?

7. How do adult developmental stages relate to career plans and goals?

8. How do health care reform issues affect nursing care planning?

9. What are the stages and benefits of career planning?

Study Questions

Matching: Write the letter of the correct response in front of each term.

_____ 1. Professionalism

_____ 2. Profession

_____ 3. Professional

_____ 4. Professionalization

_____ 5. Differentiated practice

_____ 6. Altruism

_____ 7. Job autonomy

_____ 8. Professional autonomy

A. Comprised of a system of roles that are socially defined

B. One educational level for one job assignment

C. The authority and accountability for one's work

D. Individual and collective authority and accountability

E. Selfless concern and service to others

F. One who is engaged in a profession

G. The extent to which an individual identifies and adheres to professional standards

H. Process in which occupations change in the direction of a profession

True or False: Circle the correct answer.

T F 9. McClure defines nursing's roles as caregiver and integrator.

T F 10. The scope of nursing is changing and evolving.

T F 11. The most important factor to consider when evaluating job possibilities is the financial remuneration and benefits offered.

T F 12. Career trajectories provide direction as to what resources, experience, and education are needed.

T   F   13. The career anchors of managerial competence, service, and identity are most representative of nursing.

T   F   14. It is important to stay abreast of changing trends in health care because new options may become available in nursing practice.

T   F   15. Career planning is a quick, easy-to-do process that requires little time, but has a big payoff.

T   F   16. Advanced practice nursing refers only to nurse practitioners who are in independent practices in rural areas.

T   F   17. Career plans or trajectories must take into consideration personal, family, and work-related needs for a successful outcome.

T   F   18. A nurse's proficiency level begins with novice and progresses through proficiency, advanced beginner, expert, and then to competence.

T   F   19. Mid-career factors include promotions, job changes, and family and personal obligations.

T   F   20. Nurses should always be aware of their professional image and market themselves as a career development strategy.

T   F   21. Advanced education and certification are two methods to demonstrate competence and quality.

T   F   22. In Kramer's phases of reality shock, the *shock phase* is characterized by a time when the nurse begins to learn to cope with the conflict in values.

REFERENCES

Benner, P. (1982). From novice to expert. *American Journal of Nursing, 82*(3), 402-407.

Fitzpatrick, J. J., & Whall, A. L. (2005). *Conceptual models of nursing: Analysis and application* (4th ed.). Upper Saddle River, NJ: Pearson Prentice Hall.

Friss, H. (1989). *Strategic management of nurses: A policy-oriented approach.* Owings Mills, MD: National Health Publishing.

Hardy, M. E., & Hardy, W. L. (1988). Role stress and role strain. In M. E. Hardy & M. E. Conway (Eds.), *Role theory: Perspectives for health professionals* (2nd ed., pp. 159-239). Norwalk, CT: Appleton & Lange.

Kramer, M. (1974). *Reality shock: Why nurses leave nursing.* St Louis: Mosby.

Larisey, M. (1996). Socialization to professional nursing. In J. L. Creasia & B. Parker (Eds.), *Conceptual foundations of professional nursing practice* (pp. 46-66). St Louis: Mosby.

Logan, J., Franzen, D., Pauling, C., & Butcher, H. (2004). Achieving professionhood through participation in professional organizations. In L. Haynes, T. Boese, & H. Butcher (Eds.), *Nursing in contemporary society* (pp. 52-70). Upper Saddle River, NJ: Pearson Prentice Hall.

McClure, M. L. (1991). Introduction. In I. E. Goertzen (Ed.), *Differentiating nursing practice in the twenty-first century* (pp. 1-9). Kansas City, MO: American Academy of Nursing.

Seyboldt, J. (1983). Dealing with premature employee turnover. *California Management Review, 25*(3), 107-117.

van Maneen, J., & Schein, E. H. (1979). Toward a theory of organizational socialization. *Research in Organizational Behavior, 1*, 209-264.

Vogel, G. (1990). Career development: An integrated process. *Holistic Nursing Practice, 4*(4), 46-53.

SUPPLEMENTAL READINGS

Arthur, D. (1995). Measurement of the professional self-concept of nurses: Developing a measurement instrument. *Nursing Education Today, 15*(5), 328-335.

Benson, E. P. (2004). Online learning: A means to enhance professional development. *Critical Care Nurse, 24*(1), 60-63.

Brechtel, R. D. (2003). Your career in nursing: Manage your future in the changing world of healthcare. *AORN Journal, 78*(6), 1026-1027.

Campbell, S. C. (2004). Continuing professional development: What do we need? *Nursing Management, 10*(10), 27-31.

Griffitts, L. D. (2002). Geared to achieve with lifelong learning. *Nursing Management, 23*(11), 23-25.

Miller, B., Adams, D., & Beck, L. (1993). A behavioral inventory for professionalism in nursing. *Journal of Professional Nursing, 9*(5), 290-295.

Chapter 3: Professional Practice and Career Development (pp. 59-82)

1. On what basis can nursing argue that it is a profession?

Four common themes are prevalent in various definitions of a profession: a specialized body of knowledge, service, autonomy, and a professional code of ethics. The nursing profession addresses all of these themes. Nurses work from a specialized body of knowledge that is learned during basic nursing education in an associate degree in nursing or bachelor of science in nursing education. This learning continues through ongoing education and lifelong learning. Service is provided to members of society to meet the health needs of all. Autonomy in nursing is exercised through independent, dependent, and interdependent actions limited by state Nurse Practice Acts and institutional policies. The American Nurses Association has defined a code of ethics, which mandates the standards of professional conduct for all nurses. Some may argue that nursing is not a profession, but a semiprofession, because of the various levels of education for entry into practice. Whether nursing is a full profession or not is unclear.

2. Do nurses need to act and look professional to give a professional impression?

How might a nurse act and look to promote professionalism? How do actions and appearance affect relationships with clients, families, and other health care professionals? What has your impression been of a nurse who acts and looks professional versus one who did not? How did this first impression affect the relationship with your caregiver?

3. Should nurses care about image and appearance? If so, why?

In the past, nurses have been viewed as obedient, passive, and selfless. Florence Nightingale helped to change this image through the promotion of a need for organized nursing education. However, today nurses continue to strive to overcome this long-standing image in spite of the need to be autonomous decision makers.

4. What is the most prevalent media stereotype of nurses today? How could this be changed?

Nurses currently are portrayed as health care providers who provide technical tasks as deemed appropriate by physician orders. They are not seen as professionals with critical thinking, educated judgment, and expertise. What are different ways that nurses as individuals can initiate change?

5. Can you design the "ideal" nursing uniform—one that nurses like and find comfortable and practical and yet that clients can identify?

What would one consider in designing an ideal uniform? What would help the client identify the professional nurse? What would be appropriate for male and female nurses? Should nursing hats be included in this uniform? Why or Why not? Would this uniform include a lab coat? If so, what does the length of the lab coat suggest to clients? What does the color or design of the fabric suggest to the client and to other health care professionals? Would the nurse have an embroidered name and credentials on this uniform? What would make this uniform unique for nursing? Should this uniform be developed as a standard for nurses worldwide?

6. Why should nurses plan a career? Why not just follow the available jobs?

Nurses should plan a career to achieve their professional and personal goals. A career is systematic, deliberate, and sequential process that involves a critical analysis of one's professional, personal, and educational endeavors. Planning a career is indicative of commitment, investment, and active involvement in the profession. In contrast, a job is a fragmented event, used to meet basic security needs.

7. Why are you motivated for a job or a career in nursing?

Examining your goals, strengths, and needs will assist in identifying your motivation for a career in nursing. Furthermore, your motivations will be instrumental in the exploring opportunities available in nursing, developing of your career goals, and establishing a career trajectory.

8. What developmental stage are you in? How does that affect your career planning?

Individuals experience the dynamic process of growth and development as they continue through the life span. As adults progress through developmental stages, changes they encounter often affect the balance between work, self, family needs, and roles. Adaptation or adjustment to these changes has an inevitable impact on career needs and decisions. Identification of your current developmental stage through periodical self-analysis will enhance your career development.

9. **How much should your employer contribute to your career development?**

Regulatory organizations and the community-at-large expect the delivery of competent, quality health care. To fulfill this expectation, professional preparation, continuing education, and/or self-directed learning must take place to remain current in professional practice. Employers and employees should collaborate to establish mechanisms that will meet employees' professional growth needs. To fulfill the employer's obligation to hire and maintain competent practitioners, the employer should support career counseling and professional development through educational and fiscal contributions.

10. **Is career planning encouraged in your employment setting? Why or why not?**

Think about your current employment setting. Are mechanisms in place to support career planning and advancement? Is tuition or financial reimbursement available for educational or continuing education programs? Do managers assist you in developing professional goals? Is environmental scanning and networking at professional meetings and activities encouraged and supported? Have monies been allocated for such activities?

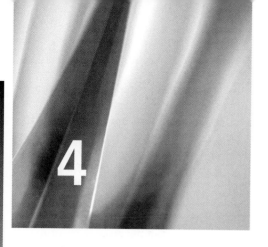

Managing Time and Stress

4

STUDY FOCUS

Time is a valuable and elusive resource to manage. Time pressures create strong demands on nurses who must make difficult choices about accomplishing goals. *Time management* is accomplishing specific activities during the time available. Successful nurses set short-, medium-, and long-term goals and objectives for time management and implement well-thought-out strategies. Those who are successful at managing time say no, control interruptions, and delegate tasks. Time management has been linked to success and the achievement of goals. Self-awareness and analysis of goals is crucial to successful time management. Those who examine their attitude about time, analyze time-wasting behaviors, and develop better time management skills are better able to meet personal and professional goals. Individuals vary in their approach to time management and their style of work. Some individuals prefer a monochromic style where they work through a project in an orderly fashion, completing each task before moving on to another. Individuals who enjoy detailed plans and scheduled are highly monochromatic, whereas individuals who approach work in an analytical and prioritized way are moderately monochromatic. Individuals who use monochromatic style tend to be individualistic and prefer an isolated and uninterrupted work environment. A polychromatic work style is characterized by doing multiple tasks simultaneous using a multidimensional, flexible, and mutually shared responsibility plan. In a highly polychromatic environment, work is done on many parts of the project simultaneously with spontaneous and adaptable changes based on the work.

No matter what style of work is preferred, managing personal and work activities will be necessary. The eight steps in the time management process are (1) analyzing current time use with logs, (2) analyzing the time logs to identify problems, (3) conducting a self-assessment, (4) setting goals and establishing priorities, (5) developing action plans, (6) implementing action plans via schedules, guides, or lists, (7) developing techniques and solutions to improve time management, and (8) following up on and evaluating time management patterns. Time management is an important aspect of controlling and minimizing stress in personal and work-related activities. Tools that can simplify your life and assist in saving time include diaries, calendars, organizers, personal digital assitants, and integrating software scheduling tools. Barriers to effective time management include procrastination, perfectionism, and not being able to prioritize. Procrastination occurs when you are not committed or are afraid of the job, it is a low-priority activity, you do not know how to do the work, or you just do not want to do it. Strategies to overcome procrastination include examining motivation and personal benefit, confronting your fears, positively reframing the task, gathering information to complete the task, or delegating it.

The management of time and use of time management strategies can increase goal accomplishment and decrease personal and professional stress. Time management strategies include taking control of your calendar, minimizing time spent on nonproductive behavior, taming the telephone through secretarial support, simplifying documentation, planning ahead, and saving time for others. Once crucial step in planning is to set aside 15 to 20 minutes each day to prioritize and organize activities. Follow your plan and ask for help when appropriate. Effective verbal and written communication saves time by avoiding the work of correcting miscommunication. Use checklists to assure accomplishment of critical tasks and to celebrate successful completion of work. Part of your list should be to maintain balance in your work. Make time for family, for friends, and for you.

Stress is part of a nurse's everyday work. *Stress* is a physical, psychosocial, or spiritual response to a stressful event called a *stressor*. *Job* or *occupational stress* is an uncomfortable sensation created by the demands of the

25

job or work of the nurse. Nurses experience stress from many sources. Common stressors include clients who are dying or in pain, emergency treatments, demanding co-workers or clients, family commitments, situations in which personal safety is threatened, downsizing, and restructuring. A classic theory that describes stress and stressors is Selye's general stress theory. *Selye's theory of stress* describes stress as a nonspecific state in which each person responds individually to stressors. Most persons respond in a fight-or-flight manner.

When stress is too great on the job, nurses may experience burnout. *Burnout* is a situation in which individuals, experiencing constant long-term stress, respond with emotional and/or physical exhaustion, decreased productivity, and overdepersonalization. New graduates also can experience stress caused by incongruity between their values of idealism and those of the actual work environment, called *reality shock*. New graduates often become disillusioned and decrease their productivity, change jobs, or return to school for a career change.

Coping effectively with stress and changes in the health care environment are essential for a satisfied, healthy, and productive employee. *Coping* is performing activities in an effort to adapt to the situation. *Cognitive appraisal* is an individual's assessment of the present stressful situation. *Stressors* can be internal or external to the nurse. *Internal stressors* can be the personal conflicts of balancing family, work, and social events. *External events* can include the work environment. Individuals react differently to stressors. Some may deny the existence of the stressors, whereas others become optimistic that they will handle the stressful occurrence. *Mediators* are supportive mechanisms that individuals use to cope effectively and include social support, coping behaviors, and biological and psychological reactions to internal or external stressors. *Personal hardiness*—a characteristic of commitment, control, and willingness to accept a challenge—has been postulated as being important in handling stress. Those nurses who are hardy are better able to manage their stress.

Hardy (1978) identified different types of role stress. *Role stress* occurs when individuals are unclear about their job obligations or they feel their obligations are impossible to meet. *Role strain* is a subjective feeling of distress arising from a response to outside forces. *Role ambiguity* occurs when role expectations are unclear to the nurse. *Role conflict* occurs when role expectations are incompatible with each other. *Role incongruity* occurs when role expectations are incompatible with the professional values of the nurse. *Role overload* occurs when a nurse cannot possibly complete all assigned activities in the scheduled timeframe. *Role underload* occurs when nurses with advanced training are not able to use their skills to the fullest extent.

Nurses must learn positive coping skills and adaptation strategies to function effectively in their personal and work lives. Individuals who cope effectively reduce their emotional distress, solve their problems, and maintain positive self-esteem. Nurses must examine stressful situations carefully and look out for their best interests. Coping strategies include spending time on recreational activities, creating a personal support network, being involved in a professional association, negotiating or resigning, walking away from problematic situations to reflect, complying when necessary, and modifying rules. Organizations that are attuned to employee well-being organize comprehensive stress management plans to benefit their workers. Strategies to improve well-being include physical activity, nutritional control, environmental control, and support groups.

Nurses have the responsibility for taking care of themselves and others to maximize health and wellness. When nurses become aware of staffing shortages, dangers to personal safety, poor interdepartmental relations, or inadequately designed team situations, they have an obligation to inform their managers of these problematic situations. Being part of a team that takes stressors and turns them into opportunities for innovations or learning boosts employee morale and satisfaction. Leaders and managers have a responsibility to empower nurses to complete their assigned work and to be creative and innovative in the workplace. To be effective, they need to facilitate professional development of staff, promote positive organizational cultures, design work structures that encourage team building, and provide adequate resources for optimal client care. Organizational structure can be designed to reduce paperwork, optimize environmental conditions, encourage participative decision making, and change workloads to facilitate client care and enhance nurse job satisfaction. Strong leadership promotes innovation and creativity, decreases stress, and generates a sense of community and organizational commitment.

LEARNING TOOLS

Self-Assessment: Managing Time

Organizing one's time is crucial. Time is a valuable asset. In the Western culture, we believe that time comes and goes; once it is gone, we cannot recover the moment. For individuals to manage time effectively, they first must determine what personal and professional goals are important for them to accomplish. This self-assessment includes three parts: identifying and prioritizing personal and professional goals, logging activities and amounts of time for each, and identifying and prioritizing activities.

Part 1

Directions

In the following blank lines, identify and prioritize by ranking five personal and professional goals for three time periods. The task of identifying and prioritizing your personal and professional goals is time-consuming and difficult but essential for you to manage your time effectively. Annually you should revisit your list and update the list and congratulate yourself on accomplishments.

1-Year Personal Goals	5-Year Personal Goals	Lifetime Personal Goals
1.	1.	1.
2.	2.	2.
3.	3.	3.
4.	4.	4.
5.	5.	5.

1-Year Professional Goals	5-Year Professional Goals	Lifetime Professional Goals
1.	1.	1.
2.	2.	2.
3.	3.	3.
4.	4.	4.
5.	5.	5.

Part 2

Directions

For a 24-hour period, in a small notebook write down all activities that you complete and the time you engaged in the activity. After you have made a 24-hour record, determine the number of minutes engaged in each activity. A sample log appears below.

This activity is useful in at least three ways. First, it identifies any time robbers such as interruptions, unproductive meetings, telephone solicitations, unorganized activities, and time wasters that may be filling your day. Secondly, it shows you what activities you chose to spend your time doing. That way you can compare these activities to your personal and professional goals to see whether they are congruent or whether you

Time Started	Time Completed	Activity	Total Time in Minutes

need to reprioritize your activities. Finally, it shows you your style of time management. Are you managing a crisis constantly? Are you spending all of your time in professional activities? How much personal time do you have?

Part 3

Directions

Identify those personal and professional activities that are most important to you and prioritize them.

This is an easy task because you have already established your goals. Now, make a daily or weekly list of activities that you need to accomplish and check them off as they are completed. This checklist should be a tool and should not become the center of time management. Below is an example of a checklist. You may rank your activities according to their priority or star those that are most critical to complete first.

This activity helps to organize your daily and weekly workload into a manageable list.

Activities to Accomplish	Date to Be Completed	Check When Completed
1. _____	_____	_____
2. _____	_____	_____
3. _____	_____	_____
4. _____	_____	_____
5. _____	_____	_____
6. _____	_____	_____
7. _____	_____	_____
8. _____	_____	_____
9. _____	_____	_____
10. _____	_____	_____

Self-Assessment Stress Test*

Purpose

To assess your level of stress.

Directions

Check each event that you have experienced during the past 12 months.

Event	Value	Score
Death of spouse	100	_____
Divorce	73	_____
Marital separation	65	_____
Jail term	63	_____
Death of close family friend	63	_____
Personal injury or illness	53	_____
Marriage	50	_____
Fired from work	47	_____
Marital reconciliation	45	_____
Retirement	45	_____
Change in family member's health	44	_____
Pregnancy	40	_____
Sex difficulties	39	_____
Addition to family	39	_____
Business readjustment	39	_____
Change in financial status	38	_____
Death of close friend	37	_____
Change to different line of work	36	_____
Change in number of marital arguments	35	_____
Mortgage or loan over $100,000	31	_____
Foreclosure of mortgage or loan	30	_____

*From Holmes, T. H., & Rahe, R. H. (1967). The social readjustment rating scale. Journal of Psychosomatic Research, 11, 213-218. Copyright 1967 by Elsevier Science Inc.

Change in work responsibilities	29	_____
Son or daughter leaving home	29	_____
Trouble with in-laws	29	_____
Outstanding personal achievement	28	_____
Spouse begins or stops work	26	_____
Starting or finishing school	26	_____
Change in living conditions	25	_____
Revision of personal habits	24	_____
Trouble with boss	23	_____
Change in work hours or conditions	20	_____
Change in residence	20	_____
Change in schools	20	_____
Change in recreational habits	19	_____
Change in church activities	19	_____
Change in social activities	18	_____
Mortgage or loan under $100,000	17	_____
Change in sleeping habits	16	_____
Change in number of family gatherings	15	_____
Change in eating habits	15	_____
Vacation	13	_____
Christmas season	12	_____
Minor violations	11	_____
TOTAL POINTS		_____

Scoring

Add up your score of stress-related events that occurred during the last 12 months. If your score falls at 150 points or less, you are fairly safe from developing a stress-related illness. If your score falls between 151 and 299, you have a 50% chance of developing a stress-related illness; and if your score is 300 or more, you have an 80% chance of developing a stress-related illness.

CASE STUDY

Kelsey Cobb, a clinical nurse on a 18-bed protective care unit in a community hospital in Rock Springs, Wyoming, has worked for the hospital for 20 years. She has observed many changes at the hospital, but lately there are several changes occurring at once with restructuring, quality improvement processes, downsizing, and the addition of unlicensed assistive personnel. Nurse Cobb has been feeling physically exhausted and depersonalized, and her productivity is declining. She feels helpless and would like all the changes to stop so that she could just provide good individualized client care. Lately, co-workers have noticed that Nurse Cobb does the minimum possible to get by and leaves promptly at the stroke of 3 PM when her shift ends.

Case Study Questions

1. What syndrome is Nurse Cobb experiencing?
2. What is causing her to feel helpless and to begin to decompensate?
3. What can Nurse Cobb do now to help herself function effectively when providing client care?

LEARNING RESOURCES

Discussion Questions

1. What are effective coping strategies for nurses to use to stay healthy and deliver optimal client care?
2. What is occupational or job stress? What causes job stress? How can nurses work effectively when experiencing job stress?
3. What is Selye's general stress theory? Describe how this theory is applicable to nursing.
4. What is the difference between reality shock and burnout? Describe and give an example of each.
5. How can nurses be proactive and use stress to their benefit? Give an example.

Study Questions

True or False: Circle the correct answer.

T   F   1. Job satisfaction is a predictor of anticipated turnover or the intent to stay.

T   F   2. Role underload is when there is not enough for a nurse to do on a shift.

T   F   3. Cognitive appraisal is rationalizing stress in an attempt to cope.

T   F   4. The goal of time management is to use every minute possible in the day to accomplish work-related activities.

Matching: Write the letter of the correct response in front of each term.

_____ 5. Stress

_____ 6. Stressor

_____ 7. Burnout

_____ 8. Reality shock

_____ 9. Role incongruity

_____ 10. Role ambiguity

_____ 11. Hardiness

_____ 12. Role overload

_____ 13. Role underload

_____ 14. Role strain

A. Occurs when nurses with advanced training are not able to use their skills to the fullest

B. When a nurse cannot possibly complete all assigned activities in the scheduled timeframe

C. When role expectations are incompatible with the professional values of the nurse

D. When role expectations are unclear to the nurse

E. Subjective feeling of distress arising from responses to outside forces

F. New graduates' experience of incongruity in their values of idealism in the work environment

G. Long-term success resulting in exhaustion or decreased productivity

H. Characteristics of commitment, control, and willingness to accept a challenge

I. A stressful event

J. A physical, social, or spiritual response to an event

REFERENCES

Hardy, M. E. (1978). Role stress and role strain. In M. E. Hardy & M. E. Conway (Eds.), *Role theory: Perspectives for health professionals* (2nd ed.). Norwalk, CT: Appleton-Century-Crofts.

SUPPLEMENTAL READINGS

AbuAlRub, R. F. (2004). Job stress, job performance, and social support among hospital nurses. *Journal of Nursing Scholarship, 36*(1), 73-78.

Caine, R. M., & Ter-Bagdasarian, L. (2003). Early identification and management of critical incident stress. *Critical Care Nurse, 23*(1), 59-65.

Cericola, S. A. (2000). Stress: A self-management approach and nursing care plan for nurses. *Plastic Surgical Nursing, 20*(1), 29-33.

DelBel, J. C. (2003). De-escalating workplace aggression. *Nursing Management, 34*(9), 30-34.

Furlow, L. (2003). Cut the clutter with cycle time reduction. *Nursing Management, 34*(3), 42-44.

Chapter 4: Managing Time and Stress (pp. 83-108)

1. **Why is self-management so important to time management?**

   Self-management allows an individual to control the time management process. Individuals who develop their own time management strategies are empowered to select approaches that will maximize available resources to achieve personal and professional commitments and goals. Selecting specific, measurable, and realistic activities that are personally relevant increases the likelihood that effective and efficient time management strategies will be implemented and actualized.

2. **What strategies of time management work best for nurses?**

   Time management strategies that work best for nurses include analyzing the workday and prioritizing the workload. Depending on the individual situation, available resources, and safety concerns, different strategies may be selected and implemented. Time may be managed successfully through the use of checklists, delegation, planning ahead, and by dividing large projects or tasks into smaller, more manageable undertakings. Time management strategies may differ depending on the practice setting. For example, in home health care, Sherry (1996) identified six time management strategies: take control of your calendar, minimize time spent in office, tame the telephone, simplify documentation, plan ahead, and save time for others.

3. **What sources of stress do you find to be the most important influences in your life and work?**

   Nurses face many sources of stress in their personal and professional lives. The sources of stress that are the most influential affect your ability to control a given situation or circumstance. Sources of personal stress may include concerns related to child care, fatigue, or financial obligations. Workplace stresses may include issues related to role expectations, interpersonal communication, environment, client care situations, or knowledge deficits.

4. **What coping strategies are most useful for stress reduction? Why are they helpful?**

   An individual's personality characteristics, perceptions of the external environment, and past experiences with similar stressors determine which coping mechanisms they select as most useful. Coping mechanisms are used to maintain or regain equilibrium in order to adjust to stressful situations. Effective coping mechanisms reduce emotional distress, enhance problem resolution, and facilitate self-esteem. Examples of coping strategies include humor, complying, resigning, using a support network, spending time with hobbies, exercising, meditation/prayer, and using relaxation techniques.

5. **To what extent should employers pay for stress management programs for nurses?**

   Human resources are the largest fiscal expenditure for organizations. Work-related stress can lead to job dissatisfaction, poor performance, and high turnover rates. High turnover rates result in increased personnel costs from new employee recruitment and orientation. Employee-oriented organizations establish stress management programs to minimize occupational stress so as to foster job satisfaction, productivity, and retention. The implementation of long-term stress management initiatives such as ensuring adequate staffing, correcting problems in the physical environment, and facilitating positive communication are positive strategies that can be implemented by nurse managers to decrease work-related stress.

6. **Why should nurses manage their own stress?**

   The health care environment is stressful, with high client condition severity levels, inadequate staffing, specialty care requirements, ethical dilemmas, and dangerous situations that jeopardize individual safety. In addition, each professional nurse has her or his own personal stressors. Taking steps proactively to manage and minimize the stress in your personal and professional lives will enhance your level of productivity and satisfaction.

7. **Why should nurses promote reality shock support for new graduates?**

   New graduates often experience personal and professional stressors as they make the transition from student to professional practitioner. Novice nurses in their first year of professional practice may experience disillusionment, dismay, and incongruence with organizational values. Experienced nurses can assist, mentor, and counsel new graduates to recognize stressors and to develop effective stress management strategies.

8. **What can nurses do to manage stress in work teams?**

Identification of stressors, effective communication, conflict resolution, and group support minimize stress in work teams. As the work team becomes more knowledgeable about stressors, collaboration occurs to design effective strategies to reduce stress in the work environment. Nurse managers can nurture and mentor teams, provide strong positive leadership direction and encourage creativity to assist with stress management.

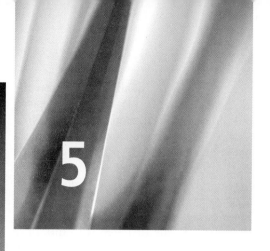

5

Health Policy, Health, and Nursing

STUDY FOCUS

Policy is an important aspect of the economics and regulation of health care services. Nursing and nurses' involvement in policy is important to influence the access, quality, and cost of health care to citizens. Political, social, and economic changes in the United States are creating major changes in health care delivery systems. Nurses must articulate clearly what nursing is, what services they provide, and at what costs in order to compete in a competitive health care environment. Changes in reimbursement methods, increasing demands for services by consumers, and the competition for market share demand that nurses provide accessible, quality services at reasonable costs. Nursing leadership must be active in legislation for health care providers and services. They also must influence policy on reimbursement for nursing services and clearly articulate the role of nursing in health care delivery. Nurses must be involved in setting policy.

Policy is the development of value statements and of setting goals and direction. To be effective in shaping policy, nurses must be actively engaged in *politics,* a process used to influence the allocation of scarce resources in setting health policy. *Policies* are choices made about goals, priorities, and ways of allocating resources. *Public policies* are authoritative decisions that are made in the legislative, executive, or judicial branches of government (Longest, 2002). *Health policy* is the set of public policies that pertain to health and illness. *Politics* is the process of influencing the allocation of scarce resources or the use of power for change. The policy-making process is influenced by values and analysis. The dominant values in the United States are individuality and competition, whereas nursing values include caring, collaboration, and collectivity. Analysis is done to provide data for policy-making decisions. Hanley (2002) proposed a five-step policy analysis framework. The five steps include defining the problem, identifying policy alternatives,

projecting consequences for each option, specifying criteria to evaluate each option, and recommending the optimal solution. One strategy that aids decision makers in determining how much health improvement can be achieved per dollar invested is *cost-effectiveness analysis* (Allred, et al., 1998).

Public policies take many different forms, but *laws* are perhaps the best known form. *Rules and regulations* are important to guide the implementation of laws. Factors that drive public policy making often are related to market failures. In a freely competitive market, the following conditions exist (Longest, 1997, 2001):

- Buyers and sellers have adequate information to make informed choices.
- No one buyer or seller dominates a market.
- Sellers can enter the market easily.
- Sellers' products can be substituted for their competitors.
- A balance exists between supply and demand of a product or service.

When market failures occur, the government has choices in responding to the imbalance. They may do nothing, try to improve the working of the market, require people to behave in a certain way, provide incentives, or engage directly in the provision of goods or services. Overall, the health care industry does not operate as a free market.

The three major players in policy making are interest groups, executive agencies that have administrative responsibility over the related policy area, and congressional committees and subcommittees that have legislative authority in these policy areas. An *interest group* is an organization of people with similar policy goals who try to influence governmental policy. Four strategies that interest groups use to influence the public policy-making process include (1) lobbying, (2) litigation, (3) electioneering, and (4) influencing public opinions (Longest, 1997). *Lobbying* is interest groups influencing the views of individual representatives, senators, or key members of the executive branch on specific issues. *Lobbyists* are hired to communicate with policy makers for the purpose of influencing their

33

decisions to be favorable to the lobbyist's viewpoint. Guidelines to influence policy effectively include organizing, doing your homework, framing your arguments to appeal to the specific audience you want to persuade, concentrating your resources, acting in a timely fashion, and obtaining the best data available to support your policy position. *Electioneering* is a strategy to elect or retain in office the policy makers who are sympathetic to the interest of the group's members. *Litigation* is a strategy to use lawsuits to challenge existing policies or alter specific implementation of policies. *Shaping public opinion* is actively seeking public support for your position. Surviving the policy agenda depends on technical feasibility, value acceptability within the policy community, tolerable cost, anticipated public agreement, and elected officials receptiveness to it (Milstead, 1999). Two models for policy formulation are (1) the Kingdon (1995) model, which describes the constant interaction between participants in the process and the policy issues, and (2) the stage-sequential model, which describes the specific steps of identifying policy problems, formulating policy, implementing programs, and evaluating policy.

Public policy is formulated through governmental activities. The policy-making process occurs in three phases and generally is initiated by a small but powerful group, by a widespread problem that affects a large group, or by the media. The first phase is policy formulation, which involves agenda setting and developing legislation. During policy formulation, much debate and input is generated with special interest groups and other influential leaders to encourage legislation or to prevent a bill. The three types of committees in Congress are oversight, appropriation, and authorization committees (Wakefield, 1999). The second phase is policy implementation, which is when the legislation is implemented. At this phase the law is vague and the details of implementation must be established. The third phase is policy modification. In this phase changes are made as the legislation is being formulated or during implementation. The legislation frequently is modified based on competing viewpoints from multiple constituents. Health policies fall within two broad categories: (1) allocative and (2) regulatory (Block, 2004). Allocative policies are designed to provide benefits to one group of individuals or organizations at the expense of others to meet specific policy (Longest, 2002). Regulatory policies influence the actions, behaviors, and decisions of others through a directive approach. The five categories of regulative health policies are (1) market-entry restrictions, (2) rate or price-setting controls on

health service providers, (3) quality controls on the provision of health services, (4) market-preserving controls, and (5) social regulation (Longest, 1997). *Policy analysis* is the systematic study of the content and anticipated or actual effects of existing or proposed policies.

Legislation at the federal level must go through a multistage process to become law. The process has many steps, in any of which the bill can die, be modified, or approved. The first step is to introduce a legislative proposal, also called a *bill*. Anyone can have input into the drafting of the bill, but only a member of Congress can sponsor the legislation. The member of Congress who is sponsoring the bill introduces it to his or her chamber where the bill will be numbered and referred to a standing committee. Hearings then are held, and the bill is marked up. The committee reports back to the chamber, and the bill is placed on the legislative agenda and then debated. During this process, the bill can stand as is or be amended. The bill will pass or be defeated. If the bill passes, it goes to the other chamber for a similar process. If both chambers approve the bill, it is sent to the president, who may choose to sign it, veto it (a two-thirds vote of both houses overrides a presidential veto), or hold it (it will become law within 10 days).

Nurses must be politically active to have an impact on their own opportunities and on client welfare in health policy. Activities that nurses can pursue include calling their legislators, writing letters clearly articulating their expectations and positions, and joining professional organizations to ensure a collective, united voice. Supporting local and state activities, assisting during a campaign for a state representative, voting, and rallying others to vote, forming and participating in a protest rally, and helping draft legislation are other useful activities to influence the legislative process.

Other essential activities include assisting in writing professional position papers through the American Nurses Association and conducting and sharing essential nursing research studies with legislators who support key issues. Nurses can stay abreast of current legislative activities by reading the newsletters of professional organizations and professional journals, reading newspapers, watching news on the television, and networking with colleagues. Major changes are occurring in health care. Nurses must be instrumental in formulating legislation to ensure nursing's position in the health care delivery system. Nurses must use the sources of power effectively to influence policy. *Legitimate or positional power* is based on an individual's social or organizational position or formal power of authority. *Reward or coercive power* is the ability to reward compliance or punish noncompliance. *Expert power* is holding expertise or information that is valued by others. And *referent power* is the circumstance in which a person, organization, or interest group engenders admiration, loyalty, and emulation from others to such an extent that they gain the power to exert influence. Hersey and colleagues (1979) identified two additional power sources: information and connection power. *Information power* is when one person has special information another desires, and *connection power* is the perceived privileged connections with individual or organizations.

Nurses comprise the largest group of health care providers in the United States. The size of the profession creates the opportunity for significant influence in public health policy. Examples of issues on the nursing policy agenda include the nursing and faculty shortage, quality care, and staffing ratios. The key to successful legislative action is perseverance and dedication. Nurses undergo four phases of political development: (1) buy-in, (2) self-interest, (3) political sophistication, and (4) leading the way (Longest, 2001). Nurses and nursing organizations must unify and speak with a single voice. We must be politically savvy to shape and influence health policy.

LEARNING TOOLS

Self-Assessment

Purpose

To become aware of the strategies for nurses to become politically active in improving health policy.

Introduction

There are many activities in which you can engage to become politically active and to support a specific health policy. One strategy is to call your legislators and discuss the importance of a bill or issue. You can provide specific details about why it is important and how it will benefit the public. For example, if the issue is providing reimbursement for nurse practitioners, essential points to discuss are the importance of eliminating financial barriers and improving access to care for families in your state. You also can provide references from nursing research articles about the increased quality, access, and decreased costs for care provided by nurse practitioners to support your position. Additional strategies to support nurse practitioners are referring clients to them, personally seeking care from them, and talking to the community about the important role nurse practitioners play in the health care delivery system. An example of the format and content of a letter to a legislator is depicted on p. 36.

Follow up with the legislator by providing a written letter addressing specific points, support for laws on the reimbursement of nurse practitioners and reasons why this is important. Include any resources that might help support your case for expanded reimbursement for nurse practitioners.

Directions

1. Identify an issue about which you are concerned and would like to see changed or supported by your legislator.
2. Call the legislator, and discuss the issue with him or her.
3. Then send a follow-up letter detailing your position, and include any documents of support. A sample letter is provided, showing you the components to include in the letter to your legislator. It is important to send a typed letter.

CASE STUDY

Jason Jarovich is a registered nurse on a 45-bed obstetric unit in a large teaching hospital in Birmingham, Alabama. Nurse Jarovich is a primary nurse for mothers and infants. He always completes a nursing care assessment and then follows up by making a telephone call to track the client's progress. Nurse Jarovich has a population of clients who are indigent and frequently request additional teaching on parent/child care activities. He is concerned that the mothers do not have the support or information available to them to provide the best possible care for their infants. Nurse Jarovich conducted a research study on a subset of his clients and divided the group into two. One group received home visits and assistance with nutritional needs, and the other only received a follow-up questionnaire and a single visit to evaluate the parent/child interaction. Nurse Jarovich noticed a marked improvement in the infants in the first group. The infants were more responsive, were more advanced in their activity level, and were all within normal limits for weight gain. The infants in the other group, however, were less active and less responsive, and 30% were underweight for their age. Nurse Jarovich decides that he needs to find a way to support mothers who needs assistance. He becomes politically active to garner support for his interventions.

35

Case Study Questions

1. What should Nurse Jarovich do to garner support for his ideas?

2. How can his research assist to support his ideas?

3. How long a process is it to change or implement a new program with state or federal moneys?

LEARNING RESOURCES

Discussion Questions

1. What changes in the delivery of health care to clients have occurred as a result of the national health care reform initiatives in the United States?

2. What can nurses do to become politically active and have a strong voice in health care policy?

3. In what phases of the policy-making process can nurses initiate changes to improve the health of the public?

4. Does nursing have a strong special interest group in Washington?

5. Describe the multistage process of how a bill becomes law, and identify strategies nurses can use to initiate or enhance legislation.

6. What are two public health issues that are important to consumers? Why are these issues important to consumers?

Study Questions

True or False: Circle the correct answer.

T   F   1. The three phases of policy making are policy formulation, policy implementation, and policy modification.

T   F   2. Policy issues are raised only when they affect the small but powerful groups in the United States.

T   F   3. Policy making is an analytical process based solely on objective data.

Date

Name
Title
Address

To: Name

In this section clearly identify what you expect of the legislator. *Example:* I would like you to support legislation and policies to remove barriers to equitable reimbursement for nurses in (identify your state).

Describe why it is important for your legislator to support your issue. *Example:* A nurse practitioner is a registered nurse who has successfully completed a graduate program in a nursing specialty and functions in an expanded practice role. These nurses are able to provide primary care to communities, increasing accessible, affordable, quality health care.

At this point, it is useful to cite statistics or research about the cost, quality, or outcomes nurse practitioners are able to provide. *Example:* I have enclosed two studies that demonstrate the benefits for the clients of nurse practitioners who provide care. These studies show that the cost of care to clients is decreased, risk factors are identified, and lifestyle modifications are implemented to improve health outcomes. In this section summarize your request, restate what you expect, and close the letter. Example: I look forward to your support for equitable reimbursement for nurses in (state). Nurse practitioners increase access to care and provide high-quality, holistic health care at a reasonable cost.

Sincerely,

Name, Credentials

T	F	4.	Nursing research should be an important component of the policy-making process.
T	F	5.	Politics is the same thing as power.
T	F	6.	An allocative health policy ensures that objectives are met.
T	F	7.	Ethical decisions should remain separate and not be discussed when public policy is set.
T	F	8.	A white paper usually is drafted by a professional organization to define its position clearly on a specific topic.
T	F	9.	Politics is the attempt to influence the allocation of scarce resources.
T	F	10.	The terms *public policy* and *health policy* can be used interchangeably.
T	F	11.	Position papers are designed by professional organizations to keep their members informed of new activities.
T	F	12.	Nurses have been instrumental in influencing public policy and routinely are sought for advice on legislative activities.
T	F	13.	The public policy-making process is cyclical.

REFERENCES

Allred, C. A., Arford, P. H., Mauldin, P. D., & Goodwin, L. K. (1998). Cost-effectiveness analysis in the nursing literature, 1992-1996. *Image, 30*(3), 235-242.

Block, L. E. (2004). Health policy: What it is and how it works. In C. Harrington & C. I. Estes (Eds.), *Health policy: Crisis and reform in the U.S. health care delivery system* (4th ed., pp. 4-14). Boston: Jones and Bartlett.

Hanley, B. E. (2002). Policy development and analysis. In D. J. Mason, J. K. Leavitt, & M. W. Chaffee (Eds.), *Policy and politics in nursing and health care* (4th ed., pp. 55-69). Philadelphia: W. B. Saunders.

Hersey, P., Blanchard, K. H., & Natemeyer, W. E. (1979). Situational leadership, perception, and impact of power. *Group Organizational Studies, 4,* 418-428.

Kingdon, J. W. (1995). *Agendas, alternatives and public policies* (2nd ed.). New York: Addison-Wesley Longman.

Longest, B. B., Jr. (1997). *Seeking strategic advantage through health policy analysis.* Chicago: Health Administration Press.

Longest, B. B., Jr. (2001). *Contemporary health policy.* Chicago: Health Administration Press.

Longest, B. B., Jr. (2002). *Health policy making in the United States* (3rd ed.). Chicago: Health Administration Process.

Milstead, J. A. (1999). *Health policy and politics: A nurses' guide.* Gaithersburg, MD: Aspen.

Wakefield, M. (1999). Government response: Legislation. In J. A. Milstead (Ed.), *Health policy and politics: A nurse's guide* (pp. 77-103). Gaithersberg, MD: Aspen.

SUPPLEMENTAL READINGS

Beu, B. (2002). Nurse reinvestment act; contacting elected officials; legislative priorities; perioperative nurse week. *AORN Journal, 76*(4), 692-695.

Kitchen, L. (2004). To impact political policy, first prepare. *Nursing Management, 35*(1), 14-15.

Landreanau, K. J. (2003). Cost issues related to American healthcare policy. *Nursing Forum, 38*(1), 17-22.

Sarikonda-Woitas, C., & Robinson, J. H. (2002). Ethical health care policy: Nursing's voice in allocation. *Nursing Administration Quarterly, 26*(4), 72-80.

Steele, S., Rocchiccioli, J., & Porche, D. (2003). Analyzing and promoting issues in health policy: Nurse manager's perspective. *Nursing Economic$, 21*(2), 80-83.

Chapter 5: Health Policy, Health, and Nursing (pp. 109-130)

1. What are the major health care values of nursing?

The nursing profession subscribes to numerous health care values, including caring, collaboration, and collectivity. Client advocacy and accessibility to health care are hallmarks of professional nursing values, standards, and practice.

2. What role do consumers play?

Historically, consumers have not been active participants in decisions related to health care legislation and politics. As consumers become more knowledgeable, lack adequate health care coverage, and experience spiraling health care costs, their influential role in health care decision has escalated. Consumers are demanding health care reform, improved health care benefits, and a political voice in policy formation.

3. Is caring a health care policy? Why or why not?

Caring is an influential element in the formulation of health care policy. Although caring is not legally mandated, it is a powerful factor in the legislation of policies that govern the distribution of health care resources. Professional nurses bring caring to the legislative arena through political activism and client advocacy for accessible, equitable, and affordable health care.

4. What kind of public policies govern your life? Govern nursing practice?

Your private life is governed by the legislative system, which includes laws, taxes, and ordinances. Licensure, practice standards, and each of the Nurse Practice Acts in each state regulate your professional nursing practice. Organizational policies, procedures, and protocols also influence the practice of professional nursing practice. Accreditation standards and infection control guidelines, as well as national and international health initiatives, have an effect on the delivery of nursing services.

5. Which branch of government is responsible for the health of the citizens?

All branches of government (legislative, judicial, and executive) have a responsibility for the health of citizens. The legislative branch creates bills to enact laws that affect health care. The judicial level oversees civil and criminal cases that influence the direction of health care, and the executive level participates in policy development and enactment, such as Medicaid/Medicare programs and health care reform.

6. Should illegal aliens be included in health care policy and benefits?

The issue of health care benefits for illegal aliens is an ethical and financial dilemma. One position espouses that illegal aliens should not be included in health care policy or be entitled to health care benefits. Some believe that because health care services are supported financially by taxpayer dollars, illegal aliens should be exempt from receiving health care. This sentiment holds true for those who are cognizant of the scarce resources available to meet the needs of the nation's citizenry, as well as legal aliens. Still, some argue that health is a universal benefit that transcends legality and citizenship.

7. Why are the professional issues in nursing that are important enough to be on the public policy agenda? Which ones are?

Nurses introduce policies on public health issues that advocate for the welfare of society. Nursing has been a strong proponent for universal access for all citizens, long-term care, and client rights. Current issues related to professional nursing practice include the nursing shortage, (which includes the shortage of nursing faculty as well), client safety issues (which includes minimum nurse staffing ratios, and outlawing of mandatory overtime), scope of practice, Nurse Reinvestment Act, prescriptive authority, reimbursement for advanced practice roles and speciality roles, and multistate licensure.

8. Why is politics useful to nurses? What strategies are most successful?

Politics is a useful tool for nurses to use as they strive toward fulfilment of professional and personal goals. Politics may be used to influence the allocation of scarce resources, implement change, and develop care delivery systems that enhance accessibility and availability of services. Nurses may select a cadre of political strategies such as voting, campaigning, community activism, and protests to influence public health policy.

9. **Why can nurses be influential in policy and politics? How does this happen?**

Nurses possess the knowledge and political skill to affect public policy. Inasmuch as nursing is the largest group of health care providers, their collective voice can be used to shape policy and politics. Nurses can establish relationships with elected officials, community leaders, and public policy makers. Nurses can lobby Congress, form political action committees and coalitions, and work with professional associations to stay informed of nursing and health care issues. Nurses also can hold political office to promote political agendas that advance the health of all persons.

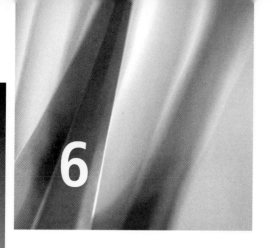

6

Critical Thinking Skills

STUDY FOCUS

The health care environment is turbulent, constantly changing, and chaotic. The health care environment has moved from a process-focused orientation in care delivery to an outcome-based orientation in which the nurse is expected to make autonomous practice decisions and meet best practice standards. Nurses, as knowledge workers, encounter environmental stressors that require critical thinking skills for high-quality decision making. According to Benner (1984), nurses go through five stages of competence: novice, advanced beginner, competent, proficient, and expert. *Critical thinking* is reasoning that generates and examines questions and problems and is central in making sound clinical judgments. Critical thinking is a reflective intellectual process to identify and challenge assumptions and explore and imagine alternatives (Brookfield, 1991). The development of critical thinking dates back to Socrates, who developed a questioning approach to thinking clearly with greater logical consistency. Great thinkers like Plato, Aristotle, Thomas Aquinas, Francis Bacon, and Descartes also emphasized the need for critical thinking where individuals used a systematic disciplining of the mind to guide thinking.

Critical thinking requires logic, breadth, depth, accuracy, and relevance. Critical thinking questions include *Why? What can I infer from this data?* and *What is the most fundamental issue?* Characteristics of critical thinking are disciplined, self-directed, accurate, and intellectual. The two cognitive processes used in critical thinking for nursing judgments are *analytical* and *intuitive* (Polge, 1995). Elements of purposeful critical thinking include clearly stating the problem, identifying the goal, having a clear point of view, stating the assumptions, using concepts and principles, collecting data, making interpretations and using reasoning to develop conclusions, and stating the implications and consequences (Kelley, 1999). Two common approaches to reasoning are inductive and deductive methods. *Inductive reasoning* is moving from specifics to generalizations, whereas *deductive reasoning* is moving from general to specific (El Paso Community College, 2004).

Traditional thinkers tend to maintain the status quo, whereas critical thinkers challenge and question the norm. Traditional thinkers use problem solving, whereas critical thinkers ask *why* and challenge the "routine." Traditional thinkers choose solutions that are comfortable and familiar. Critical thinkers seek alternative solutions and take risks in choosing possible solutions. Critical thinking is associated with creative thinking. Creative thinking is the formation of novel ideas, products, or services. *Three attributes of creative thinking* are that knowledge is received as a whole, awareness of knowledge is immediate, and knowledge is acquired independent of linear reasoning (Benner & Tanner, 1987; Polge 1995). *Creative problem solving* is oriented toward achieving goals in novel ways (LeStorti et al., 1999). Creative problem solving is based on the principles of deferred judgment and divergent-convergent thinking sequence. *Deferred judgment* refers to the temporary suspension of criticism or evaluation of an idea. *Divergent-convergent thinking sequences* are an opening up of potential possibilities with the selection of the best option.

A *problem* is a deficit or surplus of something that is needed to achieve one's goals. We encounter problems daily in our personal and professional lives. Some situations produce problems (a *difficulty*), some problems create conflict (a *dilemma*), and sometimes an individual's solution does not take a logical path (a *paradox*). Solving problems effectively is important to making good client care decisions. *Problem solving* is a process to identify obstacles that inhibit accomplishment of a specific goal. Solving problems is a rational-logical thought process. In nursing, problem solving often occurs in the context of caring for clients, team leadership, case management, and client advocacy. Nurses may use the *nursing process,* which is a framework for solving nursing problems. The *general framework for*

41

problem solving includes seven steps (Davidhizer & Bowen, 1999; Finkelman, 2001). The first step is defining the problem by clarifying the task and describing it in a single sentence. The second step is gathering information from a variety of sources and analyzing that data. The third step is determining the overall goal or desired outcome to guide decision making and actions toward the desired outcome. The fourth step is developing potential solutions to make the best choice. The fifth step is considering the consequences for each of the identified potential solutions. Making the best decision is the sixth step. Finally, implementing the solution, evaluating its effectiveness, and taking necessary corrective action occurs.

The *Kirton adaptation-innovation theory* identifies two types of problem-solving styles: adapting and innovating. *Adaptors* use more traditional approaches to problem solving. They do not seek out problems to solve but do resolve the problems they confront. In contrast, *innovators* seek novel situations, challenge rules, and create solutions. They discover problems and attack them vigorously. Problem solvers typically assess problems by their urgency and their immediacy. Some persons envision problems on a time continuum. On one end of the continuum is a potential problem, which may emerge at any time; in the middle are actual problems that require prompt attention; and on the far end are critical problems, which are extremely urgent and require crisis intervention.

Many strategies can be used to solve problems. Some of the most common problem-solving strategies include direct intervention, indirect intervention, delegation, purposeful inaction, and consultation or collaboration. *Direct intervention* involves you personally doing a task or activity. *Indirect intervention* requires good interpersonal skills such as negotiation, conflict resolution, persuasion, and confrontations to influence others to carry out activities or resolve the problem. *Delegation* is used to assign the responsibility of an activity or task to another for the purpose of workload distribution. *Purposeful inaction* is consciously ignoring or choosing not to make a choice with the hope that the problem may go away with time. Inaction can be useful in some situations. *Consultation or collaboration* is exchanging information with peers and colleagues to solve a problem.

In today's health care environment, team-based approaches to client care are commonplace. Nurses must learn to function and solve problems effectively in group environments. Dailey (1990) describes the following nine-step problem-solving procedure to solve problems in group/team settings:

1. Identifying problems

2. Determining perceptions

3. Determining the underlying causes of problems

4. Assessing the magnitude of the problem

5. Constructing a plan

6. Implementing a plan

7. Test-piloting the plan after discussing it with the team

8. Tracking effectiveness by creating indicators

9. Publicizing results

Nurse leaders must encourage critical thinking, questioning, and brainstorming to move the organization forward and to deliver quality care to clients. Many tools can be used for solving problems; among them are *gap analysis,* determining the difference between the ideal and real situations; affinity maps; and relationship diagrams.

LEARNING TOOLS

Self-Assessment: Problem-Solving In-Basket Exercise

Purpose

To identify and improve diagnostic reasoning and clinical decision making skills.

Introduction

Nurses are confronted daily with multiple problems, not only in their personal lives but also in their professional work. Diagnostic reasoning and clinical decision making are skills all registered nurses need. In-basket exercises are useful for improving skills.

Directions

1. Read the memos on p. 43 and then identify which problem type they are: potential, actual, or critical.

2. Take the critical problem you identify, and use the six-step problem-solving process to work through it.

You arrive on the unit, check your mail, and find the following memos:

Memo 1

From: Nancy, Head Nurse, 4 West
To: Sue, Staff Nurse
Re: Quality Improvement

Sue, as the 4 West representative to the hospital's quality improvement team, one of your responsibilities is to monitor documentation on the nursing flow chart and alert and assist nurses to comply with our unit standards. In the most recent report, I noticed that 4 West has a poor rate of compliance. Please attend to this situation immediately.

(What type of problem is this? _____)

Memo 2

From: Jon, Personnel Director
To: Sue, Staff Nurse, 4 West
Re: Health Insurance

Sue, it has come to my attention that two of your health insurance enrollment forms were incorrectly completed. We have submitted the required data, and you have insurance coverage, but the records should be completed properly sometime in the future.

(What type of problem is this? _____)

Verbal Report 3

Sylvia stops you in the hall and tells you that Mrs. N's family is displeased with her care. They are demanding to speak to someone in charge. Sylvia is in a hurry to get home because she has a sick child and quickly leaves.

(What type of problem is this? _____)

Determine the most critical of the three problems identified. Write the name of the problem below. Then use the problem-solving process to resolve it.

Problem-Solving Steps

Decision Name: _____

1. Define problem. _____

_____

2. Gather information. _____

_____

3. Determine the overall goal or desired outcome. _____

_____

4. Develop solutions. _____

_____

5. Consider consequences. _____

_____

6. Make a decision. _____

_____

7. Implement and evaluate solution. _____

_____

CASE STUDY

Beth Martin is a nurse manager for the cardiac intensive care unit in a large teaching hospital in Birmingham, Alabama. She enjoys challenges, pushes her staff to maximum productivity, and works at least 10-hour shifts. If the organizational rules are in her way, she challenges them and works toward an innovative solution to the problem. Nurse Martin enjoys novel situations rather than routine or day-to-day challenges. She seems to thrive on unique problems and designs creative solutions to solve them. The staff on the cardiac intensive care unit like Nurse Martin's style and support her in her efforts.

Case Study Questions

1. According to Kirton's adaptation-innovation theory, what type of problem-solving style is Nurse Martin exhibiting?

2. Describe the similarities and differences of adaptors and innovators.

LEARNING RESOURCES

Discussion Questions

1. What is the association between critical thinking and creative problem solving and how can these strategies be used in solving health care problems?

2. In what situations would a nurse use the problem-solving process as opposed to the team problem-solving process?

3. How do the steps of the problem-solving process, the nursing process, and the team problem-solving process differ? How are they similar?

4. What are some strategies that can be used to solve problems? Give examples of a situation in which these strategies would be useful.

5. Is it important for nurses to have diagnostic reasoning and clinical decision-making skills? If yes, why?

6. Should nurses consider the economic implications when providing client care?

Study Questions

True or False: Circle the correct answer.

T   F   1. Problem solving is a high-level skill used only by health care professionals.

T   F   2. Adaptors seek solutions to problems in accepted ways.

T   F   3. Innovators focus on resolving problems.

T   F   4. The first step in the problem-solving process is to define the problem.

T   F   5. The team problem-solving method is a slow process and a poor method for making decisions.

T   F   6. Critical thinking and creative problem solving are the same.

T   F   7. The two cognitive processes used in critical thinking for nursing judgments are analytical and intuitive.

T   F   8. Problem solving is a rational-logical thought process.

T   F   9. It is inappropriate for a manager to use indirect intervention to solve problems.

T   F   10. Purposeful inaction is a valuable tool in most situations.

T   F   11. Creative thinking is described as follows: knowledge is received as a whole, awareness of knowledge is immediate, and knowledge is acquired independent of linear reasoning.

T   F   12. A critical thinker preserves the norm or status quo.

Matching: Write the letter of the correct response in front of each term.

_____ 13. Problem solving

_____ 14. Actual problem

_____ 15. Adaptor

_____ 16. Innovator

_____ 17. Delegation

_____ 18. Potential problem

_____ 19. Critical problem

_____ 20. Critical thinking

_____ 21. Creative problem solving

A. A situation that is highly urgent and needs crisis intervention

B. A situation that is tenuous, and difficulties can occur at any time

C. A situation that occurs in real time and needs prompt action

D. Assigning responsibilities and tasks to others

E. Using tried and accepted solutions to problems

F. Using innovative, creative solutions to problems

G. Using a process to identify obstacles and to achieve goals

H. Reasoning that generates and examines questions and problems

I. A novel approach to thinking to accomplish a goal

REFERENCES

Benner, P. (1984). *From novice to expert: Excellence and power in clinical practice.* Menlo Park, CA: Addison-Wesley.

Benner, P., & Tanner, C. (1987). Clinical judgment: How expert nurses use intuition. *American Journal of Nursing, 87*(1), 23-31.

Brookfield, S. D. (1991). *Developing critical thinkers: Challenging adults to explore alternative ways of thinking and acting.* San Francisco: Jossey-Bass.

Dailey, R. (1990). Strengthening hospital nursing: How to use problem-solving teams effectively. *Journal of Nursing Administration, 20* (7/8), 24-29.

Davidhizer, R. E., & Bowen, M. (1999). There are solutions to problems. *Health Care Manager, 18*(1), 14-19.

El Paso Community College. (2004). Think bank. El Paso, TX: El Paso Community College/The Texas Collaborative for Teaching Excellence. Retrieved May 17, 2005, from *www.epcc.edu/Special/Critical/home.htm*

Finkelman, A. W. (2001). Problem-solving, decision-making, and critical thinking: How do they mix and why bother? *Home Care Provider, 6*(6), 194-197.

Kelley, T. A. (1999). Critical thinking for case managers. *Inside Case Management, 6*(5), 10-12.

LeStorti, A. J., Cullen, P. A., Hanzlik, E. M., Michiels, J. M., Piano, L. A., Ryan, P. L., et al. (1999). Creative thinking in nursing education: Preparing for tomorrow's challenges. *Nursing Outlook, 47*(2), 62-66.

Polge, J. (1995). Critical thinking: The use of intuition in making clinical nursing judgments. *Journal of the New York State Nurses Association, 26*(2), 4-9.

SUPPLEMENTAL READINGS

Edwards, S. (2003). Critical thinking at the bedside: A practical perspective. *British Journal of Nursing, 12*(19), 1142-1149.

Ignatavicius, D. D. (2001). Six critical thinking skills for at-the-bedside success. *Dimensions of Critical Care Nursing, 20*(2), 30-33.

Lunney, M. (2003). Critical thinking and accuracy of nurses' diagnoses. *International Journal of Nursing Terminologies and Classifications, 14*(3), 96-107.

Martin, C. (2002). The theory of critical thinking of nursing. *Nursing Education Perspectives, 23*(5), 243-247.

Ruthman, J., Jackson, J., Cluskey, M., Flannigan, P., Folse, V. N., & Bunten, J. (2004). Using clinical journaling to capture critical thinking across the curriculum. *Nursing Education Perspectives, 25*(3), 120-123.

Chapter 6: Critical Thinking Skills (pp. 131-148)

1. **How can critical thinking and problem solving be used in nursing practice?**

   Critical thinking and problem solving are cognitive skills used every day in nursing practice in a variety of situations and settings. For example, they can be used to assess the situation, determine the problem, plan the course of action, and evaluate the outcome. These intellectual processes guide the nurse in determining the complexity, urgency, and focus of the problem and in developing alternative and creative solutions.

2. **Identify a problem with which you are dealing now. What approaches might you use to solve this problem?**

   How one feels about a problem is influenced by one's education, experience, perspective, and socialization. Moreover, the approach selected to solve a problem may be influenced by one's personality-related problem-solving style that influences how one acquires, stores, retrieves, and transforms information (Kirton, 1989). The Kirton adaptation-innovation theory (1989) identified two types of problem solving styles: adaptors and innovators. Adaptors seek solutions to a problem using conventional approaches, whereas innovators create novel and different approaches to problem solving. Innovators question current practices and promote change.

3. **How do you tend to respond to a problem? Emotionally? Logically? Why is it important to identify your habitual responses to problems?**

   Because emotional responses to a problem may be rooted in fear, anger, or resentment, they may not adhere to a sound or rational process. However, logical responses do follow a rational approach to problem solving that includes gathering information, defining the problem, developing solutions, considering the consequences, making a decision, and implementing and evaluating the solutions. Understanding one's problem-solving style increases self-awareness, knowledge, and the opportunity for incorporating alternative approaches to one's problem-solving repertoire.

4. **What strategy do you tend to use for problem solving? What are other strategies you would like to use?**

   Individuals tend to use strategies that have been successful in the past. No matter what your particular strategy, some alternatives to consider are direct intervention, indirect intervention, delegation, purposeful inaction, consultation, and collaboration. Direct intervention involves direct, personal involvement, whereas indirect intervention involves only circuitous involvement. Similarly, delegation involves allocating certain responsibilities to others, whereas purposeful inaction is the conscious, deliberate decision to not act. Lastly, consultation or collaboration problem-solving strategies involve the active participation of peers and colleagues to identify solutions and to solve problems creatively. Evaluate your problem-solving strategies and try others to optimize decision making.

5. **How do leaders/managers facilitate critical thinking and problem solving?**

   Nurse managers and leaders can facilitate critical thinking and problem solving by creating a work environment in which each person feels valued. Managers use questioning and brainstorming techniques to encourage the development of ideas and to facilitate critical thinking. Mistakes are analyzed for process improvement rather than punitive action.

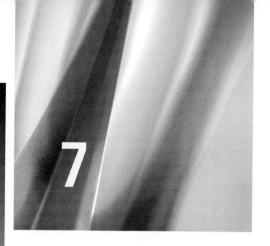

7

Decision-Making Skills

Influential leaders make effective decisions that optimize organizational productivity, resources, and market share. A *decision* is selecting among competing alternative solutions. *Decision making* is behaviors exhibited in selecting from among competing alternative solutions and then implementing activities to accomplish the goal. Decision making deals not only with problems but also with opportunities, challenges, and leadership initiatives. Decision making is a subset and vital component of problem solving. Identifying a course of action is the purpose of decision making. Factors that influence decision making include values, life experiences, and individual thinking preferences. *Decision making has five core elements:* identifying a problem, establishing criteria to evaluate potential solutions, searching for alternative solutions, evaluating alternatives, and selecting the best choice. The *phases of decision making* are deliberation, judgment, and choice (Schaefer, 1974). Individuals frame problems in different ways. One way is to use a systems approach like those used in quality improvement processes in which emphasis is placed on the organizational process and group problem solving. Another method of framing a problem is to view the decision as individual rather than organizational. In an individual problem, all responsibility, accountability, and decision-making authority rests with one person.

The basic elements of problem solving and decision making are identifying the problem and making the decisions. According to Wren (1974), the following *10 steps are included in the decision-making process:*

1. Becoming aware of a situation
2. Investigating the nature of the situation
3. Determining the objectives of the solution
4. Determining alternative solutions
5. Weighing the consequences and relative efficiency of each solution
6. Evaluating various alternatives

7. Selecting the best alternative
8. Implementing the decision
9. Evaluating the solution
10. Correcting the solution based on evaluation

Six common distortions in decision making are (1) anchoring, (2) status quo, (3) sunk-cost, (4) confirming-evidence, (5) framing, and (6) estimating and forecasting.

Desired decisions can be categorized into the endpoint of minimal or optimal. *Minimal decisions* use basic requirements and meet minimum standards. These decisions often are referred to as *satisfying decisions* because they satisfy basic requirements. Alternatively, *optimizing decisions* are evaluated carefully, competing alternatives are weighed, and the best choice is selected. Optimizing decisions often result in positive outcomes, client and staff satisfaction, and enhanced financial stability for the organization. Individuals sometimes have difficulty thinking creatively or stepping "out of the box" to design innovate solutions.

Nurses use the decision-making process for individual, clinical, and organizational problem solving. *Clinical decision making* or *clinical judgment* is decision making based on nurse and client interaction and goal setting. Some nurses use diagnostic reasoning in their practice. *Diagnostic reasoning* is a four-step process that includes attending to available cues, activating hypotheses, gathering data, and evaluating hypotheses with data until a diagnosis is reached (Elstein et al., 1978). *Organizational decision making* is assessing and solving systems problems to attain agency goals. *Ethical decision making* is examining conflicts among ethical principles, resource allocation decisions, and values.

Administrative decision making is common under conditions of uncertainty; high risk; and allocation of human, financial, and/or material resources. *Four types of administrative decision-making strategies* include satisfying, incrementalism, mixed scanning, and optimizing (Janis & Mann, 1977). *Satisfying* is

47

getting by, selecting a solution that is good enough. *Incrementalism* is a slow, step-by-step approach to solving an immediate problem with progress toward an optimal course of action. *Mixed scanning* combines an opportunistic approach to problem solving with the goal of optimizing the results. *Optimizing* entails choosing the course of action with the highest payoff. To diagnose the problem or situation when making decisions, it is important to examine the *seven problem attributes*. They are the quality of the decision, sufficient information/expertise, structure of the problem, acceptance/commitment of followers, probability an autocratic decision will be accepted, motivation of followers, and conflict about the preferred solution. Leaders may choose to use a variety of decision-making styles. These styles include authoritative or autocratic, consultative or collective-participative, facilitative, or delegative (Hersey et al., 2001). To implement a the select solution requires many steps. The steps to move the decision to action are collect information, process information into advice, make the choice, authorize the implementation, and execute what is to be done.

One may engage in many different strategies when making decisions. Formal decision strategies include trial and error, pilot projects, problem critique, creativity techniques, the decision tree, the fish bone or cause-and-effect chart, group decision making, cost-benefit analysis, and worst-case scenarios. *Trial-and-error strategies* involve selecting the first available solution and trying it on the problem. Many times this approach results in poor outcomes. *Pilot projects* are minirepresentations of a formal project. One unit is selected to implement the project, thereby minimizing risk and providing an opportunity to identify problems. *Problem critique* is a technique in which a decision maker describes a potential solution for the problem to a friend or colleague, and then the other person critiques the solution. *Multiple creativity techniques* include nominal group, Delphi, and brainstorming. The goal of creativity techniques is to identify as many potential solutions as possible without threatening individuals or critiquing responses. A *decision tree* is a graphic model of the options, outcomes, and risks of a problem. *Critical paths* are examples of decision trees. *Fish bone* or *cause-and-effect charts* are graphic figures, diagrammed as a sentence is, with horizontal and slanted lines. The diagram represents the product, process, and outcome. Fish bone charts are used to diagnose causes of production problems. *Group decision making* is a process that engages the group to take ownership for organizational problems. Group decision-making models include a rational model based on economic perspectives and maximum utility; political model based on power and influence; process model

that uses standard operating procedures and guidelines; and a garbage can model characterized by difficult problem identification and solutions under uncertain circumstances. *Cost-benefit analysis* is the process of identifying the costs and benefits of a solution to determine the fiscal, human, and material impact. Driving and restraining forces also are identified. *Worst-case scenarios* typically are used when money or prestige is at stake. Decision makers examine all possible events that could go wrong in order to determine a course of action that will protect the organization.

Nurses also may use the tools of perception and innovation in their decision making. These tools enable nurses to break out of their traditional decision-making strategies by finding novel solutions that provide a high payoff. Computerized decision making offers a tool for analyzing the decision process and potential solutions. Perception affects how one views the solution. Reframing one's perception of the problem or solution can create a new method to solve problems and may lead to the creation of a new device or new business. Innovations are those activities that have not been tried before in the same form. Reframing problems and solutions is a key strategy to change the way we perceive and select solutions. Sources of innovative opportunity include the unexpected; incongruity; innovation based on process needs; changes in the industry structure or market structure; demographics (population changes); changes in perception, mood, or meaning; and new knowledge.

Leadership is needed in designing decision support tools enabled by automation to standardize customized performance measures and quality outcome data. Effective leaders will be able to manage the concerns about health care error and client safety issues in the U.S. health care system by evaluating systems and creating new methods to ensure the safe delivery of quality health care. Malloch (1999) identified seven steps to determine an optimal course of action. Individuals should (1) clarify the situation, (2) identify goals, (3) select measures, (4) identify options, (5) consider trade-offs, (6) select the most congruent option for the goals, and (7) evaluate the choices. Nurse executives make routine and operational decisions, which carry minimal to moderate risk, and nonroutine and strategic decisions, which are complex and novel and involve higher risk and a dynamic set of decision activities using intuition and political knowledge (Nagelkerk & Henry, 1990). Nurse leaders must set priorities, apply complexity and chaos theory to decision making, and use pattern recognition in managing and leading their organizations. Complex social organizations produce patterns that may be difficult to recognize. Patterns known as attractors keep complex organizations stable in the face of change. Attractors emerge as the result of formal and informal rules, management control, flow of information, and system constraints. Negative patterns can create randomness and instability. Managers can tune parameters to increase stability. Examples of parameters include information flow, rules, diversity of ideas, control, and constraints.

Leaders will facilitate decision making in organizations and will use mistakes or errors in judgments as learning lessons. They will structure the environment for quality care delivery and continually engage staff in problem solving and innovation for optimal client care. One method to stabilize systems is to standardize the care provided. Standardization limits the number of unpredictable variables and reduces complexity. Developing, through an interdisciplinary process, standards of clinical practice is useful as a decisional aid for nurses. Nurses who are innovative will engage in future think, will mobilize energy and resources, will anticipate trends, and will plan for the future. Steps to optimize a course of action include the following: clarify the situation, identify goals, select measures, identify options, consider trade-offs, select the most congruent option for the goals, and evaluate the choice (Malloch, 1999).

LEARNING TOOLS

Group Activity: Understanding Decision Making

Purpose

To identify the different types of decisions and to determine which decision situations are more appropriate for individual and group decision making.

Directions

For the three decision situations described, identify the type of decision (administrative, clinical, or ethical) and who the appropriate decision maker is (individual or group).

Decision 1

Mr. Smith is in a nursing home. He is 72 years old and had a cerebral vascular accident 3 months ago that left him comatose. Mr. Smith has a feeding tube, and tube feedings are given regularly. Mrs. Smith visited today and stated that she does not want you to give him tube feedings anymore because he would not want to live "like this." What should you do?

Type of decision _____

Decision maker _____

Decision 2

Mr. Jones returned from surgery 8 hours ago. He had a left total knee replacement and now is complaining of excruciating pain. He is requesting pain medication. What should you do?

Type of decision _____

Decision maker _____

Decision 3

You are the team leader on an orthopedic unit for the 3-to-11 shift. All the nurses have been complaining of being overworked. At 11:35 PM, all the nurses are gathered at the exit waiting for you. They are upset and demand that something be done about the chronic short staffing. What should you do?

Type of decision _____

Decision maker _____

As a nurse, you will be confronted with the need to make many different decisions. Determining quickly which decisions you can act upon by yourself and determining which ones need to be handled by a group is crucial to your success.

CASE STUDY

Dawn Bohuise is a nurse manager for the operating room of a small community hospital in Oshkosh, Wisconsin. She is required to make many administrative decisions daily. Nurse Bohuise prefers to make administrative decisions by using a step-by-step approach to solving immediate problems, using solutions that fit into her long-range goals. For example, staffing problems have arisen in the operating room. Nurse Bohuise's long-range goal is to have a mix of technicians and registered nurses in the operating room to provide quality perioperative care. Today, Nurse Bohuise will begin discussing her plans with the staff but in the meantime will cover the staffing need with an experienced registered nurse from intensive care to assist in covering the holding room area. Nurse Bohuise's experience suggests that taking small steps to solve a problem is useful and allows time to reflect on opportunities and barriers.

Case Study Questions

1. In administrative decision making, there are four strategies commonly used to make decisions. Which is Nurse Bohuise using?

2. Describe the other administrative decision-making strategies.

3. What style of decision making is Nurse Bohuise using? What style is most effective for this situation?

LEARNING RESOURCES

Discussion Questions

1. How can you use the tools of perception and innovation in your nursing practice?

2. What is the difference between an individual and organizational problem? Give an example of each.

3. Describe the formal strategies of decision making, and provide an example of a situation in which each would be useful.

4. Discuss the problem-solving and decision-making processes. Are there similarities? Differences?

5. What types of decisions should clinical nurses make? To whom should a clinical nurse turn for assistance in decision making?

Study Questions

True or False: Circle the correct answer.

T F   1. Clinical decision making is the same thing as diagnostic reasoning.

T F   2. Organizational decision making focuses on system problems.

T F   3. Ethical decision making is influenced by each person's values.

T F   4. Administrative decision making focuses on clinical problems.

T F   5. Critical pathways are a form of a decision tree.

T F   6. Group decision making tends to be more effective for system problems.

T F   7. In most cases, satisfying leads to effective decision making.

T F   8. Administrative decisions tend to be clearcut and easy to solve.

T F   9. Decision-making strategies are interchangeable and can be used effectively in any situation.

T F   10. Pilot projects are full-scale implementations of a solution.

Matching: Write the letter of the correct response in front of each term.

_____ 11. Trial and error

_____ 12. Pilot projects

_____ 13. Problem critique

_____ 14. Creativity techniques

_____ 15. Decision tree

_____ 16. Fish bone

_____ 17. Group decision making

_____ 18. Cost-benefit analysis

_____ 19. Satisfying decision

_____ 20. Optimizing decision

A. The leader calls the group together to discuss and participate in solving a problem

B. A formal process of examining the driving and restraining forces

C. Graphic figures used to help assess potential causes of introduction problems

D. Experiments using a solution on a limited basis to identify problems

E. The first solution that seems promising is tried

F. Graphic model depicting options, risks, and outcomes

G. A one-on-one approach in which two individuals sit down and discuss a problem

H. Openly generating ideas and solutions with all ideas considered

I. Selecting a decision that is adequate to meet the required objective

J. Selecting the best option after reviewing competing alternatives solutions

REFERENCES

Elstein, A., Shulman, L., & Sprafka, S. (1978). *Medical problem-solving: An analysis of clinical reasoning.* Cambridge, MA: Harvard University Press.

Hersey, P., Blanchard, K. H., & Johnson, D. E. (2001). *Management of organizational behavior: Leading human resources* (8th ed.). Upper Saddle River, NJ: Prentice-Hall.

Janis, I., & Mann, L. (1977) *Decision making: A psychological analysis of conflict, choice, and commitment.* New York: Free Press.

Malloch, K. (1999). The performance measurement matrix: A framework to optimize decision making. *Journal of Nursing Care Quality, 13*(3), 1-12.

Nagelkerk, J., & Henry, B. (1990). Strategic decision making. *Journal of Nursing Administration, 20*(7/8), 18-23.

Schaefer, J. (1974). The interrelatedness of decision making and the nursing process. *American Journal of Nursing, 74*(10), 1852-1855.

Wren, G. (1974). *Modern health administration.* Athens: University of Georgia Press.

SUPPLEMENTAL READINGS

Currey, J., & Botti, M. (2003). Naturalistic decision making: A model to overcome methodological challenges in the study of critical care nurses' decision making about patients' hemodynamic status. *American Journal of Critical Care, 12*(3), 206-211.

Elstein, A. S., & Schwarz, A. (2002). Clinical problem solving and diagnostic decision making: Selective review of the cognitive literature. *British Medical Journal, 324,* 729-732.

Genrich, S. J., Bandks, J. C., Bufton, K., Savage, M. E., & Owens, M. U. (2001). Group involvement in decision-making: A pilot study. *The Journal of Continuing Education in Nursing, 32*(1), 20-25.

Hoffman, K., Donoghue, J., & Duffield, C. (2003). Decision-making in clinical nursing: Investigating contributing factors. *Journal of Advanced Nursing, 45*(1), 53-62.

Manias, E., Aitken, R., & Dunning, T. (2003). Decision-making models used by 'graduate nurses' managing patients' medications. *Journal of Advanced Nursing, 47*(3), 270-278.

Chapter 7: Decision-Making Skills (pp. 149-178)

1. What is your typical or preferred decision style?

Hersey, Blanchard, and Johnson (2001) outlined four decision styles:

1. *Authoritative or autocratic:* The leader makes the decision without input from others.
2. *Consultative or collective:* The leader seeks input before making the final decision.
3. *Facilitative:* The leader and followers work together to form a shared decision.
4. *Delegative:* The leader gives up control to the group. The group makes the decision.

The selection of a given decision style depends on the presenting problem and the individuals involved in the situation. An effective decision maker has an array of decision approaches on hand to optimize positive outcomes.

2. How does clinical decision making differ from managerial decision making?

Although both forms of decision making involve the collection and processing of information and the selection and evaluation of an action, the focus of the decision differs between clinical and managerial decision making. Clinical decision making focuses on client issues or problems and nursing interventions. The sophistication of clinical decision making differentiates the professional nurse from the technical nurse. Managerial decisions focus on the resolution of organizational problems or the achievement of organization goals. An example of a managerial decision is the containment of costs while maximizing health care delivery.

3. How are problem solving and decision making related in nursing?

Nursing uses problem-solving and decision-making skills for client care outcomes. These cognitive skills routinely are incorporated into the practice of clinical and managerial nurses. All nurses collect information, draw conclusions, derive a course of action, and evaluate outcomes. Clinical nurses use these cognitive strategies to select the best nursing intervention, whereas nurse managers incorporate them in organizational decisions. Problem-solving and decision-making strategies are integral to maximizing client outcomes and achieving organizational goals.

4. What important decisions do nurses make? On which ones do they collaborate?

Nurses make many important decisions relative to the provision of care and care management. For example, nurses devise an array of strategies to optimize client recovery, mobility, and self-care; maintain airway patency and hemodynamic stability; and prevent the development of decubitus ulcers. Nurses collaborate on complex client care issues that require the talents and perspectives of a variety of health care professionals in order to maximize client outcomes. More specifically, nurses collaborate with the colleagues from the disciplines including medicine, social work, pharmacy, and pastoral services to address complicated and difficult client care problems. Nurse managers collaborate with other disciplines to achieve organizational goals, implement multisystem change processes, and to improve service delivery and client outcomes.

5. What strategies work best for clinical decision making? For managerial decision making?

Several decision-making strategies have been identified: trial and error, pilot projects, problem critique, creativity techniques, decision tree, fish bone or cause-and-effect charts, group problem solving and decision making, cost-benefit analysis, scenario planning, and worst-case scenario. Because trial and error is considered a poor and risky option, the adept problem solver rarely selects it. Pilot projects are limited experimental trials used to develop an optimal and alternative solution to a problem, whereas cost-benefit analysis involves listing the positive and negative aspects of a given outcome to assist with decision-making. Critical pathways, decision trees, and algorithms are commonly used protocols that guide the nurse through the decision-making process. These tools describe activities that must occur to achieve a desired and predictable outcome. However, a caveat to remember is that the decision rendered may only be as good as the critical pathway, decision tree, or algorithm from which it was derived. Nurse managers select the best strategy considering the individuals involved and the given situation. For example, fish bone or cause-and-effect charts may be an effective strategy for nurse managers to select in examining possible causes related to production, whereas cost-benefit analysis may be an appropriate strategy to enlist when deciding budgetary issues. Scenario planning is used in group setting to brainstorm on the future. This is a beneficial strategy to use in a constantly changing environment. The development of worst-case scenarios helps to identify potential risks.

6. How can information processing help decision making by nurses?

Professional nursing practice applies nursing expertise and knowledge to solving problems and making decisions relative to client care and care management. Nurses make decisions based on data collection, classification, storage, retrieval, and analysis (information processing). Using this process, nurses can develop creative solutions to issues and problems related to client care. Quality decisions depend on the data collected at the beginning of the problem-solving process. Therefore, it is imperative that nursing data be identified clearly, that definitions and measures be described clearly, and that data sets be standardized and accessible to support fiscal and clinical decisions. Client care outcomes depend on quality data.

7. What resources are available to assist with decision making?

Several resources are available to assist nurses with decision making, such as quality improvement techniques and decision-making strategies. One's personal, professional, and organizational values and the values of professional organizations and institutions also may assist with decision making.

8. What creative or innovative ideas do you have?

Creative ideas are central to innovations in nursing and health care. Innovative nurses examine situations from novel and different perspectives and devise creative and proactive approaches to a problem or dilemma. Nursing is replete with ingenious and resourceful minds that have potential to be on the forefront of clinical and organization changes to propel us into the future as a strong and powerful profession. We all have a contribution to make. What is yours?

9. What if ...? Describe an innovative strategy.

Nurses should look for creative and innovative answers to health care issues. Drucker (1986) discussed the following seven sources of innovative opportunity that nurses could monitor:
1. The unexpected
2. Incongruity
3. Innovation based on process need
4. Changes in the industry structure or market structure
5. Demographics (population changes)
6. Changes in perception, mood, or meaning
7. New knowledge

Huber provides an example of a nurse implementing an innovative strategy. A nurse was caring for a client with fragile skin who required a bandage. The client refused the bandage because it was difficult to remove without hurting her skin. The nurse developed a bandage designed for ease of pull from the end, thus preventing skin trauma caused by the client's need to start the bandage removal by "picking at the ends with her fingernails."

Chapter **7 Decision-Making Skills**

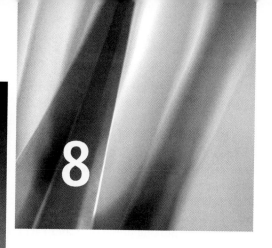

8

The Health Care System

Countries create centralized or decentralized infrastructures for the delivery of health care services. The United States has a decentralized, complex, fragmented, costly health care system. Nursing is an integral part of the health care system and serves as the backbone or core function. Understanding the health care system is important for providing high-quality care at a reasonable cost to consumers. A *health care system* is composed of structures, organizations, and services designed to deliver professional health services to consumers. Nursing services are a subset of the health care systems; and as such, there exists interrelatedness and interdependence with other services. The health care system has transformed from a weak and minor enterprise to a vast, sprawling empire. The government has a major role in the financing and delivery of services in the U.S. health care system (Feldstein, 1994). Starr (1982), in his book *The Social Transformation of American Medicine,* eloquently describes the paradigm shift from family-based home care to hospital-based care. Advanced medical knowledge and technology were a catalyst for this change. Providing further support for hospital-based care was the birth, in 1929, of modern health insurance. The creation the first Blue Cross plan was for teachers to receive hospital services.

Health care is becoming increasingly complex, turbulent, and chaotic. Strong nurse administrators are needed who can manage complex health care systems through interdisciplinary collaboration. A nurse administrator combines clinical, administrative, financial, and operational skills to manage problems and provide high-quality, cost-effective health care in acute and primary settings. The two roles that nurses assume are direct care providers and care managers. Nurses are central to health care organizations and orchestrate continuity of care for clients. Nurses facilitate environmental factors, foster interdisciplinary collaboration, and distribute resources in providing direct care and case management to clients.

The U.S. health care system often is characterized by a lack of central planning, direction, and control. The system is a blending of public and private stakeholders. The four basic functional components of the health care system are financing, insurance, delivery of care, and payment. The U.S. health care system has four distinct phases. First is the development of hospitals and the institutionalization of health care that occurred from 1850 to 1900. Second is the introduction of scientific methods that occurred from 1900 to 1940. Third is the growing interest in the social and organizational structure of health care that occurred from 1940 through the 1980s. Fourth is the limited resources, growth restrictions, and reorganization of the methods of financing and delivery of care. The current emphasis in the U.S. health care system is on chronic illness and how genetics, personal lifestyles, and environmental hazards influence health, homeland security, quality care, and the aging workforce. Another important issue in health care includes individual health care privacy and portability for which the Health Insurance Portability and Accountability Act (HIPAA) in 1996 was passed to protect the public. This legislation ensured the portability of health insurance and required the protection of individual health information. Issues that must be addressed in the future include the integration of complementary and alternative medicine, costs of medical malpractice, quality, access, and costs of health care.

Health care is moving from physician-dominated control to a multidisciplinary approach. Nurses constitute the largest group of health care providers in the United States. Nurses are well positioned to deliver population-based health care and fill care coordinator roles. Education for physicians has changed significantly based on the recommendations set forth in the Flexner Report published in 1910 with sponsorship from the Carnegie Foundation for the Advancement of Teaching. Flexner concluded there was an oversupply of poorly trained physicians who were educated by a number of deficient medical schools (Starr, 1982). In the 1870s,

55

nursing schools were being established, with student nurses providing a source of low-cost labor. In the 1930s, improvements of coursework and the focus on education led to improvements in nursing programs. During this time, hospital nursing replaced private duty nursing as the major form of nursing employment.

The Hill Burton Act of 1946 created a federal state-matching program to fund the construction of hospitals. To support physician and nurse education, the Health Professional Education Assistance Act of 1963 and the Nurse Training Acts of 1964 and 1971 were passed. In the 1970s, health systems agencies and certificates of need were implemented to alleviate concerns regarding rising health care costs and lack of accountability. Health care agencies were required to obtain a certificate of need from health systems agencies to purchase and operate costly medical equipment such as for magnetic resonance imaging. Integrated health care systems are merging to meet economic and community-based needs. These systems are interactive and interdependent health care units established through mergers, partnerships, and acquisitions. Integrated health care systems are formed in an attempt to increase efficiency and decrease cost by organizing a collection of health care providers to work interdependently and function as an open system that adapts quickly to changes. All health care systems consist of five major components: production of resources, organizational structure, management, economic support, and delivery of services (Roemer, 1986). The five leading types of health care organizations are hospitals and other acute care institutions, ambulatory care, long-term care facilities, home health agencies, and mental health facilities (Kovner, 1990). With integrated health care systems, many of the health care organizations are partnering, merging, or acquiring facilities to compete effectively and provide community-based services.

Four key functions that help to explain health care delivery are (1) financing, (2) insurance, (3) delivery method, and (4) payment. Health care systems are being held accountable for the cost of services to provide quality care to clients. In the past, health care providers charged fixed fees for services provided. To contain costs, managed care systems were created. *Managed care systems* are health plans that offer a set group of health services for a set fee per client per year. In managed care, the term *per member* (or *enrollee*) *per month* refers to capitated payment. Managed care is not without problems: restricted choice in providers and services and financial incentives for physicians have created public fears. The emerging health care reform is targeting community-based health care systems to meet service needs at the local level. The building blocks of community health care management systems include population-based planning, integration of service systems, and continuous quality improvement.

In hospitals, prospective payment systems such as diagnosis-related groups were put in place to limit and reduce costs for Medicare clients. The federal government funds two major programs: Medicare and Medicaid. *Medicare* is a two-part program of assistance with health care costs for individuals over 65 years of age and those who are disabled. Medicare Part A covers hospital costs and some nursing home care, and Part B covers physician services. *Medicaid* is a joint federal and state program administered by the states to pay for indigents' health care.

Despite efforts to contain costs, the total health care expenditures continue to rise at an alarming rate. The three categories of greatest total expenditure for health care are hospital care, physician fees, and prescription drugs. Prescription drugs have been growing at double-digit rates over the past few years as higher-priced drugs and consumer demand have fueled an increased prescription demand. Widespread concern exists that health care expenditures will continue to climb as the number of older citizens and cases of chronic illnesses increase. Changing ethnicity patterns, accelerating use of high technology, and escalating numbers of those infected with human immunodeficiency virus are also factors. Nurses will be challenged to provide community-based care to all clients, contain costs, and provide high-quality care. Quality measures and agencies have been created to monitor the quality and outcomes of care provided. Examples are the Health Plan Employer Data and Information Set of the National Committee on Quality Assurance, the Quality Initiative, and the Joint Commission on Accreditation of Healthcare Organizations. New roles are emerging for nurses with advanced practice degrees to perform primary care with emphasis on disease prevention, health promotion, and integration of health services across the continuum. The nurse administrator's role is changing and requires skills in population-based care management across the life span. Evidence-based practice focuses on theory and research.

LEARNING TOOLS

Group Activity: Understanding Health Care Systems

Purpose

To help you understand the U.S. health care system and to describe the impact of economics and governmental regulation on health care. The cost of health care in the United States, the methods of controlling costs through integrated health care systems, and the role of nursing in a changing health care environment will be examined.

Directions

1. Divide the study group into three smaller groups.

2. Assign each group to one of these topics: cost of health care in the United States; methods of controlling costs through integrated health care systems; or the role of nursing in providing access to care for clients, containing costs, and ensuring high-quality care.

3. Each group should identify important points for the assigned topic (refer to the Huber textbook Chapter 2 for base information).

4. Provide 25 minutes for group discussion, and then have each group summarize its recommendations for large group discussion.

The study group leaders should serve as facilitators and should summarize information.

CASE STUDY

Health care has become a big business in the United States and is competitive in providing cost-effective care to clients. Stiff competition for market share and costs are weighed carefully before services are provided. Nurses are now in a position where they are expected not only to provide high-quality care at reasonable costs but also to make recommendations that decrease costs while maintaining exemplary client care. Many factors influence the cost of health care for individuals. The three categories with the highest total expenditures include hospital costs, physician fees, and prescription drugs. Other factors that influence costs include the aging population, changing ethnicity patterns, and the increasing incidence of chronic illness. Government regulation, administrative costs for insurance handling, the lack of practice standardization and defensive medicine, and the overcapacity of hospital beds create further cost burdens in the United States. In addition, increasing consumer demands, the lack of healthful lifestyle practices, and new diseases and treatments contribute to rising costs.

Case Study Questions

1. How can nurses affect the cost of client care without compromising quality?

2. What strategies can nurses use to improve client care outcomes?

3. What cost factors do nurses control? Over what cost factors do nurses have influence?

4. What could happen to the profession of nursing if nurses elect to ignore cost factors?

LEARNING RESOURCES

Discussion Questions

1. Can the five leading types of health care organizations (acute care, ambulatory care, long-term care, home health, and mental health facilities) form an integrated health care system? What are the advantages or disadvantages of integrated health care systems?

2. What is Medicare? What is Medicaid?

3. Health care expenditures continue to rise. What will happen to U.S. businesses if the cost of health insurance benefits continues to escalate?

4. Are nursing positions safe from downsizing and reductions in staff as health care agencies continue to cut costs? What strategies should nurses use to show their effect on client outcomes?

5. How will the role of nursing change as acute care agencies decrease in size and number and community-based care increases?

6. How can nurses use information from other disciplines to enhance their practice?

Study Questions

Matching: Write the letter of the correct response in front of each term.

_____ 1. Health care system

_____ 2. Integrated health care system

_____ 3. Medicare

_____ 4. Medicaid

_____ 5. Diagnosis-related group

_____ 6. Prospective payment system

_____ 7. Managed care

A. A payment system in which prices are set before the service is provided

B. Federal government health care payment system for individuals over age 65

C. Federal and state health care payment program for indigent care

D. Structure and services to deliver health care to clients

E. Multiple agencies linked together to provide seamless health care

F. Categories of care based on severity of illness grouped according to medical conditions

G. Health plans that offer a set group of health services for a set fee per client per year

True or False: Circle the correct answer.

T   F   8. Nurse administrators must balance access, cost, and quality to ensure excellent health care.

T   F   9. Managed care indicates that one health care provider delivers all care to a caseload of clients.

T   F 10. Frequently, hospital bills contain extra health care charges.

T   F 11. Nursing care is the highest category in the gross national product of total health care expenditures in the United States.

T   F 12. The cost of prescription drugs grew at double-digit rates over the past few years.

REFERENCES

Feldstein, P. (1994). *Health policy issues: An economic perspective on health reform.* Ann Arbor, MI: AUPHA Press/Health Administration Press.

Kovner, A. (1990). *Health care delivery in the United States* (4th ed.). New York: Springer.

Roemer, M. (1986). *An introduction to the U.S. health care system* (2nd ed.). New York: Springer.

Starr, P. (1982). *The social transformation of American medicine.* New York: Basic Books.

SUPPLEMENTAL READINGS

Jackson, P. L. (2002). A systems approach to delivering clinical preventive services. *Pediatric Nursing, 28*(4), 377-381.

Jardin, K. D. (2001). Political involvement in nursing: politics, ethics, and strategic action. *Association of Operating Room Nurses. AORN Journal, 75*(5), 614-628.

Lang, N. M. (2003). Reflections on quality health care. *Nursing Administration Quarterly, 27*(4), 266-272.

Niessen, L. W., Grijseels, W. M., & Rutten, F. H. (2000). The evidence-based approach in health policy and health care delivery. *Social Science and Medicine, 51,* 859-869.

Ziel, S. E. (2004). Guard against HIPAA violations. *Nursing Management, 35*(4), 26-27; 84.

Chapter 8: The Health Care System (pp. 179-204)

1. What are several major challenges confronting the U.S. health care system?

Rising costs of general health care, new technology resulting in higher costs for consumers, increased demand for health care providers because of the aging Baby Boomer population, inconsistency in quality from setting to setting, high error rates, and little attention to prevention are challenges facing the U.S. health care system. Health care costs continue to increase for the business sector as health insurance premiums are skyrocketing. Medical malpractice insurance premiums also are becoming more and more expensive. Finally, the lack of prescription coverage for the senior population is one of several major challenges confronting the U.S. health care system.

2. What role does politics play in the U.S. health care system?

The government has involvement in many areas of health care at the federal, state, and local levels. Laws that affect health care are passed through federal, state, and local officials. Strong lobbyists in Washington, D.C., who represent many large professional organizations such as the American Medical Association, the American Hospital Association, and America's Health Insurance Plans influence these laws. The American Nurses Association and American Public Health Association Funding, among others, also influence public policy. Funding also is regulated by the government for certain health care programs such as Medicare and Medicaid. Some research also is funded by the government through various agencies.

3. How might an emphasis on preventive services affect the U.S. health care system?

Health care forecasters predict that most health care will be directed at the ambulatory care setting rather than acute care. The use of evidenced-based practice for medicine, nursing, and other health care providers may provide better outcomes in the management of health promotion and disease prevention and better outcomes for those with chronic illness. This may decrease admissions to the acute care setting, which would decrease overall health care costs.

4. What role(s) do nurses play in decreasing fragmentation of health care services?

Nurses are managers and coordinators of care. Nurses must understand how a health care system functions in order to coordinate care within and across the care continuum. Health promotion, disease prevention, and management of chronic conditions rely on the expertise and coordinating actions of nurses.

5. How are workforce shortages and quality of care interrelated? Which should be the main focus of resources?

Workforce shortages such as the nursing shortage can result in decreased access and decreased quality of care. As a result of these shortages, costs increase. The focus of resources should be providing optimal care at the lowest cost, which may help to change the major focus of health care in the United States to health promotion and disease prevention.

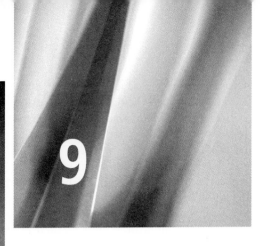

Organizational Climate and Culture

STUDY FOCUS

Leaders in health care organizations face a competitive marketplace and must be skilled in demonstrating efficiency in the provision of care, quality patient outcomes, and cost-effective performance. To accomplish organizational objectives, they must be able to influence and set a positive work culture. Nurses are positioned strategically to influence the organizational culture by virtue of their pivotal role in care delivery. Nursing encompasses two major components: caring for the sick and tending the environment in which caring takes place (Diers, 2002). Functional health care environments are characterized by open communication and collaboration.

A *hospital* is an organizational structure that exerts a powerful effect on care delivery and quality outcomes. A *nursing unit* is a structure embedded within the larger hospital or other health care organization. The nursing unit is an organizational structure that exerts a powerful effect on care delivery and quality outcomes. *Hospital culture* is composed of subcultures comprised of many different departments and groups. *Subcultures* are smaller entities of a whole organization; an example is a nursing unit. A subculture may be designated as a "work group culture." *Organizational culture* is something an organization has and something that it is (Mark, 1996). Culture is one means of achieving organizational success and realizing competitive advantage (Peters & Waterman, 1982). *Culture* is shared beliefs and values. *Climate* is the perceptions individuals hold about a particular unit or environment. Climate is evident in staff perceptions of policies, practices, and goal achievement. Organizational culture is rooted in anthropology, psychology, sociology, and management theory. Organizational culture is an amalgamation of symbols, language, assumptions, and behavior acquired by an organization. *Explicitly,* culture can be seen through policies, procedures, organizational charts, and written vision and mission statements. *Implicitly,* culture is the unwritten rules and norms that pervade the work environment.

The *mission statement* is a snapshot of strategic priorities and is another way to understand the values of the organization. Organizational culture is a shared value system, whereas unit culture is a set of actions devised by a group to manage a specific subunit. Unit culture is a set of actions devised by a group of nurses to deliver and manage care within a specific unit. *Magnet status* of hospitals is one way that excellence in organizational culture and climate is acknowledged. Magnet hospitals value nurse autonomy, effective communication, and practice excellence and furnish adequate resources to deliver superior patient care. Magnet status is the gold standard; it is a symbol of excellence. In day-to-day practice, nurses establish social norms for groups to hold together a collective vision of excellence. They establish practice patterns that formalize reporting, caregiving, and professional practice. They communicate these values and expectations through a socialization process. *Socialization* is a process used to communicate expectations of knowledge, skills, and behaviors to potential group members for the purpose of belonging and participating. *Professional socialization* is an unconscious process through which professional occupational identity is internalized as values and norms. A unit team forms a social group that holds a collective vision of excellence. Nursing leadership with staff input establishes practice patterns derived from expert knowledge. Embedded in the caregiving relationship is a core of responsibility and obligation (Benner et al., 1996).

Examining the culture and function of an organization improves nurses' effectiveness by providing useful information about the interpersonal and political forces in the organization that influence productivity and work operations. Assessing organizational culture is an important aspect of a nurse's role. Gaining an appreciation of cultural influences will improve a nurse's effectiveness by providing information about the interpersonal and political work environment.

61

Each organization has rituals, traditions, values, rules, and a structural component. Those shared beliefs, values, and practices that exist in an organization are organizational culture. Those perceptions that individuals hold about the environment are the organizational climate. Organizational culture is a more complex phenomena. Organizational culture often is subtle, and effective leaders will build the type of culture conducive to excellence in patient care. Leaders build and influence culture by providing rewards and penalties, but a group also may try to exert influence on its environment. Organizational culture serves four major functions. The first is to provide a sense of identity for group members. The second is to promote a sense of commitment to the group. The third function is to enhance the stability of the group environment. The final function is to help the group to make behavior understandable.

Several elements compose the culture of organizations, including stories, myths, rituals, and ceremonies, as well as metaphors and analogies. These elements provide concrete examples, guidance, and communication for a culture. Stories often describe heroes or conflicts. Myths are rich descriptions of events that provide inspiration and enhance belief. Rituals are embedded customs that socialize new members, provide clear messages to members, and stabilize the culture. Ceremonies entail pomp and circumstance and are functions that benefit members and the group. Metaphors and analogies are used to explain complex phenomena by simplifying the explanation using information the member knows.

Culture can be implicit or explicit. An explicit culture is more formal with rules, policies, and procedures clearly written and communicated. Norms and values are established. Implicit culture, however, is subtle and difficult to identify. Knowledge is not verbally shared, there are informal work rules, and persons do not openly communicate their values and traditions. How then, can a nurse identify the culture on a unit? A cultural checklist is a beneficial tool to analyze organizational culture. The checklist should include the following: image, deportment, status symbol and reward systems, subcultures, environment and ambiance, communication, meetings, rites, rituals, and ceremonies, and sacred cows. Assessing organizational culture is an important first step in understanding how the organization functions. Once an analysis is completed, a nurse may choose to change or build the culture to incorporate positive values and beliefs. The strategies for building culture emphasize a basic framework of support. The first step is to start building from wherever the group is currently and to work from there.

Establish personal contact, use all communication channels, and facilitate open dialogue and discussion with the group. Identify shared values and goals so the focus and desired outcome are clear. Jointly determine strategies and take action.

Positive work group cultures are important for nurse satisfaction and retention. Clinical nurses can work together to build networks and support systems for enhancing positive work environments and tackling thorny issues. Building positive cultures increases productivity and morale while improving quality patient care. Effective leaders strategically influence organizational culture to enhance patient-centered care and partnerships in a healthy work environment. A leader's primary task is to create a vision so convincing that the entire team is inspired to engage and move forward. Key areas in the nursing leader's role is staff recruitment and retention, welcoming new staff, orientation, celebrating and recognizing staff accomplishments, and facilitating change and promoting a learning environment. A leader who desires to build culture would do the following:

- Identify the desired change.
- Assess current status of the group.
- Create a shared need and group commitment to change.
- Use appropriate communication skills and personal contact to establish open discussion.
- Identify shared values and mission so the group knows where it is going.
- Determine strategies.
- Develop an action plan for change.

Leaders support key values and characteristics while trusting the knowledge and skill of their staff. A thorough understanding of unit and organizational culture is a powerful diagnostic tool that may be used to identify troubled units and high performance areas.

Current issues and trends include a nursing shortage, crisis in our health care system, and patient safety issues. There have been several landmark studies related to patient safety including *To Err Is Human: Building a Safer Health System* (Kohn et al., 2000) and the Institute of Medicine reports *Crossing the Quality Chasm* (2001) and *Keeping Patients Safe* (2004). In addition, *Health Care at the Crossroads: Strategies for Addressing the Evolving Nursing Crisis* (Joint Commission on Accreditation of Healthcare Organizations, 2002) and the Robert Wood Johnson Foundation report *Health Care's Human Crisis: The American Nursing Shortage* (Kimball & O'Neill, 2002) are important documents depicting the nursing shortage and strategies to increase the number of nurses.

LEARNING TOOLS

Group Activity: Organizational Culture Analysis

Purpose

To examine the unit where you wish to practice when you complete your educational requirements. Use the following Organizational Culture Checklist to analyze

This data will provide you with information useful in determining the type of unit where you wish to work.

CASE STUDY

Christy Sanonski is a registered nurse on a 58-bed neurosurgical unit for a large community hospital in

ORGANIZATIONAL CULTURE CHECKLIST	
Aspects of Culture	Questions for Assessment
Image	How do the nurses dress? Casually or formally? What symbols or slogans are used? Is the unit aesthetically pleasing?
Deportment	What is the level of courtesy shown to patients' families? Are males and females treated equally? Are all health care workers treated with respect?
Status symbols	Are the nurses' parking and lounges comparable to physicians' and administrators'? Is there an elitist attitude? If so, by whom? Are offices and equipment comparable?
Subcultures	Do nurses from the same cultural background tend to form friendships with each other more easily? Are there cliques on the unit? Are new employees welcomed by the group?
Environment and ambience	How well is the physical structure maintained? Is the decor attractive and ambiance well kept? Is there space for classrooms and lounges? Are rooms reserved for special groups?
Communication	How does the CEO communicate to staff nurses? Does the vice president of nursing make rounds on all units? How does the nurse manager share information with employees? Does the important communication take place in formal meetings or informally in groups?
Meetings	Who participates in which meetings? How are participants for meetings selected? How are decisions made in committee? Where are meetings held? Are refreshments provided?
Rites, rituals, and ceremonies	How are holidays celebrated? Is longevity recognized? What events and ceremonies are celebrated and recognized? What are the policies for orientation and termination?
Sacred cows	Who are the heroes/heroines? What subjects are taboo? Are there policies that are untouchable?

the organization (the checklist has been adapted from the elements described by del Bueno & Freund [1986]).

The information you gather from your cultural assessment will provide you with a basic understanding of the culture of the organization. You will be able to tell whether the culture is explicit or implicit. You will be able to tell whether the organization is formal or informal, how policies and procedures are made, and the nature of interpersonal interactions among staff.

Portland, Oregon. She is working on a project concerning organizational cultural assessments as part of the requirements for her master's degree in nursing. Nurse Sanonski has discovered tension among the staff about their new roles after an organizational redesign. There is much resistance on the part of the staff members about "letting go" of their old responsibilities and taking new ones. Nurse Sanonski carefully examines the written communications including memos, policies, procedures, and job descriptions. She notices that many of the documents have not changed since the organizational redesign. Traditionally, the hospital has relied heavily on written documents to provide stability and guidance for the staff. Now, staff are feeling insecure and reluctant to change. What should Nurse Sanonski do?

Case Study Questions

1. Has the organizational culture where Nurse Sanonski works been explicit or implicit?

2. What organizational viewpoint is most evident in this culture?

3. What strategies should Nurse Sanonski take to realign the organizational culture?

4. What critical cultural elements must Sanonski examine?

LEARNING RESOURCES

Discussion Questions

1. To do an in-depth cultural assessment of an organization, how long would it take, and what criteria would you use to evaluate the organization?

2. What strategies could a nurse use to change or build organizational culture?

3. What is the nurse's role in building organizational culture?

4. What is the difference between implicit and explicit culture? Which type of culture is easier to analyze?

5. What is the nurse manager's role in influencing the unit culture? What strategies may be useful in producing the desired cultural change?

Study Questions

True or False: Circle the correct answer.

T   F   1. Climate may be called the "personality" of the organization.

T   F   2. Examining an organizational culture improves nurses' effectiveness by increasing understanding of the interpersonal and political forces at work in the organization.

T   F   3. As a shift in health care delivery occurs from acute care to community-based care, the number and variety of jobs for nurses has decreased.

T   F   4. Culture is a form of external group control and is based on beliefs about organizational survival.

T   F   5. Culture enhances the stability of the social system.

T   F   6. Culture is the perception that individuals have about the organization.

T   F   7. Climate is the shared beliefs, values, and assumptions that exist in an organization.

T   F   8. Stories are important elements of culture because they describe conflicts and the tradition of heroes in organizations.

T   F   9. Greater resistance is seen with strong hierarchical values, a command-and-control orientation, and strong reliance on rules.

T   F   10. Magnet hospital status is a designation of excellence in practice, communication, and adequate resources.

Multiple Choice: Circle the correct response.

11. Susan, a registered nurse on the neurosurgical unit, is assessing organizational manifestations by cultural level. When she assesses the visible level, what is Susan examining?
    A. Balance of cost, quality, and access to care
    B. Physical space and social environment
    C. Guidelines of the organization
    D. Values of what ought to be in the organization

12. Susan is teaching a continuing education class on organizational culture. Which of the following definitions should she use to define organizational culture?
    A. Shared beliefs, values, and assumptions that exist in an organization
    B. Perceptions that individuals have about the environment in the organization
    C. Gives meaning and significance to activities in organizations
    D. Every organization's values, rituals, and rules

REFERENCES

Benner, P. A., Tanner, C. A., & Chesla, C. A. (1996). *Expertise in nursing practice.* New York: Springer Publishing Company.

del Bueno, D., & Freund, C. (1986). *Power and politics in nursing: A casebook.* Owings Mills, MD: National Health Publishing.

Diers, D. K. (2002). *Between practice and ....* Unpublished dissertation, University of Technology, Sidney, Australia.

Institute of Medicine. (2001). *Crossing the quality chasm.* Washington, DC: National Academies Press.

Institute of Medicine. (2004). *Keeping patients safe.* Washington, DC: National Academies Press.

Joint Commission on Accreditation of Healthcare Organizations. (2002). *Health care at the crossroads: Strategies for addressing the evolving nursing crisis.* Chicago: Joint Commission on Accreditation of Healthcare Organizations.

Kimball, B., & O'Neill, E. (2002). *Health care's human crisis: The American nursing shortage.* Princeton, NJ: Robert Wood Johnson Foundation.

Kohn, L. T., Corrigan, J. M., & Donaldson, M. S. (Eds.). (2000). *To err is human: Building a safer health system.* Washington, DC: National Academies Press.

Mark, B. A. (1996). Organizational culture. In J. J. Fitzpatrick & J. Norbeck (Eds.), *Annual review of nursing research* (Vol. 14, pp. 145-163). New York: Springer Publishing Company.

Peters, T., & Waterman, R. H. (1982). *In search of excellence.* New York: Warner Communications.

SUPPLEMENTAL READINGS

Brown, R. B., & Brooks, I. (2002). Emotion at work: Identifying the emotional climate of night nursing. *Journal of Management in Medicine, 16*(4/5), 327-343.

Burton, R. M., Lauridsen, J., & Obel, B. (2004). The impact of organizational climate and strategic fit on firm performance. *Human Resource Management, 43*(1), 67-82.

Heinen, M. G. (2004). Dare to shift cultural behaviors. *Nursing Management, 35*(9), 14.

Kramer, M., Schmalenberg, C., & Maguire, P. (2004). Essentials of a magnetic work environment (Part 4). *Nursing 2004, 34*(9), 44-48.

Wooten, L. P., & Crane, P. (2003). Nurses as implementers of organizational culture. *Nursing Economic$, 21*(6), 275-279.

Chapter 9: Organizational Climate and Culture (pp. 205-218)

1. What is the relationship between an organization and its values?

The values of a given organization are a reflection of its culture and climate. Organizational values shape normative behaviors, perceptions, and social mores within the employment environment.

2. To what extent does the culture of an organization determine job satisfaction?

Organizational culture influences one's perception of the interpersonal milieu and working environment. Job satisfaction is related to the work environment. Personal congruence with the culture of the organization will affect job satisfaction positively; conversely, incongruence with the organizational culture will affect job satisfaction negatively.

3. How can you assess the culture of an organization?

Several mechanisms are available to assess the culture of an organization. One can examine the traditions, rituals, ceremonies, myths, and rules that are present within the institution. One can evaluate the physical and social environments of the organization, the values, and the underlying assumptions of acceptable organizational behavior. Lastly, one can examine the congruency of the mission statement, formal structure, informal structure, political structure, and financial structure, with organizational decisions.

4. How long does it take to truly perceive the culture?

To examine and understand the many facets of the culture of an organization is a time-intensive process. As such, it is difficult to quantify the exact amount of effort, observation, and interaction necessary really to understand the cultural milieu of an organization. One's own perspective, acceptance, and personal agenda may influence one's comprehension and evaluation of the organizational culture.

5. What are the effects of leadership on culture?

Organizational leadership can shape, sustain, or change culture. The role of the leader is to define and communicate the vision clearly through role modeling, influencing norms, and ensuring role clarity, accountability, and a work environment that promotes safe patient-centered care. Leaders can help to change the culture through the staff recruitment and retention, orientation, recognizing staff accomplishments, and promotion of a learning environment.

6. Does organizational culture reflect an individual's perception of the organization, or is it a relatively enduring characteristic?

Organizational culture develops over time and is resistant to change. Beliefs, values, and assumptions, the defining elements of a culture, are deeply embedded core convictions that require examination, reflection, and thoughtful deliberation to amend. Cultural beliefs and values endure as long as they are accepted, supported, and perpetuated by group members.

7. How can you build a culture?

Building a culture requires a framework of shared beliefs and values. To build a culture, one would do the following:

- Identify the desired change.
- Assess current status of the group.
- Create a shared need and group commitment to change.
- Use appropriate communication skills and personal contact to establish open discussion.
- Identify shared values and mission so the group knows where it is going.
- Determine strategies.
- Develop an action plan for change.

8. What is the best kind of organizational culture for nursing?

The best organizational culture for nursing is one that is respectful, supportive, and congruent with the beliefs, values, and assumptions of nursing. Organizational values similar to professional nursing values provide a work environment that provides a "good fit" for nurses. An example is the value of caring, which is reflected in the manner the organization treats its employees.

9. What unit cultural values distinguish the nursing environment found in Magnet status institutions? Why are they important?

Nursing units that develop a culture and a reputation for providing excellent patient care, such as those occurring in Magnet hospitals, are inspired in an environment that values trust, risk taking, challenging of the status quo through use of process improvement, open communication, access to information and resources, nursing autonomy, and employee worth. Organizations that support these activities encourage employee contribution, creative thinking, and innovation at all levels in the organization, helping to create centers of excellence. These activities have been shown to have a positive effect on patient and nurse outcomes. As noted by Aiken and colleagues (1994), Magnet status hospitals provided higher levels of autonomy and control of practice and fostered stronger professional relationships between nurses and physicians than did non-Magnet status hospitals. Magnet hospitals also had a significantly lower mortality rate for Medicare patients than did the non-Magnet status hospitals. These positive effects on nursing and patient outcomes attract and retain nurses.

10. **What nursing values create dilemmas?**

Dilemmas are created when a conflict exists between individual values and beliefs and organizational expectations. This disparity causes internal conflict, despair, and discord. As a result, dilemmas arise that polarize organizational and personal expectations. Examples of issues that may precipitate a conflict between nursing and organizational values include staffing, costs, and patient's rights.

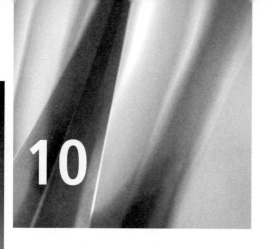

10

Mission Statements, Policies, and Procedures

Organizations are composed of a group of individuals who each have specific responsibilities to act together toward the goals of the organization. Organizational structures are designed by management to meet organizational goals efficiently and effectively and to provide direction to employees, vendors, and consumers. Thoughtful operational documents form the backbone for planning and direction. Health care organizations are complex and require professional staff to accomplish their mission. The *mission statement* of the organization describes the product or service; for health care organizations the product is client care. The organizational goal will be expressed in mission statements and carried through into policies and procedures. *Strategic plans* are a collection of written descriptions of organizational values, goals, and vision. These documents form a conceptual description of an organization and display the framework for beliefs, future plans, and operations. Themes in health care mission statements often include the provision of quality care, client satisfaction, and continuous improvement activities (Ehrat, 1994). The mission, values, and vision are the glue that hold an organization together.

An *organization* is a group of individuals with specific responsibilities who act together for the achievement of a specific purpose determined by the organization. All organizations have a purpose, structure, and collection of individuals. Organizations are social systems comprised of the (1) environment and (2) individuals. The environment is composed of the internal and external environments, roles, and goals or expectations. Individuals have their own needs, personalities, and personal agendas. At times, individuals' needs or desires may be in conflict with organizational goals. By accepting employment within an organization, employees imply that they will abide by the organizational philosophy.

Service institutions are complex. *Key aspects of effectiveness* in service organizations include quality, cost control, and access. Nurses are professional employees and serve (1) the organization as a business and (2) the client. *Strategic plans* are deliberative organizational documents developed to identify, gain consensus about, and communicate where an organization is going, over what timeframe, how it will get there, and how it will decide if it got there (McNamara, 1999a). Strategic plans may be developed for products or services, but often a business plan is used instead. The most common form of strategic planning is the goal-based form. *In goal-based strategic planning,* the goals are identified, and strategies to achieve the goals and action plans to identify who is responsible and accountability time lines are detailed. In goal-based planning, the first step is to develop a mission statement.

Organizations have mission statements to guide the institution and provide direction to employees. The *mission statement* of any organization is its purpose, function, and reason why it exists. In developing the mission statement, factors such as the products, services, markets, values, public image, and activities for survival of the organization need to be considered (McNamara, 1999b). *Vision statements* are designed to address the future of the organization and the most desirable state at some future point in time. Advantages of vision statements are that they transcend bounded thinking; identify direction; challenge and motivate; promote loyalty, focus, and commitment; and encourage creativity. *Visioning* is setting a high-level direction through turbulent times and creating a compelling picture of a desirable future state. *Core values* are strongly held beliefs and priorities that guide organizational decision making. They are anchors that relate to the mission and hold constant while operations and business strategies change. Values drive how persons act in an organization. Core values are expressed through value statements and philosophy.

A *philosophy* is an explanation of the systems of beliefs that determine how a mission or a purpose is to be achieved. A philosophy is a statement of values and beliefs. A philosophy is abstract, describing a vision and providing guidance. The philosophy of a nursing department should be congruent with the organizational philosophy and include the three vital components of client, nurse, and nursing practice. The purpose of the organization is its reason for existence. The purpose spells out the service(s) to be provided. The nursing purpose must take into consideration the organizational purpose, the state Nurse Practice Act, and legal concerns. Strategic planning efforts proceed from a focus on mission, vision, and values to identification of major strategic goals and specific action plans. This process is action planning. Action planning is establishing goals in an analytical process of deciding what the organization wants to achieve. The early phase of goal identification often entails an environmental analysis. A common method of environmental analysis is the *SWOT analysis* (strengths, weaknesses, opportunities and threats). Strengths are positive and internal; weaknesses are negative and internal; opportunities are positive and external; and threats are negative and external factors of the organizational environment. Based on the environmental scan, critical issues can be addressed and major goals set. Each major goal has objectives with responsibilities and time lines specified for tracking and evaluation purposes. The objectives are hoped-for outcomes directing activities toward organizational goal accomplishment. *Objectives* are identified outcomes directing activities toward achieving the purpose of the organization or unit (Trexler, 1987). They must be behaviorally specific statements in written format. They must be realistic, attainable, and priority-focused.

Policies and procedures are written to articulate clearly the rules of the organization that are derived from the mission statement. Policies and procedures are developed to coordinate the work of the organization. *Policies* are general guidelines that speak to repetitive problems or tasks in the organization. The policies help coordinate plans, control performance, and increase the consistency of activities. Policies are usually written, although informal policies may exist. Policies speak to all employees and not just one job category. Policies establish broad limits on and provide direction to decision making yet permit some initiative and individuality. General areas that require policies include medication error reporting and follow-up, protection of clients' or families' rights, "do not resuscitate" and end-of-life care, and personnel management and welfare. *Procedures* provide a step-by-step plan to complete a task. They are developed for those activities that recur regularly, and they provide a performance guideline for them. Procedures are written, provide a reference, and are typically in a consistent format. The procedure format includes the purpose of the activity, the individual who is responsible for performing the activity, steps in the procedure, and supplies or equipment necessary to accomplish the task. The similarities between policies and procedures are that they are a means for accomplishing goals and objectives and are important for smooth functioning of any work group or organization. The differences are that policies are general guidelines for decisions, whereas procedures give specific directions for actions.

Leadership is important to establish and implement strategic plans and vision statements. A marketing strategy called *positioning* can be used as a basis for discussion and communication. Periodic reviews are necessary to keep pace with what is or should be occurring in the work environment. Organizational documents such as strategic plans and goals direct the leader's responsibility to create a productive work environment. Leaders also must establish a positive work environment. A positive work environment fostered by a philosophy that espouses group participation and commitment is paramount to a successful, effective team. A caring approach that focuses on common elements of successful organizations, that retains employees, and that includes a managerial commitment to employees, strong leadership, and competitive salaries and benefits fosters employee commitment. A value of caring and excellence for all constituents, clients, staff, and other health care workers enhances work commitment and quality outcomes. *Caring* is defined as meaning that persons, events, projects, and things matter to an individual (Benner & Wrubel, 1988). Support for autonomy, innovation, and risk taking is embedded in a team-building philosophy.

In contrast, behaviors that reflect a lack of concern for people and a contempt for employees create barriers to developing excellence in organizations. Four ways in which contempt for others is demonstrated include (1) telling clients what they want instead of responding to the client's perceived needs, (2) casting aspersions on or depersonalizing clients, (3) lack of habitual courtesy, and (4) contempt for employees (Brown-Stewart, 1987). Contempt behaviors include consumptive, as opposed to investment, attitude toward employees; lack of orientation; ambiguity of mission, values, and job requirements; parking areas; physicians being treated preferentially; ignoring of the client's family; lack of attention to the client's comfort; amount and type of nursing staff on duty; failure to communicate; and insensitivity when creating an inconvenience. One result of organizational philosophies and cultures that create barriers to quality nursing practice is that nurses manifest a sense of job dissatisfaction, feelings of frustration or powerlessness, a feeling of not being a part of the decision-making process, and a feeling that supervisors are not empathetic. These behaviors are exhibited by preferential treatment, insensitivity, a lack

70

of communication, ambiguity in job requirements, and a user attitude toward employees.

Nurses feel strongly about job autonomy and control over their practice. They want improvements in pay, image, and working conditions. Leaders have the opportunity and the responsibility to preserve concepts of dignity, integrity, honesty, and compassion in the working environment. Open communication, trust, and mutual respect are paramount in effective working relationships. Leaders must demonstrate caring and advocacy in designing and managing services to communities.

LEARNING TOOLS

Role-Play 1

Caring Behaviors that Build Teams and Promote Commitment

Character One: Jill is the vice president of nursing and frequently makes rounds on all 15 client care units in the hospital. She is supportive of all her staff and empowers them to make autonomous decisions. Clinical and administrative staff frequently consult with her on their projects.

Character Two: Jack is a clinical nurse who was hired 3 months previously and has been doing an outstanding job with clients, but he is having some problems interacting with residents.

Character Three: Joe is a resident and has just started working with one of Jack's clients. Joe has been at the hospital for 1 year and has been short with staff on occasions.

Character Four: Sally is a nurse's aide who is working with Jack to provide supportive care to the clients.

Jill is rounding on all the units when she hears voices beginning to rise. She turns the corner to see Joe, Sally, and Jill discussing a problem in loud voices.

Role-Play Questions

1. What should Jill do? Should she intervene? If so, what should she say?

2. What strategies could she use with a caring approach to intervene?

3. How can she manage the situation to empower all of the individuals involved?

Role-Play Worksheet

Character	Student Assigned
Jill, the vice president of nursing	_____
Joe, the resident	_____
Sally, the nurse's aide	_____
Jack, the clinical nurse	_____

Which character have you been assigned?
What are your character's goals in this situation?
How can the other characters assist you in achieving your goals?
What might the other characters do to hinder you in achieving your goals?
What strategies and probes do you plan to use in this situation?

Role-Play 2

Behaviors that Create Barriers to Organizational Excellence

Using the same characters (Jill, Joe, Jack, and Sally) and the same scenario (Jill rounds the corner to discover a problem), role-play a situation using contempt behaviors that block effectiveness and increase turnover.

Role-Play Questions

1. What should Jill do? Should she intervene? If so, what should she say?

2. What strategies could she use to create a barrier and disempower employees?

3. Discuss why individuals choose to use contempt behaviors to resolve problems.

Role-Play Worksheet

Characters	Student Assigned
Jill, the vice president of nursing	_____
Joe, the resident	_____
Sally, the nurse's aide	_____
Jack, the clinical nurse	_____

Which character have you been assigned?
What are your character's goals in this situation?
How can the other characters assist you in achieving your goals?

What might the other characters do to hinder you in achieving your goals?

What strategies and probes do you plan to use in this situation?

CASE STUDY

Jacqueline Sorabond is a newly hired vice president of nursing for a 250-bed hospital in Maine. She has carefully read the mission statement of the organization and decides to make rounds on the units to see how integrated it is on the units. The mission statement describes the hospital as a community-based center of excellence that provides care to all clients in a cost-effective manner. On her rounds, she stops to talk with Debbie Yar and Karen Felp, both of whom are nurse managers. She asks them what the mission of the organization is. Nurse Yar replies that it is to provide high-quality health care, whereas Nurse Felp says that it is to increase the market share for obstetrics clients. Nurse Sorabond also asks several staff nurses about the mission statement and gets a variety of responses.

Case Study Questions

1. What purpose does a mission statement serve?

2. Is it a problem that nurse managers and clinical nurses are unable to recite or explain the mission statement?

3. What can Nurse Sorabond do to increase employee awareness of the mission statement?

LEARNING RESOURCES

Discussion Questions

1. What comprises a mission statement? How do core values, SWOT analysis, philosophy, policies, and procedures fit into organizational mission statements?

2. How does the organizational philosophy relate to the nursing philosophy?

3. Are employees obliged to agree with or carry out the mission statement? If so, why?

4. How can nurse leaders promote positive work cultures?

5. What is the clinical nurse's role in developing philosophy, core values, and objectives?

Study Questions

True or False: Circle the correct answer.

T F 1. An organization has a purpose, structure, and individuals.

T F 2. A philosophy describes the reason the organization exists.

T F 3. The purpose relates the values and beliefs of the organization.

T F 4. Objectives are outcomes that direct an activity toward goal accomplishment.

T F 5. The three core components of a nursing philosophy are the client, the nurse, and the physician.

T F 6. A policy is a step-by-step guide to solve common problems.

T F 7. A procedure is a general guideline that guides goal accomplishment.

T F 8. Caring philosophies empower individuals and assist in organizational goal attainment.

T F 9. Contempt behaviors create barriers to excellence in organizations.

T F 10. Nurses desire improvements in image, autonomy, and collaboration.

Matching: Write the letter of the correct response in front of each term.

_____ 11. Policy

_____ 12. Procedure

_____ 13. Philosophy

_____ 14. Strategic plans

_____ 15. Vision statement

_____ 16. SWOT analysis

A. Explanations of the beliefs that determine how a mission is to be achieved

B. A guideline that usually is written and formalized

C. Collection of written descriptions of organizational values, goals, and vision

D. A description of the steps to carry out an activity

E. Designed to address the preferred future of the organization

F. Organizational strengths, weaknesses, opportunities, and threats

REFERENCES

Benner, P., & Wrubel, J. (1988). Caring comes first. *American Journal of Nursing, 88*(8), 1072-1075.

Brown-Stewart, P. (1987). Thinly disguised contempt: A barrier to excellence. *Journal of Nursing Administration, 17*(4), 14-18.

Ehrat, K. S. (1994). Mission statement, goals, and values. In R. Spitzer-Lehmann (Ed.), *Nursing management desk reference: Concepts, skills and strategies* (pp. 37-59). Philadelphia: W. B. Saunders.

McNamara, C. (1999a). *Strategic planning in nonprofit or for-profit organizations.* St. Paul, MN: Carter McNamara. Retrieved July 8, 2004, from *www.managementhelp.org/plan_dec/str_plan.str_htm*

McNamara, C. (1999b). *Basics of developing mission, vision, and value statements.* St. Paul, MN: Carter McNamara. Retrieved May 17, 2005, from *www.mapnp.org/library/-plan_dec/str_plan/stmnts.htm*

Trexler, B. (1987). Nursing department purpose, philosophy, and objectives: Their use and effectiveness. *Journal of Nursing Administration, 17*(3), 8-12.

SUPPLEMENTAL READINGS

Balwin, M. A. (2003). Patient advocacy: A concept analysis. *Nursing Standard, 17*(23), 33-39.

Bart, C. K. (1998). Mission statement rationales and organizational alignment in the not-for-profit health care sector. *Health Care Management Review, 23*(4), 54-69.

Stein, P. (2004). Pushing through barriers to advocate for a patient. *AORN Journal, 80*(3), 553-558.

Telford, P. (2004). Quality of work life: A leadership imperative: One staff nurse's perspective reinforces how quality of work life and leadership relate to and impact on each other in restructuring nursing work environments. *The Canadian Nurse, 100*(6), 10-15.

Chapter 10: Mission Statements, Policies, and Procedures (pp. 219-234)

1. How do previous employee experiences color perception and attitude? Why do these perceptions linger?

The recency and vividness of the experience along with one's own values and beliefs affect how perceptions are derived and interpreted. Experiences with employees may be evoked when similar situations arise and are used as the foundation for future decisions. These perceptions tend to linger because they are salient experiences that remain accessible in and retrievable from our memories.

2. Do nurses profess loyalty to the organization/job or to the profession/work of nursing? Can an individual have loyalty to both?

Nurses' loyalty to the profession of nursing germinates early in the formal educational process. The values, beliefs, and traditions of nursing are internalized and incorporated into practice and leadership approaches. When nurses enter the institutional system, organizational loyalty is expected, requiring nurses to balance professional and organizational loyalties to find the most comfortable "fit." Similar values and beliefs support the ability of nurses to remain loyal to their profession and their organization. However, conflicts in loyalty may arise if incongruent values and beliefs are present between the organization and the profession.

3. How do you use the change process to implement a new philosophy in a preestablished work group?

Leadership involves establishing a philosophy that serves as the foundation on which innovative changes can be based, planned, and actualized. Understanding the readiness and willingness of a work group to adapt a new philosophy is key to developing strategies that will facilitate its successful implementation. Leaders can facilitate this process by motivating, guiding, inspiring, and supporting employees in the process of relinquishing old values and beliefs and shaping a new philosophy.

4. What is the "philosophy in action?" Cite some examples. Describe why this makes a difference.

Brown-Stewart (1987) described "philosophy in action" as subtle behaviors that demonstrate a lack of concern for others and an undermining of their success. Examples of such contempt behaviors include lack of habitual courtesy, withholding information, lack of education and orientation, depersonalizing clients, physicians being treated preferentially, insensitivity when creating an inconvenience, and insufficient staffing. These behaviors decrease employee satisfaction, morale, and work performance and negatively affect client outcomes and organizational accomplishments.

5. What problems are solved by having policies and procedures?

Policies and procedures, extensions of the mission statement, are standards in the form of written rules that guide decision making and performance. As such, they provide structure, consistency, and stability so that nursing functions in a coordinated fashion, decreasing the amount of chaos present in the work environment.

6. What decisions can nurses make without a written policy?

Some policies are unwritten, or are implied, by patterns of decisions that have been made already within the organization. Professional nursing judgment is used in making client care decisions. However, when management or client care issues arise outside the scope of practice or expertise of the nurse, the nurse must contact the appropriate manager or professional colleague to assist with decision making.

7. Is caring the central value for nursing? Explain.

Caring has been identified as one of the fundamental philosophical principles of nursing and often is described as the essence of nursing. Swanson (1991) defines caring as a "nurturing way of relating to a valued other toward whom one feels a personal sense of commitment and responsibility." The persons within nursing department and unit and those throughout the organization also can foster caring through valuing of each other. If caring is valued, it will be reflected in decisions, resource allocations, types of power, handling of conflict, and recognition of nurses as professionals.

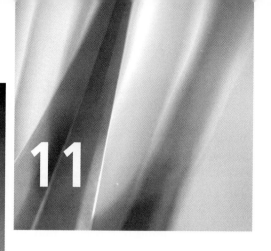

11 Organizational Structure

STUDY FOCUS

The structure of the organization provides a framework for accomplishing the work of the organization. Organizational structure is essential for the efficient and effective management of work, power, and control in organizations. The general goal of nursing is to deliver services that are caring, high quality, and cost-effective. The *structure of an organization* is the way in which personnel are divided by their tasks and are coordinated to accomplish organizational goals. Many factors are examined before organizational structures are designed. These factors include the age of an organization, its size, technology, internal and external environment, and its resources. Organizational structures may be formal or informal. *Formal structure* refers to what is clearly written into an organizational chart. *Informal structure* is the internal and external network of relationships and interdependencies around the organization. One aspect of the informal structure is the "grapevine."

Classic concepts of organizational structure include the division of labor, span of control, scalar process, and line and staff positions. The *division of labor* refers to the assignment and distribution of the work to individuals who have the authority and responsibility to complete the job. The *span of control* refers to the number of subordinates one manager oversees. The *scalar process* is the levels within the organization. *Line positions* are those in direct line of hierarchical authority and central to producing a product of the organization. However, *staff positions* are supportive and provide the expertise and knowledge to meet organizational goals.

Mintzberg (1993) has identified technology, social environment, size, and task repetitiveness as *major influences on structure.* In health care, sophisticated technologies; rapid, complex decisions; social change; generational demographics; age cohorts; and the changing professional workforce present a formidable challenge for administrators and require decentralized, autonomous teams working to promote quality client care. In general, larger organizations are slower to make decisions and are more complex to manage. Organizational size changes as it ages and evolves through a developmental process. An organization begins with a small, organic, and unelaborate structure. The second stage is entrepreneurial directed by a dynamic, powerful executive. A formalized structure emerges, and a bureaucracy begins to form. As the organization ages and grows, divisional structures develop, and finally, it may shift to a matrix structure.

Health care organizations traditionally have used one of three basic types of administrative structures: *bureaucracy, matrix,* and project team structure *(adhocracy).* Mintzberg (1993) addresses the basic coordinating mechanisms to accomplish work. They are *mutual adjustment, direct supervision, standardization of work processes, standardization of work outputs,* and *standardization of worker skills.* The more complex the environment, the more fluid and autonomous it is, needing little supervision.

Structures can be flat or tall. Tall structures are typically in a pyramid shape with the board of control at the top and the staff at the bottom. Board members typically control fiscal resources and make policy. Within each level of the pyramid, there are positions. The terms *position* and *job* often are used interchangeably; however, there is a difference between them. A *job* is composed of a collection of positions that encompass the same basic configuration of tasks. Whereas a *position* is a collection of tasks configured together, usually by one individual. Each position carries with it a degree of authority, accountability, and responsibility. *Authority* is the right to act or direct others. *Accountability* is the liability of task performance (this cannot be delegated), and responsibility is the assignment and acceptance of a task. Organizations may be centralized or decentralized. *Centralized organizations* have board members and administrators with power and authority at the top of the organization. Decentralized organizations are just the opposite.

75

They empower staff at all levels to make decisions and solve pressing problems. *Decentralized organizations* usually have flat structures with few hierarchical levels.

In turbulent environments, such as health care, decentralized structures are efficient and effective because they respond rapidly to environmental change. Nurse administrators must examine the structure and process continually to manage resources effectively and expedite the work of the organization. One method of modifying the structure is called restructuring. *Restructuring* is modifying the existing structural components of an organization; whereas *reengineering,* another method, is a radical renovation of the processes used to accomplish goals. *Job redesign* focuses on who does what tasks. Flexibility, cross-training, and productivity are key. Changing the structure of nursing organizations is essential to stay competitive and provide community-based care to clients through integrated health care systems. In the past the health care service industry has not operated as a business.

Today, health care is big business and must be responsive to cost and quality issues and changing reimbursement patterns. Organizational structures provide a framework for the division of labor and the accomplishment of work. The three types of organizations are bureaucracy, matrix, and professional team structure/adhocracy. These organizational types can be viewed on a continuum with the classic bureaucracy on one end and the delegated organizational-type adhocracy on the opposite end.

A *bureaucracy* is a tall, pyramidal, hierarchical structure in which the power is centralized at the top. In a pyramidal structure, the decision makers are at the top, and the workers are at the bottom. *Line positions* are those that are in the chain of command and that directly contribute to the product or service of the organization. The *strategic apex* is another term used to denote the top decision-making positions. The *operating core* is composed of the workers and the middle line managers coordinating the work. *Technocrats* are individuals who design, plan, change, or train others to do the work. *Support staff* provide services to enhance the technocrats' productivity.

A *matrix structure* is used for complex work environments. The matrix structure is a combination of bureaucracy and project teams. In a matrix structure, individuals may report to two or more individuals and be evaluated by them on specific components of their work. This structure is complicated and requires coordination and careful evaluation. The advantages

include maximizing the use of specialists and interdisciplinary teamwork. Its disadvantages include the need for time-consuming activities such as monitoring and evaluating multiple project teams and individuals and for ensuring optimal productivity from groups.

Project team structures or *adhocracies* are used when highly specialized professional groups practice together. Little supervision is needed, and individual workers are assigned to project teams to complete work. This structure is used by teams of specialists who are organized to complete specific jobs (Mintzberg, 1993). As project work comes into the organization, individuals are assigned according to specialty-specific expertise.

Five basic organizational types range from the most simple to the more complex. The simple structure has a wide span of control, minimal or no middle line, and no staff. The organization is typically small and new with few guidelines. A machine bureaucracy is an elaborate structure of administrative and support personnel, large units, and a pyramidal hierarchy. A professional bureaucracy has a flat structure, with few midlevel managers, but a large support staff to assist professional workers. A divisionalized form is a collection of quasi-autonomous units with a central administration. An adhocracy is a highly organic form composed of professional workers who elect to manage themselves and a flat administrative structure.

An *organizational chart* is used graphically to display the formal structure for an organization. The formal structure depicts the formal communication channels: who reports to whom and the levels of authority. The informal structure is a network within an organization that is typically oral in nature and composed of friends and co-workers who share information. The organizational chart depicts vertical or horizontal structures. Vertical structures show how tall or centralized an organization is, and horizontal structures refer to flat or decentralized organizations. Line positions are linked together by solid lines to show the flow of authority, whereas staff positions are depicted with dotted lines to show consultative relationships.

Nursing leaders are faced with a complex, turbulent, and constantly changing health care environment to manage. They are challenged to respond to client needs and health care issues and to empower employees. Three work empowerment structures are opportunity (for growth), power (information, support, and resources), and proportion (social arrangements) (Upenieks, 2002). Social structures that foster empowerment include having access to information, receiving support, having access to resources necessary to the job, and having the opportunity to learn and grow (Manojlovich & Spence Laschinger, 2002).

Nurses who lead their organizations to success also will use new or reconfigured hospital structures. The trends noted by responsive leadership teams in reconfiguration of hospital structures are flattened organizations, fluid structures, outcomes orientation, redefined staff functions with managerial accountability, reduced staff costs, subcontracting services, and refocusing on the core business. Work design, restructuring, and reengineering are strategies to reposition a health care agency in a competitive manner. Layoffs, downsizing, and substitution of assistants for registered nurses are only short-term solutions for the cost concerns of managers. Nursing leaders must take a proactive stance and provide a vision for the organization, one that combines cost and quality into an efficient, effective health care system that is grounded in positive client outcomes. Excellent leaders design organizational structures that are flexible, have few detailed rules, expand nurse autonomy, and increase diversity and the pace of change. These leaders perceive their jobs to be relevant, flexible, and visible, and they develop well-established informal alliances.

Trends in health care include the need for quantum leadership to advance health care into the next century. In *quantum leadership,* leaders focus the work on obtaining the right outcomes. The development of a futuristic infrastructure (information based), a relational and functional horizontal structure to coordinate elements and facilitate relationships at every organizational level, is key in quantum leadership. Nurse leaders must be adept at *work design* (changing the actual structure of jobs that nurses perform by measuring the workload and fitting individuals into jobs). Challenges for leaders are many and require an investment in leadership development and training and research and innovation.

LEARNING TOOLS

Group Activity: Understanding Organizational Structure

Purpose
To gain a clear understanding of the purpose and function of organizational structures.

Directions

1. Develop an interactive site with peers for the purpose of exchange information and ideas about organizational structure.

2. Appoint an interactive leader who posts the discussion topic or question. Establish a timeframe—perhaps 5 days—where each individual contributes information and comments regarding the posted topic. Through this interactive site, valuable information and research articles about organizational structure can be shared.

3. The interactive leader should summarize the major points in the discussion and then post the next topic for discussion.

Organizational Structure Topic Guide

1. Discuss the importance of organizational structure for work, power, and control elements.

2. Structure creates an environment in which practice takes place. Describe nursing administrators', nurse managers', and clinical nurses' roles in changing the organizational structure to improve client outcomes.

3. What type of an organizational structure works best in a turbulent, changing health care environment?

4. Describe activities nurses can use to create a positive work environment.

5. Describe work empowerment structures.

Group Activity: Organizational Chart Analysis

Purpose

To analyze an organizational chart to determine the channels of communication, staff and line positions, centralized versus decentralized structure, and a pyramidal or flat structure.

Directions

1. Review the following hospital organizational chart.

2. Individually or in a small group, complete an organizational chart analysis by completing the study guide questions.

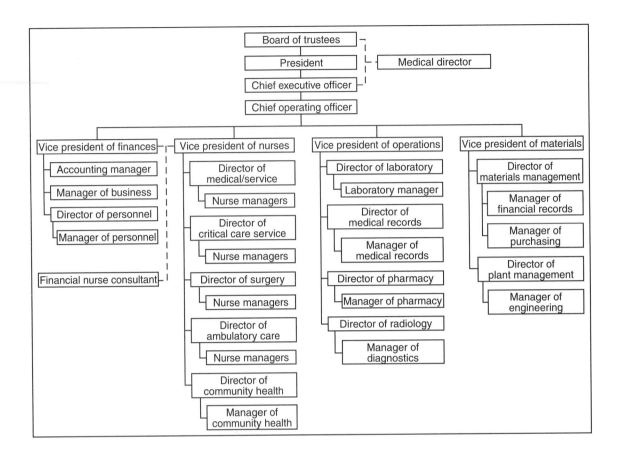

Study Guide Questions for an Organizational Chart Analysis

1. Is this a pyramidal or flat organizational structure?

2. Are communication channels simple or complex?

3. Are there any staff positions? If so, what are they?

4. How many levels are in the hierarchy?

5. Is this a centralized or a decentralized chart?

(Once you have completed the questions, review your answers with the answers below.)

Hospital Organizational Chart Answers

This is a pyramidal organizational structure with seven levels in the hierarchy. The communication channels are complex with a detailed reporting structure. It appears to be a centralized organizational structure because of the multiple levels. There are two identified staff positions, the medical director, and the financial nurse consultant.

CASE STUDY: ORGANIZATIONAL STRUCTURE

Jo Liang is a nurse manager of a 45-bed surgical unit with a position control of 58 full-time employees and that currently employs 65 individuals. Christa Ziema is the nurse educator assigned to the surgical unit. Nurse Ziema works with all of the surgical units because she is a clinical nurse specialist whose focus is surgical care. Nurses Liang and Ziema work well as a team, and they establish annual goals together and meet monthly to review progress. Nurse Liang's task is to be responsible for the fiscal and human resource management, and Nurse Ziema's responsibilities include the education of new and existing employees.

Case Study Questions

1. Is Nurse Liang in a line or staff position? Is Nurse Ziema in a line or staff position? What is the difference between line and staff positions?

2. For what tasks is Nurse Liang held accountable? For what tasks is Nurse Ziema held accountable?

3. Who has the authority to make decisions for the surgical unit?

4. Which resources can Nurses Liang and Ziema consult to determine their level of accountability?

CASE STUDY: CENTRALIZED/DECENTRALIZED STRUCTURE

Sylvia Martin is a vice president of a 720-bed acute care facility in New York. The hospital has been having severe financial problems because of the changes in reimbursement. Nurse Martin has met with the chief executive officer (CEO) and the chief financial officer (CFO), both of whom want immediate action to get the bottom line in the black. Because Nurse Martin has the largest budget with the largest number of full-time employees she is asked to make all the cuts in her department. The CEO and CFO suggested layoffs, hiring nurse extenders, and merging units to decrease the number of nurse managers in the hospital. They are not telling Nurse Martin what to do, however. If she can think of other cost cutting strategies, she is free to use them. (Nurse Martin leaves the meeting rather somber.)

Case Study Questions

1. What should Nurse Martin do?

2. Will the suggestions that the CEO and CFO made solve all Nurse Martin's problems and save money for the hospital?

3. Are the suggestions that the CEO and CFO made long-term or short-term strategies?

4. What other strategies could be used to cut costs?

LEARNING RESOURCES

Discussion Questions

1. In turbulent environments, is a centralized or decentralized structure best for accomplishing the work of the organization? Provide a rationale for your answer.

2. What are some methods nurse administrators can use to change the structure in order to deliver high-quality care to clients?

3. Describe the five basic mechanisms that organizations use to coordinate their work.

4. What is the role of the board in an organization? How can clinical nurses influence board-level decisions?

5. What is the difference between restructuring and reengineering? Give an example of each.

6. Are there differences between the health care service industry and the private business sector?

7. What type of organizational structure would be best for a highly complex, turbulent, health care environment that employs specialists?

8. What is the difference between centralized and decentralized organizations?

9. Describe the difference between a line and a staff position. Provide an example of each.

10. When would a matrix structure for an organization be useful? What are the advantages and disadvantages of a matrix structure?

Study Questions

Matching: Write the letter of the correct response in front of each term.

_____ 1. Line position

_____ 2. Staff position

_____ 3. Authority

_____ 4. Accountability

_____ 5. Responsibility

_____ 6. Scalar process

_____ 7. Span of control

_____ 8. Reengineering

_____ 9. Centralized

_____ 10. Decentralized

_____ 11. Bureaucracy

_____ 12. Matrix

_____ 13. Adhocracy

_____ 14. Pyramidal

_____ 15. Techno-structure

_____ 16. Support staff

_____ 17. Operating core

_____ 18. Horizontal structure

_____ 19. Machine bureaucracy

A. The creation of levels of authority in a hierarchy

B. The number of workers supervised by a manager

C. A position that provides expertise and knowledge for accomplishing organizational goals

D. The right to act or direct others

E. The liability associated with task performance

F. The allocation or acceptance of tasks

G. When the power to make decisions is concentrated at the top of an organization

H. When the power to make decisions is filtered down toward the individual worker

I. Direct line of hierarchical authority

J. Changing the operational process of an organization

K. A collection of semi-autonomous units linked by a central administrative structure

L. A large administrative and support staff and a tall hierarchy

M. Few administrative layers between top administrators and workers

_____ 20. Divisionalized
form

N. Those who perform the work of the organization by providing the service

O. Individuals who perform activities that enable individuals to do the direct work of the organization

P. Analysts who design, plan, change, or train individuals to do the work of the organization

Q. Tall, with a wide base and narrow apex

R. A complex combination of a hierarchical structure with project teams

S. Tall, hierarchical, centralized structure

T. Flat, decentralized structure with project teams

True or False: Circle the correct response.

T   F   21. The scalar process is the number of subordinates any one manager manages.

T   F   22. It is important for clinical nurses to influence top executive officers in areas of access, quality, and costs.

T   F   23. Job redesign examines flexibility, cross-training, and productivity issues.

T   F   24. Long-term solutions to cost containment include layoffs, downsizing, and substituting assistants for registered nurses.

T   F   25. Work design is changing the structure of jobs.

REFERENCES

Manojlovich, M., & Spence Laschinger, H. K. (2002). The relationship of empowerment and selected personality characteristics to nursing job satisfaction. *Journal of Nursing Administration, 32*(11), 586-595.

Mintzberg, H. (1993). *Structure in fives: Designing effective organizations.* Englewood Cliffs, NJ: Prentice-Hall.

Upenieks, V. (2002). What constitutes successful nurse leadership? A qualitative approach utilizing Katner's theory of organizational behavior. *Journal of Nursing Administration, 32*(12), 622-632.

SUPPLEMENTAL READINGS

Alfred, F., Stange, K. C., McDaniel, R. R., & Aita, A. (2003). Understanding organizational designs of primary care practices. *Journal of Healthcare Management, 48*(1), 45-61.

Batson, V. (2004). Shared governance in an integrated health network. *Association of Operating Room Nurses, AORN Journal, 80*(3), 493-520.

Lopopolo, R. B. (2002). The relationship of role-related variables to job satisfaction and commitment to the organization in a restructured hospital environment. *Physical Therapy, 82*(10), 984-1000.

Telford, P. (2004). Quality of work life: A leadership imperative: One staff nurse's perspective reinforces how quality of work life and leadership relate to and impact on each other in restructuring nursing work environments. *The Canadian Nurse, 100*(6), 10.

Chapter 11: Organizational Structure (pp. 235-254)

1. What purposes does the structure of an organization serve?

Organizational structure serves to provide order, distinction, and a framework for goal attainment. Nurses are to control behavioral variations among individuals, avoid chaos, direct the flow of information, determine employee positions, and provide an efficient work flow.

2. What elements of organizational structure are found in nursing organizations?

The elements of organizational structure include division of labor, hierarchy of authority, rules and regulations that govern behavior, span of control, and lines of communication. All of these elements are present in nursing organizations.

3. What elements are most important for nursing practice?

When identifying the elements of organizational structure that are important to nursing practice, one must consider what elements facilitate care delivery. Rules and regulations provide functional boundaries that govern behavior. The division of labor provides for delegation of responsibilities, and the lines of communication delineate line and staff reporting structures and direct the flow of information.

4. What factors need to be assessed before changing the organizational culture?

An organizational structure is a significant element in the culture of an organization. Before initiating any type of change process, one must have a thorough understanding of the existing structure. Assessment of the complexity of the organization; the level of specialization of the workforce; the degree of centralization of services; and the formalization of policies, procedures, rules, and regulations is essential.

5. How do nurses foster or hinder restructuring?

Organizational restructuring changes roles, jobs, and positions in nursing; therefore it elicits opposition and support. Opposition to restructuring is not surprising, especially with the history of downsizing of the registered nurse workforce now being viewed as shortsighted. Yet enhanced opportunities for nurses in a restructured health care environment include case management, care coordination across settings, advanced practice, and autonomous clinical practice.

6. What changes are needed in nursing organizations? Why?

Traditionally, nursing organizations have been bureaucratic. To be successful in a health care reform climate, nursing organizations must change to become more cost-effective, efficient, innovative, and flexible structures that respond quickly to a dynamic and turbulent environment. Nursing organizations must change or risk becoming bureaucratic relics.

7. How are the structures of community agencies the same as or different from hospitals?

In the past, hospitals often would have bureaucratic structures because of their size and complexity. However, today many hospitals are moving to a matrix structure. In a bureaucratic structure, services provided may be diverse, with multiple divisional lines and levels of authority. A board of directors heads the structure in hospital organizations as it does in community agencies. In a matrix structure, interdisciplinary teams work to become more integrated across care delivery systems. Although community agencies that are linked to state and federal agencies are complex bureaucratic entities, those linked with local government tend to resemble a matrix structure.

8. What coordinating mechanisms are used in nursing and health care organizations?

Five basic mechanisms are used in nursing and health care organizations to coordinate their work: mutual adjustment, direct supervision, standardization of work processes, standardization of work outputs, and standardization of worker skills.

9. How effective are the coordinating mechanisms used by nursing?

The effectiveness of coordinating mechanisms in nursing varies. The process of mutual adjustment or informal communication among peers for problem resolution has been used effectively since the inception of nursing practice. Direct supervision was effective before the advent of primary care nursing. However, during the decade of popularity of primary care nursing, delegation skills were lost and nurses only now are regaining them through education and experience. Nursing has been coordinating work through the use of critical paths or plans of care. Standardization efforts within organizations and national credentialing bodies are improving as demands for validation of competencies, cost containment, and quality increase.

10. **How have authority, responsibility, and accountability been used in nursing practice? What feelings do they create?**

Organizational authority is used to fulfill the responsibilities of a professional role in a specific job, whereas professional authority is used to practice professional nursing. Each nurse who fulfills a position accepts responsibility to complete the work and maintains accountability for the quality and quantity of the assigned work. These three elements of professional practice may generate mixed feelings. Authority may produce feelings of power and esteem, whereas responsibility and accountability may generate feelings of uncertainty and fear.

11. **Is power in nursing centralized or decentralized?**

Decentralization of power in nursing has become more common over the years. Decentralized structures improve quality and lower costs by placing the decision-making authority closer to work processes. With increasing demands on health care entities to lower costs and improve quality, the trend to create infrastructures that decentralize the decision-making power in nursing will continue into the future.

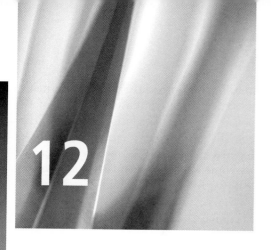

12

Decentralization and Shared Governance

A crisis is looming in health care with a growing disparity between the supply and demand of registered nurses and the aging of the Baby Boomers. Increasing demands are being placed on the health care system in response to the technical and social transformation, maturing technology, and more educated consumers. Clinical care is becoming more mobile, fast-paced, and consumer driven. Traditional hierarchical organizational structures are being reconfigured to empower nurses to make decisions at the point of care regarding client care in the practice environment. *Shared governance,* a model of organizational decision making premised on a decentralized organizational structure in which staff nurses are empowered through autonomy and accountability, is one model of empowering nurses to make decisions at the point of care regarding client care and the practice environment. The work in a hospital is guided by the philosophy. The philosophy serves as the framework that shapes the direction and development of the institution. Organizations that invest in knowledge that increases the productivity of human capital will experience productivity increases (North, 1990). The *organizational chart* is a visual representation of the horizontal and vertical reporting structure in a health care agency.

The information age has created new demands in response to the revolution of technology and information processing. Centers of excellence are able to respond to changes proactively in an efficient and effective manner, empowering employees to make innovative decisions promptly. Decision-making authority in an organization is an essential component of job and professional autonomy. Decision-making power can be *centralized,* with a few administrators at the top, or *decentralized,* with the power passed on to the individuals that decisions affect directly. Centralization and decentralization can be ranges on a continuum with centralization at one end and decentralization at the opposite extreme. Decisions can be viewed as more

or less centralized or decentralized. There is rarely a situation in which all decisions are exclusively centralized or exclusively decentralized. *Vertical decentralization* is the distribution of formal power down the chain of command, and *horizontal decentralization* is the distribution of formal power outside the chain of command where support staff participate in the decision-making process. (When an administration centralizes the structure, it is controlling decision making and holding power at the top of the organization. In contrast, an administration that decentralizes decision making empowers employees at all levels of the organization to participate.) Those managers who disperse authority have more time to devote to planning and evaluation strategies. In a decentralized structure the span of control is wider for each manager. Institutions using decentralized structures develop synergy. *Synergy* is the result of departments working together to accomplish a goal that often yields greater output than if departments work independently. *Governance* is the structure, process, and whole system by which a group functions and makes decisions. *Information asymmetry* is the imbalance of the level of knowledge about a specific topic or area. Those with specialized knowledge, such as cardiac care, are in a better position to make decisions about care for this type of client.

During turbulent times, in complex environments, and with professional staff, decentralization is a useful tool to ensure that the organization stays flexible, innovative, and committed to solving complex, multidisciplinary problems. Participation in decision making at all levels fosters autonomy, accountability, and worker responsibility.

Communication to and from individuals is important in decentralized organizations. Nurse administrators are experimenting with many different models of participatory decision making to empower nurses to provide quality care to clients. Shared governance is one professional practice framework that espouses an accountability-based governance structure. *Shared governance* is a system that fosters creativity and flexibility by empowering nurses to make autonomous clinical decisions through formal processes. The major nursing service components of shared governance include practice, quality, education, and peer governance.

Shared governance was first implemented in the late 1970s as a method to improve nurse satisfaction, improve retention, and enhance the recruitment of clinical nurses. Difficulties in establishing a shared governance environment commonly occur in a bureaucratic organization because of the complicated communication networks, rigid reporting structures, and elaborate policies and procedures that govern employee behavior. Another common problem in implementing shared governance is the difficulty of making a true change instead of a cosmetic or name change. It is much easier for an administration to use the terminology but retain all authority and decision-making power.

The implementation of shared governance in an organization creates a constant tension between organizational and professional goals. Nurses exert their influence or control by clearly defining and articulating their scope and standards of practice, their nursing care delivery system, their knowledge specialization, their knowledge and resource development priorities, and their self-evaluation or peer evaluation. Shared governance as an accountability-based model provides a mechanism for registered nurses to make decisions regarding nursing practice, quality of client care, education, nursing peer issues, and issues in the work environment. Shared governance leads to empowerment and professional autonomy (Porter-O'Grady, 2003). *Empowerment* is a process by which nurses recognize that they have power and authority to make decisions regarding their practice. To support shared governance, an infrastructure and culture must be implemented to sustain the model. Strategies to empower nurses include education, leadership, support and resources, coaching, and mentoring. Fostering the development of leadership behaviors in staff nurses will lead to empowerment and autonomy of nursing staff. Specific training on role in committee work, setting agendas, developing consensus, dealing with conflict, and conducting meetings is valuable for effective shared governance. Key elements for successful implementation of shared governance include a client focus, participation in decision-making, consensus management, free expression, individual accountability, proper timing, and a sense of cohesion through a common language (Herrick, 1998).

Three major models of professional governance are the councilar model, the congressional model, and the administrative shared governance model. The *councilar model* has committees that are elected and have clearly defined authority and function. The councilar model typically has at least one committee on each of the following: practice, education, management, and quality improvement. The *congressional model* includes officers and an elected cabinet and is modeled after the national governmental structure. The *administrative shared governance model* divides administration and clinical into two separate components and identifies the authority for each. Committees and forums are held jointly, and decisions are made at the level at which the actual work takes place. The administrative and council structure have decision-making power.

Changes in health care delivery require responsiveness to new client care demands on an ongoing basis. Clinical nurses are being held accountable for their actions and must take responsibility in designing and delivering care. Health care organizations will continue to change to maintain their viability and increase their market share, causing mergers, consolidations, multisite systems, and integrated health care networks.

Nursing leaders are challenged to restructure roles to decentralize authority to the point of service, empower clinical nurses, increase multitasking, develop work processes that support client-care delivery, and design new skill mixes. Three key criteria for which administrators will be held accountable include (1) delivering care within financial resources, (2) providing high-quality services, and (3) satisfying consumer and provider service demands. A major leadership challenge will be to develop a culture of success in the organization. Governance issues will be fluid as innovations in integration within, between, and among organizations occur through partnering, strategic alliances, and vertical integrations.

Shared governance is one of the best-practice options in the nurse leader's toolbox (Herrin, 2004). The rewards of shared governance include empowerment, autonomy, commitment, and improved outcomes for clients and organizations. Shared governance assists in establishing a culture of individual professional accountability and autonomy. A bond is forged between the nurse and the organization when accountability, partnership, equity, and ownership are shared (Porter-O'Grady, 2003). Savvy leaders use strategies that empower staff such as shared governance and the "forces of magnetism." The forces of magnetism address the following (McClure & Hinshaw, 2002):

- Quality of nursing leadership
- Organizational structure
- Management style
- Personnel policies and programs
- Professional models of care
- Quality of care
- Quality of improvement

- Consultation and resources
- Autonomy
- Community and the hospital
- Nurses as teachers
- Image of nursing
- Interdisciplinary relationships
- Professional development

Many benefits accrue to nurses, the organization, and clients when staff are empowered through shared governance models. Leaders who are visionary encourage expert nurses to think outside of the box and support them in occasional failures. Strong leaders advocate for their professional nursing staff and clients. They design shared governance models and seek Magnet hospital designation. Research supports this practice and demonstrates that Magnet-designated hospital systems have better recruitment and retention of professional nurses and better client outcomes and satisfaction (Scott et al., 1999).

LEARNING TOOLS

Group Activity: Analysis of Organizational Structure

Purpose

To analyze an organization to determine whether it is a centralized or decentralized organization and to determine whether a shared governance framework is established.

Directions

Select a health care organization with which you are familiar and complete the Governance Study Guide.

Governance Study Guide

1. Where is the power in the organization?

_____

2. How much authority does each manager have?

_____

3. Who has what decision-making responsibility?

_____

4. How many levels of hierarchy are there in the organization?

_____

5. Do clinical nurses make autonomous clinical decisions?

_____

6. Are clinical nurses elected or appointed to organizational committees?

_____

7. Do clinical nurses participate in hiring, evaluating, and scheduling decisions?

_____

8. How are clinical nurses' innovative ideas encouraged and received by administration?

_____

9. How are assignments made on the nursing units?

_____

Upon completion of the Governance Study Guide, design an organizational structure that facilitates employee participation. This exercise will help you determine the type of organizational structure with which you are comfortable and will give you ideas about the type of work environment you might look for when seeking employment.

Remember that a more decentralized structure enables clinical nurses to participate at all levels of decision making. Communication is horizontal and vertical, and innovations are encouraged.

CASE STUDY

Joyce Vanhusen has been a vice president of nursing at a 600-bed community hospital for 15 years. She has established a hierarchical nursing service and decides it is time to cut out some of the unnecessary organizational layers to contain costs. Ms. Vanhusen announces at the monthly management meeting in May that it is imperative that nursing management downsize. She says she will be consulting with several individuals to make the best possible and least painful choices. Ms. Vanhusen also announces that she has developed a shared governance model and provides a handout of the committee structure for the nursing service department. She directs the managers to tell the employees that they are now working in a shared government environment and to solicit volunteers for the committees. Managers should submit volunteer names to the executive secretary.

85

The secretary will notify the appropriate committee members when problems arise and arrange for them to meet.

Case Study Questions

1. Did Ms. Vanhusen implement a shared governance framework?

2. How is participation in decision making encouraged at all levels in the nursing department?

3. What benefits are there to espousing a shared governance framework?

LEARNING RESOURCES

Discussion Questions

1. Discuss the disadvantages and advantages of centralized and decentralized organizational structures.

2. How do changes in health care influence the type of governance model a hospital will choose to implement?

3. Compare and contrast the three major types of governance models.

4. What is meant by "only a cosmetic change occurred when shared governance was implemented"?

5. What is the clinical nurse's role in a shared governance model?

Study Questions

True or False: Circle the correct answer.

T   F   1. The congressional model uses a council format and separates the clinical and administrative tracts.

T   F   2. The administrative model elects a president and cabinet of officers who represent each nursing unit.

T   F   3. The councilar model is composed of councils with elected positions.

T   F   4. All clinical nurses are in favor of a shared governance system where accountability and decision making are encouraged.

T   F   5. Implementation of shared governance systems is costly and requires considerable time and effort.

T   F   6. Nurse leaders are challenged to design effective delivery systems in multihospital systems and integrated networks.

T   F   7. Centralization is the concentration of decision-making authority at the top of the organization.

T   F   8. Decentralization is dispersing decision-making authority throughout the organization.

T   F   9. An organization is centralized or decentralized.

T   F   10. Savvy administrators will decentralize during crisis and centralize during stable times.

T   F   11. Work redesign is implemented to increase nurse satisfaction.

T   F   12. Shared governance models empower nurses to provide quality care.

REFERENCES

Herrick, L. M. (1998). Shared governance in an academic health center. In J. A. Dienemann (Ed.), *Nursing administration: Managing patient care* (2nd ed., pp. 417-424). Stamford, CT: Appleton & Lange.

Herrin, D. M. (2004, January 31). Shared governance: A nurse executive response. *Online Journal of Issues in Nursing. 9*(1), Manuscript 1b. Retrieved September 15, 2004, from *www.nursingworld.org/ojin/topic23/tpc23_1b.htm*

McClure, M. L., & Hinshaw, A. S. (2002). *Magnet hospitals revisited: Attraction and retention of professional nurses.* Washington, DC: American Nurses Publishing.

North, D. C. (1990). *Institutions, institutional change and economic performance.* New York: Cambridge University Press.

Porter-O'Grady, T. (2003). Researching shared governance: A futility of focus. *Journal of Nursing Administration, 33*(4), 251-252.

Scott, J. G., Sochalski, J., & Aiken, L. (1999). Review of magnet hospital research: Findings and implications for professional nursing practice. *Journal of Nursing Administration, 29*(1), 9-19.

SUPPLEMENTAL READINGS

George, V., Burke, L. J., Rodgers, B., Duthie, N., Hoffmann, M. L., Koceja, V., et al. (2002). Developing staff nurse shared leadership behaviour in professional nursing practice. *Nursing Administration Quarterly, 26*(3), 44-59.

Hess, R. G. (2004, January 31). From bedside to boardroom: Nursing shared governance. *Online Journal of Issues in Nursing, 9*(1), Manuscript 1. Retrieved September 15, 2004, from *www.nursingworld.org/ojin/topic23/tpc23_1.htm*

Miller, E. D. (2002). Shared governance and performance improvement: A new opportunity to build trust in a restructured health care system. *Nursing Administrative Quarterly, 26*(3), 60-66.

ANSWERS TO TEXT STUDY QUESTIONS

Chapter 12: Decentralization and Shared Governance (pp. 255-270)

1. What is the relationship between decentralization and shared governance?

Decentralization occurs when the decision-making power is dispersed to many points within the organization. A shared governance model falls under the auspices of decentralization. Shared governance is one form of a professional practice model in which decision-making power is shared among staff nurses and management.

2. How are shared governance and structure related?

Although shared governance may assume different forms, it is an organizational structure. Shared governance legitimizes staff nurses' influence on the administrative decision-making process.

3. What conditions in the facility in which you are a student or employee would facilitate shared governance?

To identify conditions that facilitate shared governance, consider the factors that empower staff nurses to make autonomous client care decisions. Possible conditions that might be present include administrative support; interdisciplinary collaboration and team building; and educational offerings that prepare staff for authority, accountability, and resource management. A staff that is knowledgeable of the financial management processes of the organization and is encouraged to take an active role in the implementation of its strategic plan also facilitates the development of shared governance. What other conditions can you identify?

4. Are decentralization and shared governance characteristic of current hospital nursing organizations? Current community health and long-term care organizations?

The last decade has seen a movement toward decentralization in hospital nursing organizations. Hospitals have been the trendsetters among health care organizations to establish more participative management structures. Many institutions have implemented models of shared governance, with varying degrees of nurse autonomy and authority over practice and processes. As integrated health care systems continue to develop, shared governance frameworks will continue to emerge in community-based environments and long-term care settings.

5. Does changing to a shared governance model change nurses' roles? If so, how?

Nurses' roles in a shared governance model are expanded to accept more responsibility and accountability for decision making. Nurses not only will be expected to provide professional care but also will be instrumental in decision-making processes that affect their practice, the professional environment, and care delivery. Decisions about the acquisition and allocation of resources, educational opportunities, peer review, and quality improvement processes are examples of additional responsibilities that are a part of a shared governance model.

6. What is the governance structure of the nursing organization with which you are most familiar?

To answer this question, think about who makes the decisions in your organization. Are staff nurses involved in decisions that affect professional practice or their work environment? Is decision making mutually shared with management, or is it exclusive to management or staff? Is the scope of decision making limited to the unit, or are division-level decision-making opportunities available with input to the executive decision-making body? If a shared governance model were to be identified, would it be classified as a councilar model, a congressional format, or an administrative shared governance model?

7. What questions should be asked to determine the level of decentralization in an organization?

Some questions that will assist in the determination of where the decision-making power lies include the following: Who has the authority to make resource allocation decisions? Who makes care management decisions? To what extent do nonmanagers have power over decision-making processes? What are the lines of communication in the organization?

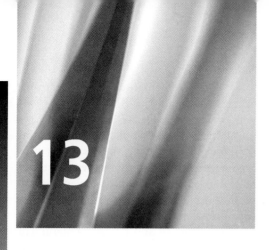

Data Management and Informatics

13

STUDY FOCUS

This is the information age. Information can be and is transmitted across the world instantaneously. Information technology has changed the way people work, play, learn, and manage their personal lives. Data is required for direct client care and for regulatory and governmental agency assessment. The Health Insurance Portability and Accountability Act was one mechanism to provide adequate protections to ensure the confidentiality of data. Computer applications in nursing administration are best understood from the intersection of three areas: (1) nursing administration, (2) informatics, and (3) effectiveness research. The *computer* is a tool to manage complexity and to control and coordinate large volumes of data (Mowry & Korpman, 1986). Accurate and timely data are essential to make decisions about client care and organizational management (Newbold, 1998). Computer applications in nursing administration are tools to make effective decisions to enhance quality client care. Nursing must develop or use existing standardized nursing databases to make meaningful comparisons across clinical sites. Computer applications have provided an efficient and effective method of acquiring financial data to evaluate outcomes of care.

Computers are the tools for managing data. *Informatics* is a combination of computer and information science. *Nursing informatics* is the management of nursing data, information, and knowledge as it is applied to nursing care delivery. *Effectiveness research* is the use of large data sets applying epidemiological methods to evaluate relationships. *Management information systems* (MISs) are integrated to collect, store, retrieve, and process data. Ten criteria for an effective MIS are the following: informative, relevant, sensitive, unbiased, comprehensive, timely, action-oriented, uniform, performance-targeted, and cost-effective (Austin, 1979). A *clinical data repository* is a physical or logical compilation of client data pertaining to health. Related terms include information warehouse or data repository. Data are stored longitudinally over several episodes of care. The primary purpose of a data repository is to facilitate easy retrieval of data (American Nurses Association, 1997).

Automated information systems are useful for collecting clinical data to direct client care and manage care processes. Great strides have been made in medical data collection and analysis, but nursing lags behind in the development of support systems because of lack of consensus on how nursing knowledge is represented and on how nurses make decisions. The standardization of a nursing data set is essential to capture the contributions that nurses make to client care. Reimbursement decisions are made based on hard data that are easily retrievable and show positive outcomes. *Four domains of nursing data* needs include the client data, provider data, administrative data, and research data. Nurses must define their data elements clearly, identify linkages between and among data sets, and design a clear coding system to ensure usable data sets. The determination of data elements and engineering technology are important aspects of nursing informatics.

The American Nurses Association recognized informatics as a nursing specialty in 1992. Data are defined as discrete, objective entities. *Information* is data that is organized, structured, and interpreted. *Knowledge* is the synthesis of information to identify relationships. The roles of the nursing informatics specialist is participating in the analysis, design, and implementation of information and communication systems; engaging in effectiveness research; and educating nurses on informatics and information systems.

Currently, 13 standardized terminologies are recognized by the American Nurses Association. The approved classifications include North American Nursing Diagnosis Association Inc. (NANDA), nursing interventions classification system (NIC), nursing outcomes classification system (NOC), nursing management minimum data set (NMMDS), home health care classification (HHCC), OMAHA system, Patient Care Data Set (PCDS), SNOMED CT, Nursing Minimum

Data Set (NMDS), International Classification of Nursing Practice (ICNP), ABC Codes, and Logical Observation Identifier of Names and Codes (LOINC) (Nursing Information & Data Set Evaluation Center, 2004). Different types of terminology structures exist. The most commonly used terminology structures are classification systems. Concept-oriented or reference terminologies are used as structure for documentation in modern computer database systems. A reference terminology model depicts the system of concepts that provides the structure for the organization of documentation terms (Bakken et al., 2001). The International Standards Organization (ISO) Technical Committee ISO/TC 215 Health Informatics workgroup met to design an integrative evolving multidisciplinary terminology standard. The ISO RTM for Nursing Action is comprised of six categories—action, target, recipient of care, means, route, and site (International Standards Organization, 2002)—to describe nursing interventions.

The first electronic health record was designed in 1965. Electronic health records are designed to provide a longitudinal account of care, an information system that tracks care in a variety of settings, and a tracking mechanism of care across settings and time. The purpose of an electronic health record is to document client care in a single repository as a clinical, financial, and legal record. The advantages of an electronic health record include readily available access to longitudinal records linked over time, access to real-time availability, legible records, triggers, and reminders. Barriers to the use of an electronic health record include readiness, security, confidentiality issues, complexity, and volume of data. The development and use of electronic health records may include systems that alert clinicians to abnormal data, contain clinical decision support systems, and link knowledge bases. In 2004 the position of national health information technology coordinator at the Department of Health and Human Services was created. The goal is for each American to have an electronic health record by 2014. Work is being done on developing an interoperable electronic health record system, the standardized vocabulary, SNOMED CT, is available as a free download from the National Library of Medicine (U.S. Department of Health and Human Services, 2004). With the use of an electronic health record, a reduction in errors in the health care system is anticipated. An integrated electronic health record combines pharmacy, laboaratory, and clinical information systems, allowing the implementation of computerized provider order entry, decision support systems, and medication administration systems. It is estimated that a nationwide implementation of an electronic health record system could save $12.7 billion to $36 billion annually (Staggers et al., 2001).

The result of computerized applications to nursing administration for nurse leaders is the designing of an integrated management information system that uses standardized nursing language and data elements for comparative purposes. To advocate the inclusion of essential nursing data elements in national databases is crucial for nursing practice and reimbursement. The uniform hospital discharge data set does not include nursing data elements because nursing lacks a standardized data set that is clearly defined, valid, and reliable. Nurses are challenged to identify and validate a standardized nursing data set to ensure inclusion in national data sets.

The creation of nursing outcome databases are critical for the following two reasons (Iowa Intervention Project, 1997):

1. Nurses must be able to measure and document how nurses influence client outcomes.

2. The study of nursing-sensitive outcomes will allow comparisons between interventional strategies and advance the science of nursing care delivery.

The *Nursing Minimum Data Set* is a collection of essential nursing information for comparisons across client populations. The three categories of data elements in the NMDS are (1) nursing care, (2) demographics, and (3) service. Data elements related to nursing care include nursing diagnosis, intervention, outcome, and intensity of nursing care (Werley & Lang, 1988). Such efforts are currently under way for nursing administration. The *nursing management minimum data set* is a database that includes 17 service-related management data elements. Data elements include cost, quality, and outcome data. The limitations of the NMMDS are that nursing practice and personnel data about individual nurses is omitted, and it lacks uniform collection practices across sites.

Nursing leadership is needed to provide innovations in data management and informatics to enhance client care. Data security and confidentiality are key components in managing information systems. A current trend in data management and informatics is the continued growth of managed care as a market force driving extensive changes in the use of information technology. The American Organization of Nurse Executives has called for redesign of work to use technology to augment nursing practice in a period of a decreasing and aging workforce. The purpose of this mandate is twofold: (1) to attract more individuals to the profession and (2) to use technology to enable nurses to remain in active caregiving roles. Tools as emerging technologies in nursing include the Internet, continuous speech recognition, wireless computing, thin-client computing, and data warehouses (Simpson, 1999).

LEARNING TOOLS

Activity: Domains of Nursing Data

Purpose
To identify essential elements in the domains of nursing data.

Directions
Using each of the four domains of nursing data listed on p. 92, identify elements in each domain that would be important to collect and analyze in a nursing information system (NIS). Review the following table for outcomes and variables in the three domains of nursing data needs; the illustration that follows this table contains proposed NMMDS elements.

Outcomes and Variables in Three Domains of Nursing Data Needs

	DOMAINS		
	Client	Provider	Administrative
Outcomes	Client satisfaction Achieved care outcomes Costs Access to care	Job enrichment Job/work satisfaction Physician satisfaction Job stress Intent to leave	Costs Productivity Turnover Income

Variables	Attitudes/beliefs
	Diagnosis, gender, age
	Marital status
	Support system
	Satisfaction
	Level of dependency
	Severity of illness
	Intensity of nursing care
		Attitudes/beliefs
		Education
		Years of experience
		Age
		Work excitement
			Agency philosophy
			Priorities
			Organizational
			  structure
			Fiscal data
			Climate
			Policies and
			  procedcures
			Conflict

Chapter **13** Data Management and Informatics

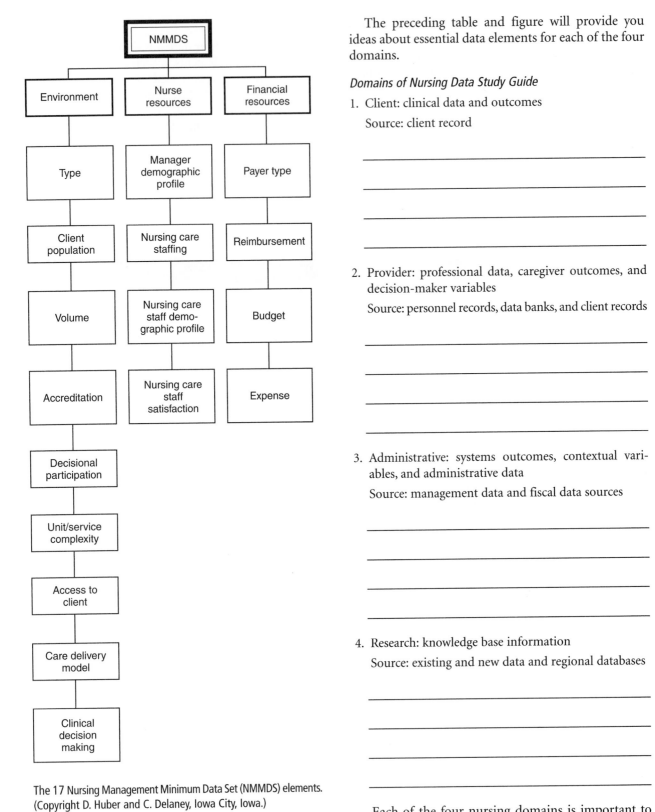

The 17 Nursing Management Minimum Data Set (NMMDS) elements. (Copyright D. Huber and C. Delaney, Iowa City, Iowa.)

The preceding table and figure will provide you ideas about essential data elements for each of the four domains.

Domains of Nursing Data Study Guide

1. Client: clinical data and outcomes
   Source: client record

   _____

   _____

   _____

   _____

2. Provider: professional data, caregiver outcomes, and decision-maker variables
   Source: personnel records, data banks, and client records

   _____

   _____

   _____

3. Administrative: systems outcomes, contextual variables, and administrative data
   Source: management data and fiscal data sources

   _____

   _____

   _____

   _____

4. Research: knowledge base information
   Source: existing and new data and regional databases

   _____

   _____

   _____

Each of the four nursing domains is important to include in the NIS and MIS. Identifying essential variables and outcome by nursing unit and by institution is critical to obtaining quantifiable comparable data. This data can be used to compare units within an institution and across institutions. The collection and analysis of basic nursing data sets are important for nursing to demonstrate nurses' unique contribution to client care.

CASE STUDY

Jackie VanMeter is a nursing director of critical care and has been asked to make recommendations for purchasing a NIS for a large teaching hospital. Ms. VanMeter is knowledgeable about clinical issues but has not had much experience with computers or information systems. She reads about NISs and MISs and wonders whether purchasing an MIS would not be a better choice for the organization. Ms. VanMeter struggles to determine which data elements are essential when purchasing an NIS.

Case Study Questions

1. Would an MIS meet the needs of a nurse administrator?

2. Is there an advantage to a nurse administrator in purchasing an NIS over an MIS?

3. What four domains of nursing data should Ms. VanMeter remember to include as criteria for selection of an NIS?

LEARNING RESOURCES

Discussion Questions

1. What is the difference between informatics and nursing informatics?

2. What is effectiveness research, and how can it be useful in nursing practice?

3. How can standardized nursing data sets help nurses gain reimbursement status for nursing services?

4. Should the NMMDS be refined, or should a new data set be designed? Why?

5. Identify benefits of an NIS for clinical nurses. Identify any barriers for clinical nurses in using an NIS.

Study Questions

Matching: Write the letter of the correct response in front of each term.

_____ 1. Nursing informatics

_____ 2. Informatics

_____ 3. Computer

_____ 4. Effectiveness research

_____ 5. Management information system

_____ 6. Computer-based client record

_____ 7. NMMDS

_____ 8. Quality improvement tools

_____ 9. Clinical data repository

_____ 10. Nursing Information and Data Set Evaluation Center

A. Tool for managing data

B. Analysis of large databases using epidemiological methods

C. Combination of computer and information science

D. Integrated system to collect and manipulate data for the purposes of directing and controlling resources

E. Management of data to support the practice and delivery of nursing care

F. Tracks longitudinal accounts of client care

G. Identifies common causes of variation and visual display of data

H. Physical or logical compilation of client data pertaining to health

I. A center that assists nurses with vendor evaluation of automated information systems or computer-based client record systems

J. Elements crucial to evaluation of nursing interventions on client outcomes

True or False: Circle the correct answer.

T   F   11. Nurses have not agreed on the basic or core data elements essential to manage a nursing service.

T   F   12. Nursing must have standardized, uniformly collected, retrievable, and comparable service-related management data elements.

T   F   13. Nursing informatics is a combination of computer and information science.

T   F   14. A management information system is defined as an integrated system for collecting, storing, retrieving, and processing a collective set of data.

REFERENCES

American Nurses Association. (1997). *NIDSEC standards and scoring guidelines.* Washington, DC: American Nurses Association.

Austin, C. (1979). *Information systems for hospital administration.* Ann Arbor, MI: Health Administration Press.

Bakken, S., Warren, J., Lundberg, C., Casey, A., Correia, C., Konicek, D., et al. (2001, September). *An evaluation of the utility of the CEN categorical structure for nursing diagnoses as a terminology model for integrating nursing diagnosis concepts into SNOMED.* Paper presented at the MEDINFO 2001, Amsterdam.

International Standards Organization. (2002). *Health informatics: Integration of a reference terminology model for nursing* (Committee Document No. ISO/TC 215N 142). Geneva, Switzerland: International Standards Organization.

Iowa Intervention Project. (1997). *Nursing outcomes classification (NOC).* St Louis: Mosby.

Mowry, M., & Korpman, R. (1986). *Managing health care costs, quality, and technology: Product line strategies for nursing.* Rockville, MD: Aspen.

Newbold, S. (1998). Information systems for managing patient care. In J. A. Dienemann (Ed.), *Nursing administration: Managing patient care* (2nd ed., pp. 323-338). Stamford, CT: Appleton & Lange.

Nursing Information & Data Set Evaluation Center. (2004). *ANA recognized terminologies that support nursing practice.* Atlanta: American Nurses Publishing. Retrieved May 28, 2004, from *www.nursingworld.org/nidsec*

Simpson, R. L. (1999). What does IT have in store for nursing? *Nursing Management, 30*(10), 14-15.

Staggers, N., Bagley Thompson, C., & Snyder-Halpern, R. (2001). History and trends in clinical information systems in the United States. *Journal of Nursing Scholarship, 33*(1), 75-81.

U.S. Department of Health and Human Services. (2004). *Secretary Thompson, seeking fastest possible results, names first health information technology coordinator.* Washington, DC: U.S. Department of Health and Human Services. Retrieved May 20, 2004, from *www.dhhs.gov/news/press/2004pres/-20040506.html*

Werley, H., & Lang, N. (Eds.). (1988). *Identification of the nursing minimum data set.* New York: Springer.

SUPPLEMENTAL READINGS

Brown, C., Bagby, R., Neiswinder, J., & Helmuth, A. (2004). Computer-based data collection boosts productivity, regulatory compliance. *Nursing Management, 35*(2), 40B-40D.

Curtin, L., & Simpson, R. L. (2001). Standards of practice for nursing informatics. *Health Management Technology, 22*(4), 52.

Preston, P. (2005). Teams as the key to organizational communication. *Journal of Healthcare Management, 50*(1), 16-18.

Sreckovich, C., & Fahnestock, M. (2002). Identifying and validating managed care data. *Healthcare Financial Management, 56*(10), 54-59.

Chapter 13: Data Management and Informatics (pp. 271-286)

1. **What restraining forces impede the use of nursing data for the analysis of nursing care?**

   Decreased reliability and validity discourages the use of nursing data for the analysis of nursing care. For instance, if a data system is not capturing key elements of care such as the severity levels when determining staffing ratios, the information may not be helpful. Cost is also an issue. Gathering data manually from client charts and then entering it into a data set can be time consuming and expensive. Also, if the chart documentation is incomplete, data interpretation will be skewed. With the current nursing shortage, nurses are too busy to take the extra time needed to gather data while caring for clients. What other restraining forces are present?

2. **What can nursing data be used for?**

   Nursing data is used to evaluate client care, provider staffing, administration of care and the organization, and knowledge-based research for evidence-based practice.

3. **What are advantages that might be seen with the implementation of an electronic health record?**

   The electronic health record has many advantages. It provides a record of the client's health that may be accessed across the continuum of care (if designed to do so). Standards of care may be programmed into the system to assist in prompting optimal care. These standards also can be used as guides for data collection. Data can be gathered easily from the clinical and business processes. Data also can reduce errors in medication administration and order entry.

4. **What difference can nurses who manage health care services make to the design and implementation of an electronic health record?**

   Early electronic health records (EHRs) were merely a word document such as the nursing flow chart or an order sheet entered into a computer. Effective EHRs are interactive. For instance, when a nurse practitioner's order for a lipid profile is entered into the computer (by the ordering provider), the laboratory automatically receives it. The pending laboratory order may appear automatically on the nurse's online worksheet or via notification that a lipid profile has been ordered. The order also may appear on the progress notes. Nurses understand how different aspects of care interrelate and can help design the EHR to meet these needs.

   Most importantly, nurse leaders also can ensure that EHR systems are selected that collect nursing data and support the work of nursing.

5. **What impact will information/communication technology have on nursing care delivery in the future?**

   The American Organization of Nurse Executives has mandated that work be redesigned to augment nursing practice through the use of technology. Advances in the integration of technology will be helpful in streamlining communication between providers, thus decreasing time spent in communication. Clinical data will be easier to aggregate for use in the management of staffing and workload and for determining the quality of care in an institution.

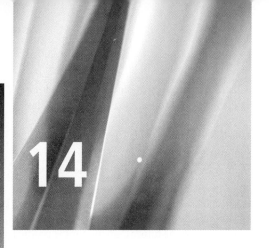

14   Strategic Management

STUDY FOCUS

Strategic management involves assessing the environment, knowing the competition, establishing successful performance, achieving targets, and evaluating success. Strategic management is important in health care to find ways to gain a competitive edge in a highly competitive environment. *Strategic planning* is a systematic process of making entrepreneurial decisions, planning for implementation, and evaluating outcomes (Drucker, 1974). *Strategic management* is a broad concept that includes strategic planning and focuses on important aspects of strategy implementation. Strategic management assists nurses in responding to turbulent changes and capturing opportunities that increase the likelihood of achieving desired outcomes.

A *strategy* is a comprehensive business approach designed to produce a successful outcome. A *tactic* is an operational choice for actions that are made to implement strategy. Strategy comes first and then tactics follow. A *strategic plan* is a written document for allocating resources to accomplish organizational goals. *Organizational vision* or *mission* is the guiding framework that describes what the organization views as its business and future direction. *Objectives* are targets that an organization wants to achieve.

Strategic management begins with the strategic planning process to establish a competitive position in the market or to address a need. Questions asked in the planning process include the following: Where are we currently? Where do we want to go? How will we get there? The components of the nursing process (assessment, planning, implementation, and evaluation) are similar to those of strategic management. The components of strategic management include developing a strategic mission or vision, setting objectives, developing strategies to achieve the objectives, implementing the strategies, and evaluating the results.

The first step of the strategic planning process is identifying the vision or mission of the organization. The mission statement reflects the vision of what the

organization seeks to do and become. The assessment of future environmental impact often is referred to as *assumptions.* Involving individuals at all levels of the organization ensures a variety of perspectives and facilitates "buy in" to the final outcome. After the mission and vision are completed (step two), the strategic goals and objectives are crafted. The objectives define the *who, what,* and *where* of the strategies to be implemented. Without strategic objectives, there is a lack of direction and often an inability to move the organization in a coordinated direction. Objectives often are written in terms of improving the financial health and improving the market position of the organization.

The third step in the strategic planning process is to develop an implementation strategy. The organizational strategy must be flexible to respond to evolving needs of customers, increasing technological advances, and changing political climate; capitalize on new opportunities; attend to market conditions; and respond to crises. The fourth step is implementing the strategy. Functions necessary for implementation include demonstrating leadership, rewarding individuals, allocating resources, formulating policies and procedures, initiating quality improvement, developing best practices, and maintaining a culture that supports strategy. The final step is evaluating effectiveness by measuring outcomes. Environmental analysis (SWOT), is a systematic examination of the *s*trengths, *w*eaknesses, *o*pportunities, and *t*hreats. Strengths and weaknesses are internal to the organization and include key areas of operations, management, products, and finances. Opportunities and threats are the external components and include industry, marketplace, economy, political climate, technology, and competition. The SWOT analysis helps build on strengths, resolves or minimizes weakness, exploits opportunities, and avoids threats.

The sections of a strategic plan include an executive summary; background; mission, vision, and values; goals and strategies; and appendixes. Strategic plans should be disseminated widely internally and externally. Implementation of the strategic plan often involves developing a business or action plan. The *action plan* includes a priority order for achieving objectives, identifying who is responsible for achieving objectives, indicating financial support, and developing a timetable to achieve objectives. The action plan is a living document. Individuals, who are passionate and committed to the process are called *champions*.

Strategic management is a leadership tool designed to provide competitive advantage for organizations. The strategic planning process creates a spirit of partnership and cooperation among internal and external organizational players. The results of planning may increase ownership, improve morale, and increase commitment by all stakeholders. Strategic plans need to be realistic and future-oriented.

Intrapreneurs are individuals in an organization who design new products or services. *Entrepreneurs* are individuals who establish their own businesses. An entrepreneurial opportunity must be a desirable future state involving change or growth, and the individual must believe that he or she can reach the goal (Stevenson & Gumpert, 1992). Business and marketing plans are essential elements of a strategic plan. In organizations, a feasibility study often is used because it is a modified business plan developed to capture internal resources. For those who plan to establish their own company, a business plan is essential. A business plan is a written document that summarizes the business opportunity and specifies the plan for capitalizing on the opportunity. Trends in health care include excellence in care delivery and attaining Magnet status. Magnet status is a designation and recognition conferred on health care agencies that attain excellence in the delivery of quality care to patients (American Nurses Credentialing Center, 2003). Strong leaders use evidence-based practice in making decisions about the health of the organization and to guide clinical practice. Savvy nurses are capitalizing on their expertise and are designing health care businesses.

LEARNING TOOLS

Group Activity: Developing a Business Plan

Nurses are becoming more entrepreneurial and are establishing businesses in communities. To be successful in developing a business, one should complete a business plan to develop strategies to compete successfully in the marketplace.

Directions

The group should decide on a health care product or service that the members would like to develop into

a business. Once the core health care business is identified, complete the Basic Elements of a Business Plan.

Basic Elements of a Business Plan

1. Executive summary: provides an overview of the business, market, and profitability of the company
2. Company description: provides a detailed description of the business
3. Industry survey: provides a description of the history, the present state, and the future demand for the product or service
4. Market research: conducts or finds information that provides data regarding the product or service that is proposed
5. Management team: identifies the individuals who will compose the management team and the strengths that they bring to the company
6. Professional assistance: identifies the types of assistance (and names of individuals) that will be needed to form the company (e.g., necessity for attorneys, technical individuals, or accountants)
7. Operational plan: outlines the time line and steps to develop the product or service, as well as who is accountable for each step and whether there are any checkpoints
8. Research and development: outlines the plans for continued research and development and who will be in charge of this component of the business
9. Overall schedule: summarizes where the master schedule is kept and who is responsible to keep activities on schedule
10. Risks and opportunities: identifies the risks and opportunities that the company faces today and the potential risks and opportunities in the future
11. Three-year financial forecast: written document that outlines the 3-year financial forecast that should be in place and the evaluation points that should be identified
12. Proposed financing: outlines where the proposed financing will come from and the plans for repayment of debt
13. Legal structure: outlines how the business will be formed and whether it will be a corporation
14. Marketing plans and research: provides the marketing plans and strategies, including which markets are targeted and what type of ongoing marketing efforts will be implemented
15. Venture capital: discusses the financial support for the development of the product or service, as well as whether any grants are available to assist with start-up costs and whether there any community support is at hand

Summary

A business plan is an important aspect of developing a new venture. Often a business plan is used to acquire financing, to provide strategic policy, and to attract key individuals with specialized expertise to the new organization. A well-written business plan provides strong data to determine the viability of the proposed business venture and provides a guide for measuring attainment of goals.

CASE STUDY

Sam Blue is a staff nurse who is employed by a large teaching hospital in Phoenix, Arizona. She works the 3-to-11 PM shift on a 65-bed medical-surgical unit. Sam is creative and enjoys patient education. Nurse Blue makes sure that every patient that she cares for begins educational activities the day they are admitted to ensure mastery of material before discharge. She has designed a novel approach to patient education for individuals who undergo a hysterectomy. Nurse Blue has designed a game for them to play, which provides postoperative care and instructions for home care. The patients all comment on how useful the game is and how much they enjoy this approach to learning. Nurse Blue's peers are requesting that she provide the games for other units, and she is receiving requests from nurses employed at other hospitals to use the games that she has designed. Nurse Blue decides that she would like to expand this concept and make the patient education games available to other hospitals.

Case Study Questions

1. Whom should Nurse Blue approach to gain support for further development of the teaching tool?

2. Is Nurse Blue an intrapreneur or an entrepreneur?

3. Should a feasibility study or a business plan be developed?

4. In what types of intrapreneurial and entrepreneurial activities can nurses engage?

LEARNING RESOURCES

Discussion Questions

1. Discuss intrapreneur and entrepreneur activities that nurses in your community have designed. In a small group setting, discuss ideas and activities that could be undertaken by nurses to develop a company or enhance the viability of an organization.

2. What is the relationship between strategic planning and strategic management?

3. Describe the strategic planning process.

4. What are the elements of a strategic plan?

5. What are the common features of strategic management?

Study Questions

True or False: Circle the correct answer.

T   F   1. A strategy is a competitive move or business approach designed to produce a successful outcome.

T   F   2. Operational effectiveness is performing similar activities better than rivals do.

T   F   3. Strategic management involves strategic planning and implementation.

T   F   4. The best strategic planning is top-down.

T   F   5. The strategic planning process is threatening to employees and creates decreased job satisfaction.

T   F   6. Entrepreneurs are employees who create new programs or ventures for the organization.

T   F   7. A close relationship exists between opportunity and individual need.

T   F   8. Tactics are operational choices for action that are made to implement strategy.

T   F   9. Strategic management is administrative, systematic, environment-related, future-oriented, and sensitive to the correct positioning of the organization.

T   F   10. A basic form of strategic planning is a detailed written business plan with a comprehensive market analysis.

REFERENCES

American Nurses Credentialing Center. (2003). The *magnet recognition program for excellence in nursing service, health care organization, instructions and application process manual.* Washington, DC: American Nurses Credentialing Center.

Drucker, P. F. (1974). *Management: Tasks, responsibilities, practices.* New York: Harper & Row.

Stevenson, H. H., & Gumpert, D. E. (1992). The heart of entrepreneurship. In W. A. Sahlman & H. H. Stevenson (Eds.), *The entrepreneurial venture* (pp. 9-25). Boston: Harvard Business School Publications.

SUPPLEMENTAL READINGS

Capper, S. A., & Fargason, C. A. (1996). A way to approach the strategic decisions facing academic health centers. *Academic Medicine, 71*(4), 337-342.

Johnson, D. E. L. (2004). What is strategic management, planning? *Health Care Strategic Management, 22*(2), 2-3.

Johnson, J. E. (1990). Developing an effective business plan. *Nursing Economic$, 8*(3), 152-154.

Milone-Nuzzo, P., & Lancaster, J. (2004). Looking through the right end of the telescope: Creating a focused vision for a school of nursing, *Journal of Nursing Education, 43*(11), 506-511.

Stark, S., MacHale, A., Lennon, E., & Shaw, L. (2002). Benchmarking: Implementing the process in practice, *Nursing Standard, 16*(35), 39-42.

99

Chapter 14: Strategic Management (pp. 287-298)

1. What is strategic planning, and how does it differ from strategic management?

Strategic planning is a process of developing an action plan for actualizing the mission. It includes the strategy, goals, and objectives, and it consists of the who, what, by when, where, and, in general terms, the costs involved.

Strategic management is the management of an organization based on its vision or mission. Strategic management is an approach to doing business that involves assessing the environment, knowing the competition, establishing successful performance, achieving targets, and evaluating success. Strategic management involves strategic planning and implementation of the plan.

2. How can nurses use strategic management to improve the care they provide patients?

Strategic management can assist nurses in making decisions about the delivery of care. New policies, programs, projects and services can be developed to meet the needs of patients as guided by the strategic plan. Nurses also can use strategic management principles to help them meet personal and professional goals.

3. What are some ways to ensure that a strategic plan actually is implemented?

Integration of the strategic plan into daily activities will help keep the strategic plan as the major focus for the institution. The development of an action plan helps to break the strategic plan into manageable parts. This helps to divide the responsibility of implementation. A workable action plan must include the following:

- A priority order for achieving the strategic objectives or outcomes
- The determination of who will be responsible for achieving these objectives
- An indication of available or necessary financial support
- A timetable when achievement of the objectives can be expected

4. What should be included in a strategic plan for nursing?

The input of nurses should be included in a strategic plan for nursing. Staff members will feel a sense of ownership in the process and pride in their accomplishments. Input into the strategic plan also provides an opportunity for recognition of the accomplishments of nurses.

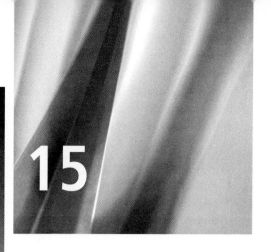

15

Marketing

STUDY FOCUS

Marketing is a concept from business administration that pertains to sales, persuasion, and image projection. *Marketing* is concerned with stimulating and meeting consumer demand. The key to successful marketing is to stimulate and satisfy buyer wants and needs. Marketing is one aspect of strategic organizational planning. For-profit businesses have used marketing as a tool for many years, and not-for-profit health care organizations now use marketing in a highly competitive, resource-constrained environment to capture and maintain market share. Kotler (1999) suggests that marketing is the art of finding, developing, and profiting from opportunities.

Some individuals feel that marketing is a negative aspect in the health care environment. They feel that marketing is a waste of scarce resources and that it relies on high-pressure sales, stimulating competition, creating unnecessary demand, and promoting low-quality products. However, marketing is an imperative for organizational survival in a turbulent health care environment. With no money, there can be no mission and the organization will cease to operate. In health care the rules of a free market do no apply because supply and demand, foundational elements of a free market, are distorted. Reasons for this include third-party payers, often the end consumer rarely acts like a typical customer, the seller of services does not have complete control of setting the price (governmental regulation), and there is almost an unlimited demand for services. *Benefits of marketing* include increased client satisfaction, improved acquisition of resources, and improved organizational efficiency (Kotler & Clarke, 1987). Marketing has helped organizations cope, grow, and thrive.

A *market* is a collection of buyers or sellers who make transactions around a specific product group. Marketing is a social and managerial process whereby individuals or groups obtain what they need and want by a process of exchange with others. *Exchange* is the act of obtaining a valued product from someone by giving something in return (Kotler, 2000). A *marketing mix* is a blend of marketing strategies used to achieve established objectives. A *marketing orientation,* also called a customer orientation, focuses energy on identification of needs and on the delivery of services that create satisfied customers. *Market share* is the percentage of the total market for the product or service that is captured by the organization. *Market research* is a systematic process for evaluating marketing problems or opportunities by conducting a study and using the data to refine or establish strategic plans (Alward & Camunas, 1991). *Needs* are basic biological, psychological, and social needs. *Wants* are desires satisfied by specific products or services that are influenced by external cues. *Products* are goods, services, or ideas that satisfy wants and needs of individuals.

Markets vary depending on the geographical location, customer orientation, and service or products produced. For nurses, the primary markets are clients, the employing organization, and physicians. For health care organizations, the primary markets are clients, employees, payers, and physicians. Marketing occurs within the context of voluntary exchange. Values are benefits derived from the exchange minus the cost associated with the product or service. A marketing orientation is the identification of customers' needs and wants and delivery of satisfactory goods in exchange for a price. *Five attributes of a marketing orientation* include a customer-oriented philosophy, integrated marketing organization, adequate marketing information, strategic orientation, and operational efficiency (Alward & Camunas, 1991; Kotler & Clarke, 1987).

The *key elements of marketing* are strategy and research. The basis of the strategic plan of an organization includes defining the business, determining the mission, and formulating long-term objectives. Marketing efforts use research tools to provide a report of the opportunities and threats, market analysis, and competitor position. Elements of environment scanning include assessing demographic and societal trends,

101

organization position, internal business performance indicators, market research, and the strength of suppliers and partners. Market strategies may be broad or narrow. *Mass marketing* aims the product to the entire market, and *target marketing* aims the product to a specific segment of the population. Three critical concepts in marketing include product differentiation, segmentation, and positioning. Differentiation does not require segmentation, but segmentation cannot be achieved without differentiation (Schnaars, 1991). Marketing strategies often are aimed at fulfilling needs.

The five-step process of effective marketing includes (1) *researching* to uncover opportunities and data, (2) identifying *segments* to target, (3) establishing the marketing *mix,* (4) *implementing* the marketing plan, and (5) *controlling* for effectiveness. The marketing mix can be viewed from the seller's and customer's points of view. The seller's point of view includes the four *P*'s of product, price, place, and promotion. The customer's point of view includes customer solutions, costs, convenience, and communication (Kotler, 2000). The *product* is the core of the business and is usually an object, service, or idea. A *core product* is what clients seek to meet basic needs; a *tangible product* has characteristics of style, quality, and brand name; and *augmented products* have added services and benefits (Alward & Camunas, 1991; Kotler, 1999).

Services are provided in a way that the other party does not become an owner of the product. Services are differentiated from products by four characteristics: intangibility, inseparability, variability, and perishability. Nurses and nursing need to capitalize on the uniqueness of the services provided. Clear articulation of the services of nurses will enhance the message and improve desired outcomes in health care. Nurses must position themselves strategically in the market.

Today's health care environment is competitive, turbulent, and constantly changing. Consumers' expectations are high, and they are more sophisticated and price sensitive than ever before. Consumers expect quick and convenient service delivery, high-quality products and services, and enhanced value. Brand loyalty is eroding, resulting in greater competition for consumer demand. Astute marketing strategies are based on customer value. Marketing strategies that are customer-oriented tend to focus on understanding customer needs, developing customer relationships, and learning how to keep and grow customers (Kotler, 1999). Critical to the success of health care organizations is the development of a marketing orientation. Nursing leaders need to develop an attractive product to market to consumer groups.

Ethical issues may arise around marketing of health care products and services. There are issues surrounding price and profit in selling health care services and protecting the public. There are ethical questions around issues such as end-of-life care, organ procurement, human genome therapy, and health care as a right and as a cost. Nurses and nurse leaders will struggle with ethical issues in health care and provide leadership in ethical decision making.

Leadership is needed in nursing to gain a competitive advantage in marketing nursing products and services to consumer groups. Strategies to cope with the rapidly changing health care environment include analyzing the business through five categories: outputs, personnel, resources, operations, and customers (Zell, 1999). Gathering and analyzing information is imperative to competing in the health care environment. A strong customer service orientation is a key to gaining and maintaining market share. Nursing also must step forward and take leadership positions in the health care market. Nursing leaders will position their health care organization strategically to earn national recognition for excellence in care. Examples of national recognition include Magnet recognition, an "America's Best Hospital's" designation by *U.S. News & World Report,* or high accreditation score from the Joint Commission on Accrediation of Healthcare Organizations.

LEARNING TOOLS

Group Activity

Purpose

To identify a potential health care product or service that could be packaged and marketed to the community. To identify the essential elements of a marketing plan and to evaluate marketing strategies for the new health care product or service.

Directions

Identify the health care product or service that you feel has business potential. Then complete the Marketing Study Guide to help you determine what work would need to be done to develop, market, and sell the product or services.

Marketing Study Guide

Section One: Four Strategic Planning Decisions that Contribute to the Development of a Cohesive Marketing Plan

1. What is the core business?

_____

2. What is the mission?

_____

3. What is the marketing strategy?

_____

4. What budget is needed?

_____

Section Two: Attributes of a Marketing Orientation

1. Is there a customer-oriented philosophy?

_____

2. Is there an integrated marketing organization?

_____

3. Is there adequate marketing information?

_____

4. Is there a strategic orientation?

_____

5. Is there operational efficiency?

_____

Section Three: Marketing Process

1. Has research been undertaken to uncover opportunities and provide data for strategic planning?

_____

2. Have the segments to target been determined? If so, what are they?

_____

3. What is the optimal tactical marketing mix?

_____

4. Has the marketing plan been implemented with specific time lines and authority checkpoints?

_____

5. What is the plan for evaluating the effectiveness of the marketing strategies, and has it been implemented?

_____

Section Four: Four *P*s of Service Business Marketing

1. What is the packaging to present the product or service and to generate interest?

_____

2. Is the price competitive?

_____

3. Is the place or location convenient and accessible?

_____

4. What are the promotion strategies to maintain and acquire more business?

_____

Section Five: Strategies Based on Customer Value

1. What are the customer's needs, and what solutions does the product or service present?

_____

2. Is the cost of the product or service reasonable and affordable to the targeted client base?

_____

3. Are the services convenient in location, hours, and accessibility?

_____

4. What are the communication strategies used to keep and grow customers?

_____

Section Six: Change

1. Are systems in place to cope and to develop a competitive advantage as change occurs?

_____

2. What are the outputs, personnel, resources, and operations that are needed to change?

_____

3. How will the change affect customers?

_____

4. What marketing strategies will be needed to make a successful change?

_____

Summary

This exercise is to assist individuals to explore entrepreneurial ideas and to determine what steps need to be taken to develop a business. Nurses have many opportunities to develop products or services in health care to meet client needs. Historically, nurses have been hesitant to establish businesses and compete in the health care market. Today, nurses are stepping forward to design products and services that are unique to nursing and satisfy consumer needs.

CASE STUDY

Shawmee Naval was hired recently as the vice president of nursing for a large health care center in Pensacola, Florida. She is impressed with the quality of health care services provided in the inpatient and outpatient areas. Ms. Naval notes extensive interdisciplinary team building, consultation, and sharing of key information throughout the organization. Clients who receive care at the community hospital rate the services as exceptional. Ms. Naval reviews trend data for inpatient and outpatient nursing services and notes a flatline trend. There is neither growth nor retrenchment in service utilization. She feels that with the outstanding health care services provided by the employees of the community health care center there should be a steady growth in utilization. Ms. Naval bases this assumption on the fact that the population in the five-county region is growing at approximately 6% annually. She contacts the media relations department for the health center and inquires about the marketing plan and strategies for the organization. The director of media relations informs Ms. Naval that there is not an active marketing campaign because the number of visits to the facility has been stable and there has been no need to spend money on marketing. Ms. Naval notes that the other health care organizations in their market area use a multitude of marketing strategies such as advertising in the newspaper, on the radio and television, providing community activities and workshops, and doing large mailings to alert consumers of new services that are being provided. Ms. Naval schedules an appointment with the chief executive officer to discuss marketing for the community health care center.

Case Study Questions

1. Is marketing effort necessary at the community health center? Provide rationale for your answer.

2. What are the steps in effective marketing?

3. What are the ethical implications for marketing health care services? What is the role of nurses in ethical decision making?

4. Who in an organization should be responsible for marketing? Is there a role for nurses in marketing?

5. Should nurses market their services to the community? Provide a rationale for your answer.

LEARNING RESOURCES

Discussion Questions

1. What strategic planning decisions contribute to the development of a cohesive marketing plan?

2. What is a core product, tangible product, and augmented product?

3. What is the marketing mix from the seller's point of view and from the customer's point of view?

4. Describe the relationship between differentiation and segmentation.

5. Describe mechanisms for recognition of excellence in health care organizations.

Study Questions

Matching: Write the letter of the correct response in front of each term.

_____ 1. Market

_____ 2. Marketing

_____ 3. Exchange

_____ 4. Marketing mix

_____ 5. Marketing orientation

_____ 6. Market share

A. A blend of marketing strategies used to achieve established goals

B. The percentage of the total market for the product or service that is captured by the organization

C. Goods, services, or ideas that satisfy wants and needs of individuals

_____ 7. Needs

_____ 8. Wants

_____ 9. Products

D. Actual or potential buyers and users of goods, services, and ideas

E. Desires satisfied by specific products or services that are influenced by external cues

F. Focusing energy on identification of needs and on the delivery of services that create satisfied customers

G. Basic biological, psychological, and social needs

H. The act of obtaining a valued product from someone by giving something in return

I. A social and managerial process whereby individuals or groups obtain what they need and want by a process of exchange with others

True or False: Circle the correct answer.

T   F   10. Marketing is a process that relates to transactions in an exchange of goods and services in a market.

T   F   11. Marketing is only used in for-profit businesses as a strategy to increase market share.

T   F   12. Marketing occurs within a framework of voluntary exchange.

T   F   13. Gathering and analyzing information will lay the foundation for proactive capitalization on change opportunities.

T   F   14. For most nurses, the primary markets are clients, the employing organization, and physicians.

T   F   15. A marketing orientation means that energy is devoted to selling products that normally do not sell well.

REFERENCES

Alward, R. R., & Camunas, C. (1991). *The nurse's guide to marketing.* Albany, NY: Delmar.

Kotler, P. (1999). *Kotler on marketing: How to create, win, and dominate markets.* New York: The Free Press.

Kotler, P. (2000). *Marketing management* (Millennium ed.). New York: The Free Press.

Kotler, P., & Clarke, R. N. (1987). *Marketing for health care organizations.* Englewood Cliffs, NJ: Prentice-Hall.

Schnaars, S. P. (1991). *Marketing strategy: Customers and competition* (2nd ed.). New York: The Free Press.

Zell, A. J. (1999). *Change: An opportunity* [online publication]. Retrieved from *www.sellingselling.com/articles/opportun.html*

SUPPLEMENTAL READINGS

Byers, J. F. (2001). Marketing: A nursing leadership imperative. *Nursing Economics, 19*(3), 94-99.

Greenawait, B. J. (2001). Can branding curb burnout? *Nursing Management, 32*(9), 26-31.

Hughes, K. (2000). Quality and marketing issues in nursing education. *Nursing Economic$, 9*(12), 763-768.

Kataoka-Yahiro, M., & Cohen, J. H. (2002). Marketing principles for a learning-service community partnership model, *Journal of Nursing Education, 41*(3), 136-138.

Pinkerton, S. E. (2002). Marketing and branding. *Nursing Economic$, 20*(1), 42-43.

Chapter 15: Marketing (pp. 299-312)

1. Do nurses have a marketing orientation? Why? Why not?

Marketing orientation (customer orientation) is defined as focusing energy on the identification of the needs and wants of customers and on the delivery of services that create satisfaction (Alward & Camunas, 1991). Nurses provide care through a customer orientation everyday whether they realize it or not. It is imperative that organizations realize the impact that nurses have on marketing orientation to the most important customer, the client. Organizations can enhance the marketing orientation by ensuring that all caregivers and support staff are informed and thoughtful about what it takes to meet customer needs.

2. What is the product of nursing? Of health care?

The product of professional nursing practice is problem resolution and quality care provision for clients. Nurses use their knowledge, expertise, and skill to identify problems, implement strategies, and coordinate services to enhance client outcomes. Although intangible, health is the desired product of the health care industry.

3. How can nurses identify market opportunities for their services? What are the next steps once those opportunities are identified?

Nurse can identify marketing opportunities by identifying and fulfilling needs, by recognizing an emerging or latent need, or by introducing a new product or service. The identification of marketing opportunities in specific areas of need or interest provides nurses with proactive growth potential. Nursing can use the marketing process strategy as follows:

- Conduct rigorous research to uncover opportunities and provide strategic planning data.
- Determine target segments and strategize the positioning of the product or service.
- Establish the marketing mix.
- Implement the plan.
- Control for effectiveness.

4. How are value and positioning important for nurses?

Identifying the total value of a product or service and promoting its value position are essential components of the marketing process. As nurses begin to identify, differentiate, and articulate the value and benefits associated with nursing service, they will be able to solidify their position as a notable business partner. The establishment of this partnership will be imperative to meet the increasing demands of consumers and health care organizations for the delivery of value-based services.

5. What role do nurses play in designing the marketing mix?

The marketing mix is an individualized blend of marketing strategies used to achieve goals. These strategies may include price, product, place; promotion, or customer solution or value, cost, and convenience; and communication. Nurses can play a role in designing the marketing mix by lowering costs through judicious use of resources (price), delivering quality nursing service (product), within the context of health care arena. As nurses communicate to consumers their ability to provide care that is cost-effective, compassionate, competent, and convenient, they will be able to assume a proactive role in the development of the marketing mix.

6. How might important target groups view nurses? How can nurses influence this perception?

Clients, physicians, and health care organizations are important target groups for nurses. Each target group may hold its own image of the nursing profession; however, the image of nursing is undergoing a metamorphosis. The expanded roles for nurses have contributed to this transformation. An increased number of nurses are being recognized for their knowledge, expertise, and contribution to the health care system. As nurses assume expanded roles such as advanced practice and case management, the image of nurses has been elevated from a subservient one to an image that reflects an autonomous, credible health care provider.

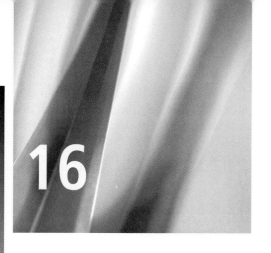

16

Models of Care Delivery

STUDY FOCUS

The goals of successful client care delivery are high-quality, low-cost care and the achievement of client outcomes and satisfaction levels. To meet these goals, the organization matches human and material resources with client health care needs. The assignment of nursing care personnel to clients is a basic function in a health care system. An *assignment* is the transfer of a task and the accountability for the resulting outcome (American Nurses Association, 1997). *Delegation* is the transfer of an assignment from one person to another, for example a registered nurse to an assistant, while retaining accountability for the outcome. The determination of the structure and method by which assignments are made are reflections of the model of care delivery. Nursing care modality or the nursing care delivery system of the organization is important in the allocation of resources and in the control of decision making about client care. The type of care modality determines, to a large extent, whether professional practice exists. Nursing care delivery systems are a mechanism to organize and deliver care to clients. The four *basic elements of nursing care delivery systems* that individuals consider when designing systems are (1) clinical decision making, (2) work allocation, (3) communication, and (4) management.

The practice model links the mission statement, professionals, and clients in the delivery of care. *Relational coordination* is management of communication and relationships among health care providers to provide quality and efficient care. Nursing care models address direct client care functions and indirect client care functions. Nurse leaders are responsible for making decisions about and designing strategies to create a climate and environmental context. Fiscal responsibility and accountability to the consumer are priorities in the setting of increasing health care costs and health care errors. The appropriate care delivery model is the one that maximizes existing resources while meeting the objective of direct and indirect client care function (Deutschendorf, 2003).

Selecting or designing a nursing care delivery system is a major task and requires a series of strategic decisions. The four *strategic decisions* needed are developing a philosophy of resource use, choosing a delivery system, developing practice expectations, and designing the role of the registered nurse. The six types of care modalities are functional, private duty, team, primary, case management, and the current evolving care delivery types. Four of these—(1) functional, (2) team, (3) primary, and (4) case management—have been used in hospitals. Private duty and case management are associated with public health, home health, and community health.

Private duty nursing, the oldest type of care modality, is a model in which the nurse cares for one client. This model is positive for the nurse and client and fosters a close relationship and increased registered nurse (RN) and client satisfaction with care delivery; however, it is costly, there is little job mobility, and job security is low. *Group nursing* originated from private duty and was an attempt to decrease costs by grouping clients in a hospital ward. The clients then paid the nurse directly. *Total client care* also originated from private duty nursing. Total client care is a method of providing total care for a group of clients during one shift. Advantages of total client care include the intensity of focus with shift-only responsibility, whereas the disadvantages include lack of communication and limited continuity of client care.

Functional nursing is the assignment of tasks to personnel prepared for that function. Examples of task assignments include medication administration, intravenous administration, baths, and vital signs. Functional nursing is efficient, but client and nurse satisfaction is low. Team nursing involves the coordination of care by an RN who assigns work to RNs, licensed practical nurses (LPNs), and nurse's aides. The assigned team members provide the majority of care to their assigned clients. *Team nursing* is cost-effective, and each member's

107

skills are used. Functional nursing was a precursor to team nursing, and with team nursing some RNs may be underutilized in their functional assignment. *Modular nursing* evolved from team nursing and clusters clients geographically with a group approach to care.

Primary nursing is the first professional practice model and designates 24-hour accountability for assigned clients from admission to discharge. The RN coordinates care and is accountable for the outcomes. The advantages to primary care include close client-nurse relationships, greater nurse autonomy, and holistic care. However, the cost of care increases with the exclusive use of a professional staff.

Case management is the coordination, monitoring, and procuring of services for the multiple needs of clients and is the fastest growing form of a "new" care delivery model. *Case management* may occur only in the hospital, based on populations, or across the health care cycle of the individual. One advantage is cost-effectiveness through a holistic approach to care. Case management in acute care settings is a system of client care delivery aimed at achieving client outcomes within effective and appropriate timeframes and resources. Structured care methodologies are streamlined interdisciplinary tools to determine best practices, assist in standardization of care, and assist with variance tracking, quality care, and outcomes research (Cole & Houston, 1999). *Critical paths* are one method to manage the care and resources of clients through a written plan that identifies key activities and treatments necessary at prescribed timeframes. Managed care is care coordination that is organized to achieve specific client outcomes, given fiscal and other resource constraints. Managed care originated from case management and is focused on specific client types and outcomes within fiscal and resource constraints.

The new *evolving types of care delivery systems* are mixed client care models. They are the second generation of professional practice models in nursing. The new evolving types tend to focus on costs, quality, and professional practice. In an era of managed care, fiscal restraint becomes a driver for restructuring, reengineering, and redesign. Concepts of accountability, cost containment, effectiveness, seamless continuum of care, integration, multidisciplinary collaboration, new roles, alteration in skill mix, and new assignments systems are key components. The new type of care delivery models emphasize partnerships and interdisciplinary teams that are client-centered. The new models are built around complex systems requiring knowledge workers to deliver high-quality integrated care. Various types of teams (cross-functional teams, self-directed work teams, multidisciplinary client care teams) are formed to complete the work required in a complex environment. Client-centered care is the resources, client care delivery system, and personnel organized to meet the client's health care needs (Maehling, 1995). Key factors in the client-centered approach are the cross-training and multitasking of team members (Higginbotham, 1999). The advantages of client-focused care redesign is that it centers systems and services closer to the client.

Managers and clinical nurses are challenged to design client care delivery systems that are cost-effective, provide quality care, and ensure client satisfaction. Important factors nurses must consider when designing care modalities are the staff, assignments, nursing and physician diagnoses, the reporting structure, decision-making autonomy, communication channels, and cost. Political, economic, and social forces are pressuring nurses to treat health care as a business with identifiable outcomes and client satisfaction. Nurses are challenged to restructure or design nursing care delivery systems to provide holistic, cost-effective client care.

Nurses must be able to demonstrate the effectiveness of a nursing care delivery system in producing financial and clinical outcomes. The central components of practice that need to be considered in the construction of a nursing care delivery model are the direct and indirect client care functions; provider roles, competencies, and experience; fiscal accountability; client characteristics and case mix severity; clinical service intensity; practice guidelines; and new medical information and technologies (Deutschendorf, 2003). In designing new emerging care delivery services, nurse leaders must use the guiding principles of nurse work as knowledge and caring, client-directed care, "critical synthesis" of knowledge, incorporation of technology, and management of care throughout the continuum (Haase-Herrick, 2004).

LEARNING TOOLS

Group Activity: Understanding Nursing Care Delivery Systems

Purpose

To examine your philosophy of nursing critically and apply it to the design of a nursing care delivery system. This exercise entails designing a professional nursing care delivery system that you feel will provide top-quality, cost-effective care to satisfied consumers by workers who enjoy their work.

Directions

First determine the four strategic decisions about resource use, delivery systems, practice expectations, and the role of the RN. The following questions will help guide your decision making:

1. What is your philosophy of resource use? Should all clients have equal access to all types of equipment, procedures, medications, and supplies? Who should determine what is to be ordered for each unit and in what quantities? Should all nurses and nurse extenders (nurse aides) have access to all supplies and resources? How will human resources be distributed?

2. What existing nursing care delivery system will you use? Or will you design or restructure an existing care delivery system to better meet the needs of your client population and organization?

3. What are the practice expectations for each level of care provider? What are the practice expectations for the management team? Will you have working managers? How does nursing interface with other health care professionals in your organization? Will your nursing care delivery system foster collaboration and consultation in a multidisciplinary team approach?

4. What is the role of the RN? Will the RN be responsible for supervision, coordination, and provision of care? What will the roles of the other health care providers be? Who will delegate work and what process will be used?

Now examine the following key components of practice when designing your nursing care delivery system:

- Composition and skill mix of your staff: What skills are needed to accomplish client care activities? How will the staff be assigned to accomplish the work?
- Nursing and physician diagnoses: What are the common medical and nursing diagnoses for your client population? How can the diagnostic needs of clients best be met?
- Reporting procedures: How will reports be given from one shift to another? What type of report will be used? How will physicians be notified of client changes?
- Communication channels: How will nurses, clients, physicians, and other health care workers communicate needs and changes in procedures? How will the manager communicate with all health care members? Will the communication network be written or verbal?
- Cost-effectiveness: How will supplies and equipment be used? What mechanisms will be in place to encourage cost-effective care? Will critical pathways be used?

After you have thought about all these questions, design a nursing care delivery system by modifying an existing one or constructing your own. This exercise will help you determine what type of care delivery structure you prefer, give you ideas to share in your work environment, and force you to analyze the use of precious resources.

CASE STUDY

Mary Jo Saur is the nurse manager of the respiratory unit in Middlesville, North Carolina. Middlesville hospital has been experiencing budgetary problems, and Nurse Saur has been instructed to cut costs in human resources. She designs a new care delivery system and informs the staff the next morning that the unit will fill all of the empty positions with unlicensed assistive personnel. Nurse Saur has made the assignments as follows:

- Two RNs are assigned to pass medications and intravenous fluids.
- Two LPNs are assigned to give baths.
- Another LPN is assigned to do treatments.
- One nurse extender (nurse aide) is assigned taking of vital signs, meal preparation, and transportation duties.
- Two RNs are floated to intensive care to work.

Case Study Questions

1. What type of care modality did Nurse Saur design?
2. What are the advantages and disadvantages of this type of care delivery system?
3. What factors did Nurse Saur need to consider?

LEARNING RESOURCES

Discussion Questions

1. What are the advantages and disadvantages of each of the six types of nursing care delivery?
2. What are the four common types of nursing care delivery systems used in hospitals?
3. What are the two common types of nursing care delivery system used in community health settings?
4. What factors should nurses consider when designing or restructuring a care delivery system?
5. What social, political, and economic factors influence the delivery of client care? How?
6. What is the clinical nurse's role in designing care delivery systems?

Study Questions

True or False: Circle the correct answer.

T   F   1. The most costly care modalities are primary and functional.

T   F   2. The two factors nurses must consider when designing a care delivery system are cost and quality.

Matching: Write the letter of the correct response in front of each term.

_____ 3. Nursing care modality

_____ 4. Private duty nursing

_____ 5. Team nursing

_____ 6. Primary nursing

_____ 7. Managed care

_____ 8. Case management

_____ 9. Functional nursing

_____ 10. New evolving type of care delivery

_____ 11. Total client care

_____ 12. Group nursing

A. A mixed model approach to provide care

B. Managing care to achieve specific client outcomes given fiscal and resource constraints

C. A system of health service delivery, coordination, and monitoring used to meet multiple service needs of clients

D. The assignment of clients to one nurse who has 24-hour accountability

E. Coordination of care with RN, LPN, and aide assignments by an RN to a group of clients

F. The assignment of tasks to RNs, LPNs, or aides

G. When nurses provide care to one or more clients for one shift

H. When clients are grouped together and cared for by one nurse

I. When one nurse provides care to one client

J. A method of organizing and delivering care to clients

REFERENCES

American Nurses Association. (1997). *Definitions related to ANA 1992 position statements on unlicensed assistive personnel.* Washington, DC: American Nurses Association. Retrieved May 19, 2005, from *http://nursingworld.org/readroom/position/uap/uapuse.htm*

Cole, L., & Houston, S. (1999). Structured care methodologies: Evolution and use in patient care delivery, *Outcomes Management for Nursing Practice, 3*(2), 53-59.

Deutschendorf, A. L. (2003). From past paradigms to future frontiers: Unique care delivery models to facilitate nursing work and quality outcomes. *Journal of Nursing Administration, 33*(1), 52-59.

Haase-Herrick, K. (2004). The nurse of the future: Fewer workers, new technologies and older patients place RNs at center stage. *Modern Healthcare, 34*(16), 18.

Higginbotham, P. (1999). Teams: The essential work unit. In S. P. Smith & D. L. Flarey (Eds.), *Process-centered health care organizations* (pp. 113-117). Gaithersburg, MD: Aspen.

Maehling, J. A. S. (1995). Process reengineering: Strategies for analysis and redesign. In S. S. Blancett & D. L. Flarey (Eds.), *Reengineering nursing and health care: The handbook for organizational transformation* (pp. 61-74). Gaithersburg, MD: Aspen.

SUPPLEMENTAL READINGS

Clark, J. S. (2004). An aging population with chronic disease compels new delivery systems focused on new structures and practices. *Nursing Administration Quarterly, 28*(2), 105-115.

Grayson, M. (2002). Forward motion. *Hospitals & Health Networks, 76*(10), 34-38.

Guo, K. L. (2004). Leadership processes for re-engineering changes to the health care industry. *Journal of Health Organization and Management, 18*(6), 435-439.

Racine, A. D., Stein, R. E., Belamarich, P. F., Levine, E., Okun, A., Porder, K., et al. (1998). Upstairs downstairs: Vertical integration of a pediatric service. *Pediatrics, 102*(1), 91-97.

Chapter 16: Models of Care Delivery (pp. 313-336)

1. **What is the role of nursing leadership in determining a model for client care delivery?**

   Nurse managers, in collaboration with nursing leadership, design nursing systems for the provision of client care and the betterment of the organization. Organizations using shared governance or other professional practice models include staff nurses in the development and selection process. The type of care delivery system defines control over nursing decision making (Manthey, 1989). Nurse managers and leaders should choose models that promote professional practice because these have implications for job satisfaction, the character of professional practice, and the amount of authority that the nurse possesses.

2. **How do nurses decide which nursing care delivery system to use?**

   Nurses involved in the selection or development of a nursing care delivery system should use a systematic assessment process that considers direct and indirect client care functions, provider roles, competencies and experience, fiscal accountability, client characteristics and case mix severity, clinical service intensity, practice guidelines, and new medication information and technology (Deutschendorf, 2003). The selection of a nursing care delivery system requires the consideration of several specific issues, including the role of the registered nurse, practice expectations, nursing interventions, staffing composition, accountability of nurses, decision making about care, end-of-shift reporting, physician-prescribed care, communication, and cost-effectiveness. A nursing care delivery system must balance nurses' needs with those of clients, physicians, and organizations.

3. **What are the structure and process variables that influence nursing practice and client care delivery?**

   Appropriate skill mix for the level of client condition severity, nurse/client ratio, use of temporary staff, workload, nursing education/experience, technology level, and continuing education are a few of the variables that can influence nursing practice and client care delivery. Process variables include availability of supplies, coordination of care planning, professional client assessment/monitoring, and effective staff communication.

4. **Why are nursing care delivery systems being revised and restructured?**

   Nursing care delivery systems are being revised and restructured in an effort to provide quality client care that is cost-effective. Restructuring must occur as a result of changes in the health care climate, consumer expectations, client characteristics, and new medical information and technology. New or modified care delivery systems are emerging to fit better with the changing social expectations and a dynamic health care delivery environment.

5. **What issues arise when the care delivery system is changed?**

   Changes in the care delivery system may threaten the balance between meeting client needs and those of the organization. Important issues surface related to the quality and cost of services, client and care provider satisfaction, and workforce composition. Other critical issues such as care provider role clarity; registered nurse preparation and delegation skills; a client-versus-task focused perspective; and the appropriate use of registered nurse skills, knowledge, and experience must be considered when the care delivery system is changed.

6. **What common themes emerge among the newest care delivery systems being developed? How do they compare with older models?**

   The newest care delivery systems attempt to reconfigure care provision within resource constraints, care needs, and current ideas about professional nursing practice. Contemporary care delivery systems emphasize outcomes management, multidisciplinary collaboration, accountability, a seamless continuum of care, new roles, alteration in skill mix, and new scheduling systems. Compared with older models, newer ones are more complex and client-centered and include a multidisciplinary team approach. Recent care delivery models emphasize the role of the professional nurse who is concerned with providing quality, cost-effective care within the context of a larger organization.

7. **What care delivery system best fits a merger of hospital and community agencies? Or are multiple care models needed?**

Which care delivery system best fits each setting in which nursing is practiced is not known. However, concepts from case management and managed care models seek to integrate services provided between the hospital and community agencies. Efforts are under way to develop a care delivery system that will provide quality care in a cost-effective manner. The restructured system must emphasize the seamless continuum of care between multiple care providers in which services are client-focused rather than hospital or agency focused. Cooperation, commitment, and collaboration are necessary to actualize this change.

8. **How should the implementation of new care delivery systems be evaluated?**

New care delivery systems can be evaluated by monitoring specific quality, financial, and client satisfaction outcomes.

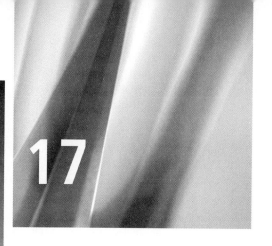

Case Management

STUDY FOCUS

Case management activities have the potential of saving money, improving effectiveness, and maintaining the quality of care (Cook, 1998). Case management is an intervention strategy used by health care professionals to advocate for clients, coordinate health care delivery, and facilitate outcomes of cost and quality. *Case management* is an interdisciplinary strategy that crosses settings and sites of health care. Case management is designed to coordinate care, decrease costs, and promote access to the appropriate type of needed services. In 1990 the Case Management Society of America, the organization that represents case managers, was founded. The case management role is one of the fastest growing roles in health care. The Case Management Society of America has promulgated the following: standards of practice, ethical statements on case management practice, and support of certification and evidenced-based practice standards. Managed health care, called *managed care,* enjoyed increasing popularity with national concern over rising health care costs and expenditures, fragmentation of care, and lack of access to care. Managed care has evolved as the economic and health service delivery strategy to manage costs and ensure access to care. By the end of the 1990s, health maintenance organizations had become the predominant form of health care coverage for businesses in the United States that employ more than 100 persons (Beilman et al., 1998; Coleman, 1999; Tahan, 1998).

Managed care is the integration and coordination of financing and delivery of health care services (Grimaldi, 1996). Managed care terminology has been applied to a wide range of organizational structures, prepayment arrangements, negotiated discounts, and prior authorization agreements for services with a focus on lowering costs and maximizing the use of resources. The three most common managed care-related organizational structures are health maintenance organizations, preferred provider organizations, and privately managed indemnity health insurance plans. Today, managed care refers to reimbursement strategies of arrangements and organizations. Managed care refers to a system that provides the structure and focus for managing the use, cost, quality, and effectiveness of health services. Managed care is the umbrella under which case management may be one cost-containment strategy. A common form of managed care financial reimbursement is capitation. *Capitation* is a fixed dollar amount paid to provide a specific set of health care services that an insured client requires (Grimaldi, 1996). The typical arrangement for capitation is a payment to a health care provider for a per-member-per-month payment regardless of the amount of care required by the covered clients.

Case management refers to client-focused strategies designed to coordinate care (Bower, 1992). The American Nurses Credentialing Center catalog defines case management as "a dynamic and systematic collaborative approach to provide and coordinate health care services to defined populations. The framework for nursing case management includes five components: assessment, planning, implementation, evaluation, and interaction" (2004, p. 10). Case management is described as a system of client care delivery that focuses on the achievement of client outcomes within effective and appropriate timeframes and resources.

Case management is the use of client-focused strategies to coordinate care (Bower, 1992). A key component of case management is interdisciplinary collaboration. Case management encompasses coordination of services and sequencing of care for optimal outcomes using available resources. In acute care settings, case management generally is used for high-risk populations. A registered nurse typically is assigned the accountability for case management of clients with a specific diagnosis-related group over the entire hospitalization. Case management also has been used in public health and by community nurses. Case management extends across the health care continuum. *Disease management* is different; it is a comprehensive,

113

integrated approach to care and reimbursement based on the natural course of a disease. The goal is to address the disease condition with maximum effectiveness and efficiency (Zitter, 1997). Disease management programs incorporate a series of clinical processes and services across the health care continuum to identify and manage a medical or chronic condition in an at-risk population to improve care, promote wellness, and manage or reduce costs (Ward & Rieve, 1997).

A *critical pathway* is a written plan that identifies key incidents that must occur at set times to achieve client outcomes within a predetermined timeframe. Critical pathways are best practice tools that identify and document the standardized interdisciplinary processes that need to occur for a client to move toward a desired outcome in a defined period of time. Many names are associated with critical pathways, such as critical path, care path, clinical pathway, clinical protocol, care track, or care step. These tools are cause-and-effect visual grids or paths to direct care toward goals. Critical pathway elements include an index of problems, a time line, a variance record, and the path or grid. Benchmarking and evidence-based practice are used to construct critical pathways. *Benchmarks* are a frame of reference against which an organization can compare itself relative to others. When differences occur between what is expected and what actually occurs on the critical pathway, a variation results. A *variation* is a deviation from what is expected. A variation may be positive or negative.

Many case management models appear in the literature. Case management exists in many contexts across many settings. Case management can be described as a system, role, technology, process, and service (Bower, 1992). As a *system,* case management is assessment and problem identification, planning, procurement, delivery, and coordination and evaluation of systems and client outcomes within effective and appropriate timeframes and resources. As a *role,* case management provides clients with a clinician who actively coordinates their care. As a *technology,* case management generates the tools to organize care and maximize activities, resources, and outcomes. As a *process,* case management focuses on health issues and client needs along the care continuum and across multiple settings. As a *service,* case management provides facilitation and gate keeping functions for clients. Two factors common across all case management models are coordination of care and advocacy. The various case management models have varying configurations, but the form of the model depends on basic client needs, level of care, the discipline and profession of the case manager, the environment in which the client lives, and the

organization for which the case manager works. Two major nursing models are identified in the literature: the New England model of acute care nursing case management and the community-based model of Carondelet St. Mary's Community Nursing Network. The New England model exemplifies an organization-specific focus. The model is best known for structuring the episode of care to balance cost, process, and outcomes. The model is a client-centered approach instituted during episodes of acute illness. Written standardized documents such as case management plans, time lines, and critical paths were developed and evolved into CareMap tools. The complete CareMap system includes variance analysis, outcome-time focus in all multidisciplinary communication, case consultation and health care team meetings that are held for clients with more-than-acceptable variance, and continuous quality improvement. In contrast, the Carondelet St. Mary's model uses professional nurse case managers, organized as a nursing health maintenance organization (HMO), at the hub of a network to broker services. This is a hospital-to-community model implemented to follow the movement of high-risk clients across the care continuum. Case managers work in long-term relationships with clients to assist them in self-care management of chronic illnesses. In addition to the nursing case management models, there are four models in social work: broker, primary therapist, interdisciplinary team, and comprehensive. Other models of case management include independent practice or private case management. The case manager has three main functions: (1) coordination, (2) advocacy, and (3) counselling (Clark, 1996).

Managed care is a broad term and can be viewed as a system that provides structure and focus for managing the use, cost, quality, and effectiveness of health services. Many disciplines lay claim to case management. The historical perspective of case management tends to be discipline-specific. Social work history indicates that case management began with Mary Richmond and the early settlement houses. The perspective of the insurance companies is that case management began with the management of catastrophic and high-cost insurance cases. In nursing, case management began with private duty nursing. With the rise of the early settlement houses and large numbers of immigrants and poor, there was a need for coordination of health care services. Public and human services in the United States were initiated in this era. Lillian Wald and Mary Brewster, nurses who were identified as social workers, founded the Henry Street Settlement in 1895. Community service coordination was a forerunner to case management and began at the turn of the century in public health programs. The term *case management* occurred in the literature in the 1970s in social welfare literature and then in the nursing literature.

The key functions of a case manager are assessment, planning, facilitation, and advocacy (Case Management Society of America, 2002). The four basic principles that guide nursing case management include coordination and integration of holistic care, promotion and preservation of health, conservation and allocation of resources, and provision of follow-up care. The six direct outcomes of case management include client knowledge, client involvement, client participation in care, client empowerment, client adherence, and coordination of care (Braden, 2002). Case management programs are based on roles and functions of case managers. Priorities for case management include a high rate of recidivism, unpredictable care needs, significant complications, comorbidities or variances in care outcomes, and high-risk profiles or high-cost cases. The general process for developing a case management program includes assessment, identification of high-volume or high-risk cases, determination of problems with high-volume or high-risk cases and set goals, formation of an interdisciplinary team, design of a critical pathway, development of a pilot program, and evaluation of the pilot. The 10-step process for developing a case management plan includes designing the format, selecting the target population, organizing the interdisciplinary team, educating the team, examining the current process, reviewing the literature, establishing the length of the plan, developing the content, conducting a pilot study, and standardizing the plan.

Nurses have two roles: (1) caregiver and (2) care coordinator (McClure, 1991). The emphasis on managed care in integrated health systems requires a new type of clinical nursing practice system. Case management is one approach to redesigning care delivery systems. Case management is a growing trend with increasing opportunities for nurses. As shifts occur in nursing care delivery systems to case management, nurses' job responsibilities and roles will shift. A trend in case management is the push for accountability and accreditation.

LEARNING TOOLS

Group Activity: Understanding Critical Pathways

Purpose
To explore the role and design of critical pathways in the delivery of health care to clients.

Directions

1. Divide yourselves into small groups of four.

2. Each small group should discuss the role of critical pathways in health care delivery, determining what types of client problems/diagnoses lend themselves to critical pathway development.

3. Select one client problem/diagnosis and sketch out a critical pathway. (Small group members should bring a critical pathway from where they work [clinic, hospital] and share it with everyone during the study session).

When each small group shares its critical pathway, compare your critical pathway with those that the hospitals or clinics where you practice use. Notice the critical steps or client points at which treatment, medical, nursing, or other health care worker intervention is required. Also note the length of time for each and the desired client outcomes. Finally, note the similarities and differences in the structure of the critical pathways among the various groups, hospitals, and clinics. Discuss and summarize these key points.

CASE STUDIES

Case Study 1

Dale Jackson is a nurse manager on a 52-bed neurological unit in a large community hospital. The administration has just informed Nurse Jackson that he needs to cut 15% from his budget for the upcoming year. He recently attended a case management conference that had a breakout session on critical pathways. At the conference the attendees discussed several strategies to conserve scarce resources. Nurse Jackson learned the general process for developing a case management program and has instituted these steps to effect change on his unit. Nurse Jackson decided to form an interdisciplinary team to design a critical pathway for the highest-volume diagnosis-related group clients for whom his staff provides services.

Case Study 1 Questions

1. What is the general process for developing a case management program that Nurse Jackson will use?

2. Will development of a critical pathway save resources on Nurse Jackson's unit?

3. What are the steps for developing a critical pathway?

4. What criteria should Nurse Jackson use for determining which critical pathway to develop?

5. Who should be involved in designing the critical pathway?

Case Study 2

Bob Jones is a family nurse practitioner who works for an HMO in Orlando, Florida. He is responsible for coordinating the care for a caseload of clients who enroll in the HMO. Nurse Jones' boss has told him that the objectives of his care coordination and delivery should focus on lowering costs with maximum value and quality outcomes. Nurse Jones is careful to refer clients only to those specialists listed on the preferred provider list because he knows that they have agreed to a discounted payment arrangement. Nurse Jones also provides holistic care with an emphasis on health promotion and wellness.

Case Study 2 Questions

1. What type of care modality is Nurse Jones using at the HMO? Is it case management or managed care?

2. What are the characteristics of case management versus managed care?

3. Can Nurse Jones refer outside of the preferred provider specialist list that the HMO provides for him?

LEARNING RESOURCES

Discussion Questions

1. What was the impetus for the development of case management?

2. Compare and contrast case management and managed care.

3. What types of case management models are there in the literature?

4. What are the four basic principles that guide nursing case management and what is the general process for developing a case management program?

5. How can critical pathways be used in organizations to improve quality and decrease costs of care?

6. What are the leadership and management challenges for nurses for designing care delivery systems in the future?

7. What is the clinical nurse's role in the provision of care, coordination of care, and the design of new care delivery systems?

Study Questions

Matching: Write the letter of the correct response in front of each term.

_____ 1. Capitation

_____ 2. Critical pathways

_____ 3. Benchmark

_____ 4. Variation

_____ 5. Disease management

A. A comprehensive, integrated approach to care and reimbursement that is based on the natural course of a disease

B. A frame of reference against which an organization can compare itself relative to others

C. A deviation from what is expected that may be positive or negative

D. A fixed dollar amount that is paid to provide a specific set of health care services that an insured client requires

E. A written plan that identifies key incidents that must occur at set times to achieve client outcomes within a predetermined timeframe

True or False: Circle the correct answer.

T   F   6. Case management is an interdisciplinary strategy that crosses settings and sites of care.

T   F   7. The case manager role has been one of the slowest growing roles in health care in the last 10 years.

T   F   8. The process of developing and using critical paths encourages critical thinking and accountability.

T   F   9. Critical pathways can and should be individualized to clients.

T   F   10. *Managed care* is a broader term than case management.

T   F   11. Nurses must document their effects on client outcomes to demonstrate that they can provide cost-effective services.

T   F   12. Case management frequently is associated with health maintenance organizations and preferred provider organizations.

T   F   13. Managed care is care coordination and delivery at the provider-client level.

T   F   14. Managed care typically is used for only high-priority clients.

T   F   15. Critical pathways are used only with case management.

T   F   16. Multidisciplinary teams are essential in a complex health care environment.

T   F   17. Case management entails providing holistic care, the conservation of resources, and care across episodes and settings.

T   F   18. Case management focuses on continuity of the plan.

T   F   19. Registered nurses are moving from a care-providing role to a care-coordinating role.

T   F   20. A current trend is the push for accountability and accreditation for case management organizations.

T   F   21. In developing case management programs, the organization and client populations should be assessed.

T   F   22. Case management is an interdisciplinary strategy that crosses settings and sites of care.

T   F   23. Benchmarks form a frame of reference against which an institution can compare itself relative to others.

REFERENCES

American Nurses Credentialing Center. (2004). *ANCC certification: Specialty nursing, nursing administration (basic, advanced) clinical nurse specialist (community health & home health).* Washington, DC: American Nurses Credentialing Center.

Bielman, J. P., Sowell, R. L., Knox, M., & Phillips, K. D. (1998). Case management at what expense? A case study of the emotional costs of case management. *Nursing Case Management, 3*(2), 89-95.

Bower, K. A. (1992). *Case management by nurses.* Kansas City, MO: American Nurses Publishing.

Braden, C. J. (2002). *State of the science paper #2: Involvement/participation, empowerment and knowledge outcome indicators of case management.* Little Rock, AR: Case Management Society of America.

Case Management Society of America. (2002). *Standards of practice for case management.* Little Rock, AR: Case Management Society of America.

Clark, K. A. (1996). Alternate case management models. In D. L. Flarey & S. S. Blancett (Eds.), *Handbook of nursing case management* (pp. 295-304). Gaithersburg, MD: Aspen.

Coleman, J. R. (1999). Integrated case management: The 21st century challenge for HMO case managers, Part 1. *The Case Manager, 10*(5), 28-34.

Cook, T. H. (1998). The effectiveness of inpatient case management: Fact or fiction? *Journal of Nursing Administration, 28*(4), 36-46.

Grimaldi, P. L. (1996, October). A glossary of managed care terms. *Nursing Management, 27* (Special Suppl. 10), 5-7.

McClure, M. (1991). Introduction. In I. E. Goertzen (Ed.), *Differentiating nursing practice: Into the twenty-first century* (pp. 1-11). Kansas City, MO: American Academy of Nursing.

Tahan, H. A. (1998). Case management: A heritage more than a century old. *Nursing Case Management, 3*(2), 55-60.

Ward, M. D., & Rieve, J. A. (1997). The role of case management in disease management. In W. E. Todd & D. Nash (Eds.), *Disease management: A systems approach to improving patient outcomes* (pp. 235-259). Chicago: American Hospital Publishing.

Zitter, M. (1997). A new paradigm in health care delivery: Disease management: In W. E. Todd & D. Nash (Eds.), *Disease management: A systems approach to improving patient outcomes* (pp. 1-25). Chicago: American Hospital Publishing.

SUPPLEMENTAL READINGS

Debusk, R. F., Miller, N. H., Parker, K. M., Bandura, A., Kraemer, H. C., Cher, D. J., et al. (2004). Care management for low-risk patients with heart failure: A randomized controlled trial. *Annals of Internal Medicine, 141*(8), 606-613.

Kalina, C. M., Haag, A. B., & Tourigian, R. (2004). What are some effective chronic disease management strategies that can be used in case management? *AAOHN Journal, 52*(10), 420-423.

Sackett, K., Pope, R. K., & Erdely, W. S. (2004). Demonstrating a positive return on investment for a prenatal program at a managed care organization: An economic analysis. *Journal of Perinatal & Neonatal Nursing, 18*(2), 117-126.

Schein, C., Gagnon, A. J., Chan, L., Morin, I., & Grondines, J. (2005). The association between specific nurse case management interventions and elder health. *Journal of the American Geriatrics Society, 53*(4), 597-602.

Whitelaw, S. E. (2004). Ehlers-Danlos syndrome, classic type: Case management. *Dermatology Nursing, 16*(5), 433-449.

Chapter 17: Case Management (pp. 337-360)

1. What are the goals of case management?

Case management is an approach to managing care and service delivery to meet client needs in the most cost-effective manner. Essential goals of case management include coordinating client-focused care, decreasing costs, and promoting access to appropriate and needed services. Another important goal of case management is the provision of follow-up care that tracks and guides service delivery across time and settings.

2. What are the goals of managed care? How do they compare with those of case management?

Managed care strives to lower costs and maximize the value of services and resources. Managed care goals are similar to those of case management in that both seek to reduce costs and conserve resources. Managed care differs from case management in that managed care goals are broader and provide the structure and focus for managing the use, cost, and effectiveness of health services for all clients. In contrast, case management goals focus on client advocacy, coordination of health care delivery, and facilitation of cost and quality outcomes.

3. What are the outcomes anticipated by case management? By managed care?

Anticipated outcomes for case management are the achievement of client outcomes within effective and appropriate timeframes and resources. Nurse case managers coordinate and integrate the seamless continuum of care to reduce fragmentation and redundancy. Managed care outcomes focus on cost control and resource conservation by monitoring client-care decisions and resource allocation.

4. How does case management affect the role of the nurse?

Case management is expanding the role of the nurse and was one of the fastest growing roles in health care in the 1990s, especially in nursing (Haw, 1996). Nurse case managers are responsible for the coordination and integration of multidisciplinary services across the continuum of care. Effective case management requires specialized knowledge and expertise, as well as advanced education, to address the complex and diverse needs of clients.

5. Who should be the case manager? Who should lead the multidisciplinary team?

Advanced practice nurses are skilled in the coordination of client care, possessing expert knowledge, experience, and education. As such, they are eminently qualified to be case managers. Given the interdisciplinary nature of case management, the advanced practice nurse is able to draw on a wealth of knowledge to coordinate efforts of the health care team to achieve desired client outcomes.

6. Does the public health model apply to hospital settings? Why or why not?

The focus of traditional public health models has been the coordination of client-centered care within the community setting. In contrast, the focus of tertiary care models has been on the treatment of acute, episodic health care conditions. As societal and economic pressures have demanded that health care organizations implement cost-effective, quality care, the hospital setting has patterned the care delivery system after the public health model.

The perspective of the public health model guides the health care organization to coordinate and integrate services across the continuum from hospital to community, thereby reducing costs and eliminating redundancy of services.

7. Do all clients need case management?

Although all clients need coordinated care, case management best serves the needs of targeted, high-risk populations. All clients do not need the close monitoring that case management provides, especially in an environment where case managers are a limited resource. A recent alternative to managing the use, cost, quality, and effectiveness of health care services has been the implementation of managed care systems.

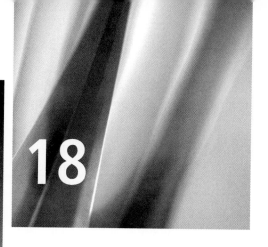

18

Disease Management

STUDY FOCUS

Disease management is an important and effective intervention to coordinate care and services for better outcomes at lower costs. Three initiatives are used in coordinating care: disease management, case management, and population health management. These initiatives have the potential of saving money, increasing effectiveness, and improving the quality of care. *Case management* is an intensive focus on an individual client with one or more health conditions. The use of case management is often for complex, high-cost, or high-volume conditions. *Disease management* is an intensive focus on disease or health condition of population groups that then is applied to individuals. Disease management is a population-based strategy for the management of groups requiring specialized health services. *Population health management* is a community-based population strategy.

Two major forces triggered the development of disease management programs: the proliferation of managed care systems and the national attention generated by the Institute of Medicine health care quality initiative *Crossing the Quality Chasm: The IOM Health Care Quality Initiative* (2004). Health plans have designed disease management programs for care coordination and service integration often to meet the needs of members who have chronic health care needs. The need to design new ways to deliver integrated health care services is being driven by the aging of the U.S. population, high pharmaceutical costs, advancing medical technology, increases in chronic health conditions, and the U.S. government budget deficits.

According to the Disease Management Association of America (DMAA; *www.dmaa.org*) "disease management is defined as a system of coordinated health care interventions and communications for populations with conditions in which patient self-care efforts are significant" (2004, p. 1). Disease management supports the provider/client care plan, emphasizes prevention using evidenced-based practice guidelines and client

empowerment, and evaluates outcomes to improve overall health. Disease management is multidisciplinary, population, or group based and covers illness and behavior health domains. The six components of disease management are (1) using a population identification processes, (2) implementing evidence-based practice guidelines, (3) designing collaborative practice models, (4) providing client self-management education, (5) collecting process and outcome measurement, evaluation, and management, and (6) designing a routine reporting/feedback loop (DMAA, 2004).

Case management is an interdisciplinary strategy that crosses settings and sites of health care. Case management is designed to coordinate care, decrease costs, and promote access to the appropriate type of needed services. In 1990 the Case Management Society of America, the organization that represents case managers, was founded. Case management is the use of client-focused strategies to coordinate care. The definition of *case management* by the Commission for Case Manager Certification is "a collaborative process that assesses, plans, implements, coordinates, monitors, and evaluates options and services required to meet an individual's health needs, using communication and available resources to promote quality, cost effective outcomes" (2004, p. 2). A key component of case management is interdisciplinary collaboration. Case management encompasses coordination of services and sequencing of care for optimal outcomes using available resources. Case management is used for high-risk populations across the health care continuum. Priorities for case management include a high rate of recidivism, unpredictable care needs, significant complications, comorbidities or variances in care outcomes, high-risk profiles, or high-cost cases.

Disease management and case management are distinct and separate strategies, but there are areas of overlap because both are interventions designed to coordinate care for better outcomes and lower costs. Case management involves work with an intensive focus on coordinating the care for individual clients for one or more diseases or health conditions. Disease management involves intensive focus on a disease or health condition with a population group. Disease management is population-based and proactive (Huston, 2001). *Health promotion* is helping individuals improve and change their lifestyles to attain optimal health in all domains of life. The *health domains* include physical, emotional, social, intellectual, and spiritual (*American Journal of Health Promotion*, 1989). Nurses are challenged to facilitate healthful lifestyles across the health care continuum. A *continuum of care* is a linkage of health services across health care delivery settings and sites.

In population-based management, there are many terms that may be new to you, including population health, population, aggregate, target population, community, and community health. *Population health* is an intervention approach to improving health for the entire population to reduce health inequities. A *population* is a group of individuals who have one or more personal or environmental characteristics in common (Williams, 1996). An *aggregate* is the members of the community who are defined in terms of geography, special interest, disease state, or other population characteristics. *Target population* is used in research for a specific population. *Population-based care management* is the integration and coordination of health services to a specified population. A *community* is a locally based entity composed of systems and organizations reflecting the group's norms (Schuster & Goeppinger, 1996). The community is the client when the focus is on the collective good rather than a single client. *Community health* is meeting the collective needs of a group by identifying problems and managing interactions within the community and between the community and the larger society. Thus the term *community* denotes a local entity, whereas the term *population* refers to an aggregate.

Chronic health conditions pose two particular difficulties for businesses: diminished productivity and greater portion of the business' revenue being diverted into health care expenditures (Javors et al., 2003). Approximately $1 trillion is spent on health care, and many of these resources go to treat chronic diseases and their complications, many of which are preventable (Javors et al., 2003). Individuals with chronic conditions cost 3.5 times as much to serve as others, and they account for a large proportion of services (Nobel & Norman, 2003). These and other forces are creating sweeping changes in disease management programs. These forces include experiencing the highest health care cost trends in a decade, continuing of a weak economy and softer labor market, increasing consumer demands, increasing expectations of higher-quality care and client safety, and rising provider costs (up to 300% variance) (Ho, 2003). Proactive outreach is a major strategy of disease management. One such outreach activity is the use of *personal health advisors* to serve as a single point of contact for care and service coordination for clients having health problems by developing trusting relationships. A related model is called the *chronic care model*. The six basic elements of this model are community, the health system, self-management support, delivery system design, decision support, and clinical information systems.

Population-based program planning models contain four *components:* contextual analysis, implementation plan, budget, and evaluation plan (Hall, 1998). The six basic *steps* of a community-focused or population-based care delivery planning are establishing the contract partnership, assessing, determining the nursing diagnosis of the problem, planning, implementing interventions, and evaluating interventions and outcomes. To determine the community health status, a systematic data collection process is needed. The five key methods of collecting data are (1) informant interviews, (2) participant observation, (3) windshield surveys, (4) analysis of existing data, and (5) surveys. The six criteria to establish *priorities* for population based care are community awareness of the problem, community motivation to resolve it, the nurse's ability to influence problem solution, the availability of relevant expertise, severity of consequences, and the speed with which resolution can be achieved (Schuster & Goeppinger, 1996).

Population-based risk assessments are important to determine how to spend scarce resources. The *levels of risk* are primary (prevention), secondary (early detection), and tertiary (management of an episode of care) (Burgess, 1999). A model of population care management contains six *levels:* population needs assessment, identification of health services, targeted health planning, wellness and prevention, care management, and case management (Qudah & Brannon, 1996). Six key success *factors* for the development and implementation of a disease management program are (1) understanding the course of the disease, (2) targeting clients likely to benefit from the intervention, (3) focusing on prevention and resolution, (4) increasing client adherence through education, (5) providing full care continuity, and (6) establishing integrated data management systems (Zitter, 1997). The four *modules* used by effective disease management programs are (1) candidate identification and stratification, (2) enrollee recruitment, (3) the intervention itself, and (4) evaluation (Nobel & Norman, 2003). The seven *criteria* used to select a condition to implement a disease management program are (1) availability of treatment guidelines, (2) generally recognized problems in therapy, (3) large practice variation and treatments, (4) large numbers of clients whose therapy could be improved, (5) preventable acute events, (6) measurable outcomes, and (7) cost savings (Gillespie, 2002).

Leadership is needed to facilitate and manage interdisciplinary and interorganizational communication for continuity of care. Three major *strategies* of disease management programs are (1) the use of an interdisciplinary team, (2) outcomes evaluation to measure results, and (3) application of information management technologies. Nurse leaders will integrate, coordinate, and advocate for individuals, families, and communities to improve continuity and enhance appropriate resource utilization. Nursing leaders in public health need to be politically competent, have business acumen, demonstrate program leadership, and be skilled managers (Misner et al., 1997). Disease management programs foster adherence and maintenance of positive self-care health behaviors. Successful leaders will foster technological innovations and the analysis and use of large databases. They will use important applications of information management technologies including predictive modeling and calculation of return on investment. *Predictive modeling* is the use of statistics to calculate expected costs based on variables (Kramer, 2004). *Calculation of return on investment* is a method of describing the impact of case or disease management in terms of a dollar calculation.

LEARNING TOOLS

Activity 1: Population-Based Program Plan

Purpose
To review the components of a comprehensive population-based program plan for identification of needed resources, community support, and evaluation.

Population-Based Program Plan

Johanna Dickenson is a registered nurse in a small rural community in central Pennsylvania. The community is very close. Major problems include a high poverty rate, teenage pregnancy, a high rate of high school dropouts, and alcoholism. She is an expert clinician and is well respected in the community. Nurse Dickenson is involved in the parent-teacher association for the local school and the women's guild at her church and is active with the local library.

Nurse Dickenson decides that she would like to institute a new community initiative on colon cancer awareness in the community. She has spoken to the church leaders, and they have provided space for her to have a screening clinic. Nurse Dickenson has met resistance from the city council for financial support for this project. The first screening clinic had a poor turnout.

Directions

1. Complete the Population-Based Program Planning Study Guide.

2. Review the foregoing scenario and evaluate the components of the integrated population-based program planning model, the steps in establishing a community-based plan, and the criteria for determining community priorities.

3. Describe why Nurse Dickenson had a difficult time in implementing her community program. What might she have done to increase the likelihood of success for a community-based program?

Population-Based Program Planning Study Guide
Components of an Integrated Population-Based Program

1. The program has a clear contextual analysis and framework.

2. The program has an implementation plan with time points.

3. The program has a budget for planning, implementation, and evaluation.

4. The program has a comprehensive systematic evaluation plan.

The completion of the components of an integrated population-based program assists the community with tackling priority community issues, having the resources to complete the project, and implementing an evaluation at the conclusion of the project.

Criteria for Determining Community Priorities

1. Is there high community awareness of the problem?

2. Is there community motivation to resolve the problem?

3. Does the nurse have the ability and expertise to influence problem resolution?

4. Is there expertise in the community to manage the problem?

5. What are the consequences of not solving the problem?

6. How quickly can the problem be resolved?

The more resources, community commitment, and expertise available, the greater the chance of success for resolving the issue. What is perceived as a priority in the community will have the greatest likelihood of success in implementation and resolution.

Developing a Community-Based Plan

1. Was a community partnership established?
2. Was a comprehensive community assessment conducted?
3. Were community priority problem(s) determined?
4. Was a planning process established, and was a comprehensive plan that included community involvement developed?
5. Was the plan implemented using time lines and responsibility points?
6. Were the interventions and outcomes evaluated based on the comprehensive plan?

By using a community-based plan that follows the nursing process, there is greater potential for success. The community-based project is identified clearly; key individuals are included; and a plan, implementation schedule, and evaluation framework are established before implementation.

Activity 2: Understanding Coordination of Care Initiatives

Purpose

To explore the role of case management, disease management, and population health management in the coordination of care.

Directions

1. Divide yourselves into small groups of four.
2. Each small group should discuss the role of case management, disease management, and population health management in coordination of care.
3. Each small group should bring an example of the use of each of the three initiatives (case management, disease management, and population health management) and share it with everyone during the study session.
4. When each small group shares its programs, compare your care coordination projects and determine in what health care settings they could be implemented. Notice the difference in client level versus group level versus community focus in programming for the different initiatives. Also note the importance of establishing desired program outcomes in terms of client, group, or community goals. Finally, note the similarities and differences in the structure of each of these initiatives. Discuss and summarize these key points.

CASE STUDIES

Case Study 1

Juanita Farzel is a registered nurse employed in a large primary care clinic in New Orleans. Part of her role is to coordinate the care in her office and to improve systems for the improvement of quality care. Nurse Farzel has noticed that the clients who have a diagnosis of diabetes mellitus are consistently failing to meet their glycemic goal of a 7.0 $HgbA_{1c}$ level even with quarterly visits to their health care provider. She approaches the leadership team with this information, and they assign her the task of designing a program to improve the quality of care for this client group.

Case Study 1 Questions

1. What type of care management program should Nurse Farzel consider?
2. What is the difference between case management, disease management, and program health management?
3. What are the components of a disease management program? What are the steps in developing a disease management program?
4. What are the benefits of a disease management program?

Case Study 2

Bonita Bell is a registered nurse in Baton Rouge, Louisiana, managing a large primary care nursing center that employs 14 family nurse practitioners, 6 medical assistants, 4 registered nurses, 4 clerical staff, and an x-ray technician. The nursing center was established in 1992 and has served the south side of the city. Nurse Bell has been tracking the number of clients registered at the nursing center and notices that there is a definite flat line for new clients. Nurse Bell reports this information at the staff meeting and discusses the need to conduct a population-based health needs assessment as part of their program planning. The team supports Nurse Bell in her efforts, and an in-depth community assessment is conducted.

Based on the community needs assessment, Nurse Bell uses criteria to establish priorities for problem resolution. She determines that the four major health needs of the population that they serve are diabetic and hypertensive management, well-child examinations, and women's health issues. Nurse Bell reports her findings to the staff. During the meeting, the staff divided themselves into four groups to design services, programs, and health seminars on the four topic areas. A marketing plan was developed, and resources were set aside to address the issues.

Within 6 months, Nurse Bell noticed an increase in new clients coming to the nursing center for services. She reported this finding to the staff, who made a commitment to involving the community in their program planning and interventions.

Case Study 2 Questions

1. What actions did Nurse Bell take to improve the position of the nursing center in the health care market?
2. What is a population-based health needs assessment?
3. What is an integrated population-based program planning model?
4. What are criteria for determining community priorities?
5. What are the basic steps of population-based care planning?

LEARNING RESOURCES

Discussion Questions

1. What is the continuum of health services?
2. What are competencies of excellent nursing leadership in disease management?
3. Compare and contrast case management, disease management, and population health management.
4. What were the forces in the last decade that were the impetus for disease management?
5. What are the benefits of disease management?
6. What is the difference between compliance and adherence?
7. What are key methods of collecting data for population-based risk identification?
8. What are the levels of risk?
9. What was the impetus for the development of case management, disease management, and population-based management?
10. Compare and contrast case management and disease management.

11. What are the components of a disease management program?
12. What were the major forces that triggered the rise and proliferation of disease management programs?
13. Discuss the rising cost of health care in the United States and strategies to restructure the health care system to be more cost efficient while improving quality care?

Study Questions

Matching: Write the letter of the correct response in front of each term.

_____ 1. Population

_____ 2. Population-based care management

_____ 3. Community

_____ 4. Disease management

_____ 5. Case management

_____ 6. Community health

_____ 7. Compliance

A. To help determine the best use of staff and clinical resources while determining the long-term health care needs of a population

B. A comprehensive, integrated approach to care and reimbursement based on the natural course of a disease

C. A group of individuals who have one or more personal or environmental characteristics in common

D. An entity with a local base that is composed of a system of formal organizations or groups that are interdependent and function to meet a variety of collective needs

E. The degree that a client continues positive health behaviors without supervision

_____ 8. Adherence

_____ 9. Maintenance

_____ 10. Population-based risk identification

F. Meeting the collective needs of the group by problem identification and management within and between the community and society

G. The degree that a client continues a negotiated treatment

H. Is a collaborative process of care coordination and advocacy to meet an individual's health needs in a cost-effective manner

I. The degree that a client initially assents to a treatment plan

J. The integration and coordination of health services to a specified population

REFERENCES

American Journal of Health Promotion. (1989). Definition of health promotion. West Bloomfield, MI: *American Journal of Health Promotion*. Retrieved May 19, 2005, from *www.health-promotionjournal.com/*

Burgess, C. S. (1999). Managed care: The driving force for case management. In E. L. Cohen & V. DeBack (Eds.), *The outcomes mandate: Case management in health care today* (pp. 13-19). St Louis: Mosby.

Commission for Case Manager Certification. (2004). *Code of professional conduct for case managers with standards, rules, procedures, and penalties*. Rolling Meadows, IL: Commission for Case Manager Certification.

Disease Management Association of America. (2004). *Definition of disease management*. Washington, DC: Disease Management Association of America. Retrieved February 7, 2004, from *www.dmaa.org/definition.html*

Gillespie, J. L. (2002). The value of disease management—part 3: Balancing cost and quality in the treatment of asthma. *Disease Management, 5*(4), 225-232.

Hall, P. J. (1998). Planning an integrated population-based program. *Journal of Nursing Administration, 28*(10), 40-47.

Ho, S. (2003). The emerging role for health plans: Info-Mediary. *Disease Management, 6*(1 Suppl), 4-10.

Huston, C. J. (2001). The role of the case manager in a disease management program. *Lippincott's Case Management, 6*(5), 222-227.

Institute of Medicine. (2004). *Crossing the quality chasm: The IOM health care quality initiative*. Washington, DC: National Academies Press. Retrieved October 2, 2004, from *www.iom.edu/-focuson.asp?id=8089*

Javors, J. R., Laws, D., & Bramble, J. E. (2003). Uncontrolled chronic disease: Patient non-compliance or clinical mismanagement? *Disease Management, 6*(3), 169-178.

Kramer, M. S. (2004, January 10). Predictive models make smart purchasers. *Business & Health*, pp. 1-4.

Misner, T. R., Alexander, J., Blaha, A. J., Clarke, P. N., Cover, C. M., Felton, G. M., et al. (1997). National Delphi study to determine competencies for nursing leadership in public health. *Image, 29*(1), 47-51.

Nobel, J. J., & Norman, G. K. (2003). Emerging information management technologies and the future of disease management. *Disease Management, 6*(4), 219-231.

Qudah, F. J., & Brannon, M. (1996). Population-based case management. *Quality Management in Health Care, 5*(1), 29-41.

Schuster, G. F., & Goeppinger, J. (1996). Population-based care management. *Quality Management in Health Care, 5*(1), 29-41.

Williams, C. A. (1996). Community-based population-focused practice: The foundation of specialization in public health nursing. In M. Stanhope, & J. Lancaster (Eds.), *Community health nursing: Promoting health of aggregates, families, and individuals* (4th ed., pp. 21-33). St Louis: Mosby.

Zitter, M. (1997). A new paradigm in health care delivery: Disease management. In W. E. Todd & D. Nash (Eds.), *Disease management: A systems approach to improving patient outcomes* (pp. 1-25). Chicago: American Hospital Publishing.

SUPPLEMENTAL READINGS

Institute of Medicine. (1999, November). *To err is human: Building a safer health system*. Washington, DC: National Academies Press. Retrieved July 14, 2004, from *www.nap.edu/books/*

Wong, J., Wong, S., Weerashinghe, S., Makrides, L., Coward-Ince, T. (2005). Building community partnerships for diabetes primary prevention: Lessons learned. *Clinical Governance, 10*(1), 6-14.

Chapter 18: Disease Management (pp. 361-382)

1. Which should come first, case management or disease management?

Case management involves work with a focus on coordinating the care of the individual client in relationship to one or more diseases or health conditions. Disease management focuses on a specific disease or health condition of a population group with application subsequently to individuals. Either can come first, depending on the health encounter of the client that drives the case management or disease management process. Case management tends to focus on an episode of a client's care such as an inpatient hospitalization requiring coordination of rehabilitative services, financial assistance, and teaching regarding rehabilitative expectations. Disease management may focus on all clients with a particular diagnosis such as that of diabetes mellitus within a particular health care system. This population of diabetic clients will require management for all issues related to diabetes such as diabetic nephropathy, peripheral neuropathy, cardiovascular disease, and other health risks caused or accentuated by diabetes. Case management or disease management can occur in any setting.

2. Should all nurses be doing population-based care management? Why or why not?

Nurses should provide optimal care for clients, but it is not cost-effective to case manage every client. Population-based risk identification and the referral of individuals into case management and disease management programs is a better use of staff and clinical resources.

3. How can nurses motivate others to facilitate coordination across organizations?

The nurse's role as coordinator of care and client advocate can work to build collaboration and integration of health care across the continuum through communication between team members. The use of client outcome data and financial data can aid in the "selling" of the benefits of case coordination across the continuum to others.

4. What is the role of informatics in disease and population-based care management?

Information gathering, information integration and analysis, and information deployment are critical in disease and population-based care management. Current research is showing that disease and population-based care management are viable programs to address cost and quality issues.

5. How are community health and population-based care management applied in nursing?

Population-based care management is defined as the integration and coordination of health services to a specified population. Community health refers to meeting the collective needs of a group by identifying problems and managing interactions within the community and between the community and the larger society. Nursing can meet the needs of clients within a population and within the entire good of the community. For instance, community health initiatives may include fluoride treatments at local schools, whereas population-based care management may focus on the care of people of Native American descent who have diabetes.

6. Why do all clients not need disease management?

Clients who are knowledgeable and have a great deal of adherence to the designed plan as a result of self-management education may not need disease management.

7. Who should do disease management?

Nurses have a leadership role and opportunity to provide disease management. As coordinators of care, masters of collaboration, and ideal client advocates, the nursing role is ideal for coordination of care across the continuum.

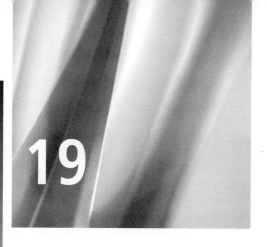

19

Patient and Family Cultural Values

STUDY FOCUS

There is a need for the U.S. health care system to meet the challenge of increasing racial and ethnic diversity. The U.S. Department of Health and Human Services acted at the end of 2000 to make cultural competence a priority in health care. They adopted the national standards for culturally and linguistically appropriate services in health care. Fourteen standards were published in the *Federal Register*. The standards include culturally competent care, language access services, and organizational supports for cultural competence. The growing appreciation for the global community has raised the awareness of cultural differences and the differing values in subcultures in local communities. For successful delivery of health care services, nurses must recognize the values of other cultures as they relate to health and take positive steps to recruit persons from other cultures to the nursing profession.

Cultural diversity is the variety and differences in the customs and practices of defined social groups. *Cultural competence* is a set of behaviors, attitudes, and policies among professionals that provide meaningful and effective interactions with clients in a cross-cultural framework. Cultural competence is providing care effectively to persons from multiple cultures in a dynamic and evolving process that embodies an evolution of knowing, respecting, and incorporating the values of others. Cultural competence involves the recognition of the importance of integrating persons with other values in the process of health care delivery. *Linguistic competence* is the provision of culturally appropriate oral and written language services to persons with limited English proficiency through qualified interpreters and translators (Agency for Healthcare Research and Quality, 2003). *Transcultural nursing* is a formal area of study and practice that focuses on cultural care, comparison of cultural variations, and the provision of culturally compassionate care (Leininger, 1997).

The demographic makeup of the U.S. population in the areas of ethnicity and age are radically changing.

Of the four major U.S. populations, the Hispanic and Asian populations continue to grow at a much faster rate than the population as a whole. Despite the rapidly changing demographic characteristics of the U.S. population, there is failure to obtain parity in positive health care outcomes for members of minority groups. In addition, the U.S. median age continues to rise, from 35.3 years on April 1, 2000, to 35.9 years on July 1, 2003 (U.S. Census Bureau, 2004). Nurses are in a pivotal role to enact changes in effectively managing quality health care and managing resources to influence vulnerable populations in communities positively. Factors related to disparities in health care are income, access to insurance, and physician decisions about referring clients for additional care. Statistics show that 86.6% of the total registered nurse population is non-Hispanic white, but 72% of the total U.S. population is white (U.S. Department of Health and Human Services, 1996). Recruitment efforts need to be aimed at attracting a diverse cultural mix of individuals into the nursing profession. Emphasis should be on culturally competent client care practices and on a culturally competent workplace environment. More role models from underrepresented racial/ethnic groups are needed in the workforce.

A critical core concept in nursing is the awareness and recognition of cultural diversity. The U.S. culture is characterized by its pluralism. As global trends in mobility, migration, cultural identity importance, and changing roles increase, there is a greater need for transcultural awareness. The first step in caring for clients is to determine how they want to be treated. Road signs to cultural competence include the use of questioning and person space in interactions. Americans perceive four space zones, as follows:

- Public (12 feet to limits of sight)
- Social (4 to 12 feet away)
- Personal (2 to 4 feet away)
- Intimate (0 to 2 feet away)

127

Nurses must have an awareness of other cultures, but they do not have to agree with all the dominant beliefs of the culture. An important step in gaining cultural competence is recognizing one's own cultural beliefs. Valuing the client's perspective and right to choose treatment options is paramount to caring for clients. Cultural assessments assist health care providers in strengthening cultural awareness, sensitivity, and competence. It has been suggested that addressing cultural issues during the delivery of health care augments efforts to improve client compliance. The six areas often included in cultural assessments are communication, interpersonal space, social organization, sense of time, environmental control, and biological variation. Cultural beliefs about health and illness are learned and transmitted via cultural environments (Davidhizar et al., 1998). The elements of a cultural assessment include cultural affiliation, health and care beliefs and practices, illness beliefs and customs, interpersonal relations, spiritual practices, and worldview and other social structure features (Rosenbaum, 1995). There are many cultural assessment tools that you may use to heighten awareness and sensitivity. One such tool can be found on the Internet (*www.med.umich.edu/multicultural/ccp/tools.htm*).

To care effectively for culturally diverse clients, nurses must use strategies to enhance cultural competence. Two such strategies are becoming cognitively aware of potential issues and building a repertoire of strategies to enhance cultural competence. Basic communication techniques such as how to address an individual properly and what a nod may mean can affect a nursing intervention positively or adversely. General guidelines for cultural competence include the following:

- Nurses' awareness that their behavior may be perceived as abrupt when it is different from the client's cultural orientation
- Being aware of the clients attitude toward suffering
- Evaluating the fit of the treatment plan with the client's lifestyle
- Anticipating that informed consent forms may be frightening
- Recognizing the client's unfamiliarity with the nurse as professional staff and expectation that care will be delivered by a physician
- Realizing that Americans emphasize the clock, whereas other cultures may not

One culturally competent model of care was developed by Campinha-Bacote (1994). This model has four components: (1) cultural awareness including sensitivity and biases, (2) cultural knowledge including worldviews and frameworks, (3) cultural skills including assessment tools, and (4) clinical encounters including exposure and practice. *Cultural awareness* is a deliberate cognitive process of becoming aware of and sensitive to the client's culture by becoming aware of one's own values and not imposing those values on others. *Cultural knowledge* is a process of obtaining information about the different worldviews of varying cultures. *Cultural skills* involve the process of learning how to do a cultural assessment. *Cultural encounter* is the process of engaging in cross-cultural interactions. Analysis of body language is helpful in understanding cultural differences. Examples include the use of silence, distance, eye contact, facial expressions, and body language.

A trend in cultural awareness is the attracting of a culturally diverse workforce. The synergy of diverse viewpoints can improve health care knowledge and delivery of services. Strategies for success with cultural diversity in the workplace include respecting differences, exploring beyond the comfort zone, withholding judgment of others, and emphasizing the positive, and practicing good communication. Diversity is the "consideration of socioeconomic class, gender, age, religious belief, sexual orientation, and physical disabilities, as well as race and ethnicity" (American Association of Colleges of Nursing, 1997, p. 1). An issue that is becoming increasingly prevalent is that health illiteracy increases with age. Language diversity is also an issue. The 2000 census showed that in addition to English, there are seven languages each spoken by more than a million persons in the United States (U.S. Census Bureau, 2004). Therefore nursing interventions aimed at effective educational and communication strategies and materials to improve health care knowledge of the elderly are essential in the delivery of services. Creative strategies such as interpreting services and information applications can be used to improve linguistic availability. Strategies to increase health care worker diversity include incorporating diversity into mission statements, career development, and management programs for minority groups.

LEARNING TOOLS

Group Activity: Characteristics of Selected Minorities

Purpose

To identify characteristics of selected minorities and to identify nursing strategies to produce positive health care outcomes for a select group.

Directions

Select three cultural groups in your geographical area that you would like to explore. Examples of dominant cultures within the United States include Mexican American, African American, Vietnamese American, Chinese, Japanese, Cuban, and Puerto Rican.

On a sheet of paper list the major characteristics that you will research. Examples of major characteristics are:

Cultural group

Language spoken

Predominant religion

Role of the family

Health care practices

Communication patterns

Risk factors

Compare and contrast the three cultural groups that you have researched. What characteristics are similar among the groups? What characteristics are different among the groups? How could you tailor interventions based on cultural beliefs to enhance positive health care outcomes?

Individual Activity: Giger and Davidhizar's Transcultural Assessment Model

Purpose

The transcultural assessment tool provides a comprehensive assessment format for culturally competent care. This assessment tool is a mechanism to evaluate cultural variables that influence health and illness behaviors.

Directions

Identify a client for whom you would like to complete a comprehensive cultural assessment. Use the following tool to identify cultural variables that will influence the nursing plan of care.

Giger and Davidhizar's Transcultural Assessment Model*

Culturally Unique Individual

1. Place of birth

2. Cultural definition

    What is …

3. Race

    What is …

4. Length of time in country (if appropriate)

------

*From Giger, J. N., & Davidhizar, R. E. (1995). Transcultural nursing: Assessment and intervention (2ⁿᵈ ed.). St Louis: Mosby.

Communication

1. Voice quality

    A. Strong, resonant

    B. Soft

    C. Average

    D. Shrill

2. Pronunciation and enunciation

    A. Clear

    B. Slurred

    C. Dialect (geographical)

3. Use of silence

    A. Infrequent

    B. Often

    C. Length

       (1) Brief

       (2) Moderate

       (3) Long

       (4) Not observed

4. Use of nonverbal

    A. Hand movement

    B. Eye movement

    C. Entire body movement

    D. Kinesics (gestures, expression, or stances)

5. Touch

    A. Startles or withdraws when touched

    B. Accepts touch without difficulty

    C. Touches others without difficulty

6. Ask these and similar questions:

    A. How do you get your point across to others?

    B. Do you like communicating with friends, family, and acquaintances?

    C. When asked a question, do you usually respond (in words or body movement, or both)?

    D. If you have something important to discuss with your family, how would you approach them?

Space

1. Degree of comfort

    A. Moves when space invaded

    B. Does not move when space invaded

2. Distance in conversations

    A. 0 to 18 inches

    B. 18 inches to 3 feet

    C. 3 feet or more

3. Definition of space
   A. Describe degree of comfort with closeness when talking with or standing near others
   B. How do objects (e.g., furniture) in the environment affect your sense of space?

4. Ask these and similar questions:
   A. When you talk with family members, how close do you stand?
   B. When you communicate with co-workers and other acquaintances, how close do you stand?
   C. If a stranger touches you, how do you react or feel?
   D. If a loved one touches you, how do you react or feel?
   E. Are you comfortable with the distance between us now?

Social Organization

1. Normal state of health
   A. Poor
   B. Fair
   C. Good
   D. Excellent

2. Marital status

3. Number of children

4. Parents living or deceased?

5. Ask these and similar questions:
   A. How do you define social activities?
   B. What are some activities that you enjoy?
   C. What are your hobbies, or what do you do when you have free time?
   D. Do you believe in a Supreme Being?
   E. How do you worship that Supreme Being?
   F. What is your function (what do you do) in your family unit/system?
   G. What is your role in your family unit/system (father, mother, child, advisor)?
   H. When you were a child, what or who influenced you most?
   I. What is/was your relationship with your siblings and parents?
   J. What does work mean to you?
   K. Describe your past, present, and future jobs.
   L. What are your political views?
   M. How have your political views influenced your attitude toward health and illness?

Time

1. Orientation to time
   A. Past-oriented
   B. Present-oriented
   C. Future-oriented

2. View of time
   A. Social time
   B. Clock-oriented

3. Physiochemical reaction to time
   A. Sleeps at least 8 hours a night
   B. Goes to sleep and wakes on a consistent schedule
   C. Understands the importance of taking medication and other treatments on schedule

4. Ask these and similar questions:
   A. What kind of timepiece do you wear daily?
   B. If you have an appointment at 2 PM, what time is acceptable to arrive?
   C. If a nurse tells you that you will receive a medication in "about a half hour," realistically, how much time will you allow before calling the nurses' station?

Environmental Control

1. Locus of control
   A. Internal locus of control (believes that the power to effect change lies within)
   B. External locus of control (believes that fate, luck, and chance have a great deal to do with how things turn out)

2. Value orientation
   A. Believes in supernatural forces
   B. Relies on magic, witchcraft, and prayer to effect change
   C. Does not believe in supernatural forces
   D. Does not rely on magic, witchcraft, or prayer to effect change

3. Ask these and similar questions:
   A. How often do you have visitors at your home?
   B. Is it acceptable to you for visitors to drop in unexpectedly?
   C. Name some ways your parents or other persons treated your illnesses when you were a child.
   D. Have you or someone else in your immediate surroundings ever used a home remedy that made you sick?
   E. What home remedies have you used that worked? Will you use them in the future?
   F. What is your definition of "good health"?
   G. What is your definition of illness or "poor health"?

Biological Variations

1. Conduct a complete physical assessment noting the following:
   A. Body structure (small, medium, or large frame)
   B. Skin color
   C. Unusual skin discolorations
   D. Hair color and distribution

130

E. Other visible physical characteristics (e.g., keloids, chloasma)

F. Weight

G. Height

H. Check laboratory work for variances in hemoglobin, hematocrit, and sickle cell phenomena if black or Mediterranean

2. Ask these and similar questions:

A. What diseases or illnesses are common in your family?

B. Describe your family's typical behavior when a family member is ill.

C. How do you respond when you are angry?

D. Who (or what) usually helps you to cope during a difficult time?

E. What foods do you and your family like to eat?

F. Have you ever had any unusual cravings for the following:

(1) White or red clay dirt?

(2) Laundry starch?

G. When you were a child, what types of foods did you eat?

H. What foods are family favorites or are considered traditional?

Nursing Assessment

1. Note whether the client has become culturally assimilated or observes own cultural practices.

2. Incorporate data into plan of nursing care:

A. Encourage the client to discuss cultural differences; persons from diverse cultures who hold different worldviews can enlighten nurses.

B. Make efforts to accept and understand methods of communication.

C. Respect the individual's personal need for space.

D. Respect the rights of clients to honor and worship the Supreme Being of their choice.

E. Identify a clerical or spiritual person to contact.

F. Determine whether spiritual practices have implications for health, life, and well-being (e.g., Jehovah's Witnesses may refuse blood and blood derivatives; an Orthodox Jew may eat only kosher food high in sodium and may not drink milk when meat is served).

G. Identify hobbies, especially when devising interventions for a short or extended convalescence or for rehabilitation.

H. Honor time and value orientations and differences in these areas. Allay anxiety and apprehension if adherence to time is necessary.

I. Provide privacy according to personal need and health status of the client (NOTE: the perception and reaction to pain may be culturally related).

J. Note cultural health practices.

(1) Identify and encourage efficacious practices.

(2) Identify and discourage dysfunctional practices.

(3) Identify and determine whether neutral practices will have a long-term ill effect.

K. Note food preferences.

(1) Make as many adjustments in diet as health status and long-term benefits will allow and that dietary department can provide.

(2) Note dietary practices that may have serious implications for the client.

CASE STUDY

Juan Torrez, a 45-year-old migrant worker, arrives at the clinic with fatigue, polydypsia, polyuria, and polyphagia. A translator is with Mr. Torrez and tells you that he works in the fields from early morning to late evening picking produce. The health care provider orders laboratory tests and determines that Mr. Torrez is diabetic. Mr. Torrez is instructed on checking his blood glucose level, is provided information in Spanish on diabetes, and is instructed on medication administration. During the instruction, Mr. Torrez gets very upset when he is told to limit his intake of beverages with sugar. He tells the translator that he only has Kool-aid in the fields because it is readily available and is provided by the employer.

Case Study Questions

1. How is your communication with the client influenced by the presence of a translator?

2. What cultural implications are apparent in this case study?

3. How will your nursing interventions be tailored to assist Mr. Torrez in managing his diabetes?

LEARNING RESOURCES

Discussion Questions

1. How can nurses use information about various cultures to influence health care service delivery?

2. What is cultural diversity? What strategies can be used to increase cultural diversity in the workforce?

3. What is the demographic makeup of the U.S. population? How does the demographic makeup in the United States compare with the demographics of the registered nursing population in the United States?

4. What should a cultural assessment include?

Study Questions

True or False: Circle the correct answer.

T   F   1. Cultural differences in ways of doing things and in beliefs about health and illness are learned and transmitted via cultural environments.

T   F   2. Examples of cultural differences include eye contact norms, gender issues, touching and physical contact, and food practices.

T   F   3. Japanese clients usually are given lower dosage levels of medications and have less tolerance for side effects.

T   F   4. Minority groups obtain parity in positive health care outcomes compared with the general overall health of the American people.

T   F   5. Cultural competence is defined as an ongoing evolution of knowing, respecting, and incorporating the values of others.

T   F   6. The four components of Campinha-Bacote's culturally competent model of care are cultural awareness, cultural knowledge, cultural skill, and cultural encounters.

T   F   7. The demographics of the U.S. population are similar to the demographics of nurses in the United States.

T   F   8. Diversity includes only race and ethnicity.

T   F   9. One of the major concerns in providing health care to the elderly population is the low literacy concerning health.

Matching: Write the correct letter of the correct response in front of each term.

_____ 10. Cultural awareness

_____ 11. Cultural knowledge

_____ 12. Cultural skill

_____ 13. Cultural encounter

_____ 14. Cultural diversity

A. The process of seeking and obtaining an educational background about the different worldviews of various cultures

B. A process of directly engaging in cross-cultural interactions

C. The process of learning how to do a cultural assessment, allowing the nurse to identify an individual client's perceptions, beliefs, and practices

D. A deliberate and cognitive process of becoming aware of and sensitive to the client's culture by becoming aware of the influence of one's own cultural values and learning to avoid imposing them on others

E. The variety and differences in the customs and practices of defined social groups.

REFERENCES

Agency for Healthcare Research and Quality. (2003). *What is cultural and linguistic competence?* Rockville, MD: Agency for Healthcare Research and Quality. Retrieved May 19, 2005, from *www.ahrq.gov/about/cods/cultcompdef.htm*

American Association of Colleges of Nursing. (1997). *AACN position statement: Diversity and equality of opportunity.* Washington, DC: American Association of Colleges of Nursing. Retrieved May 19, 2005, from *www.aacn.nche.edu/-Publications/positions/diverse.htm*

Campinha-Bacote, J. (1994). Cultural competence in psychiatric nursing: A conceptual model. *Nursing Clinics of North America, 29*(1), 1-8.

Davidhizar, R., Bechtel, G., & Giger, J. (1998). Model helps CMs deliver multicultural care. *Case Management Advisor, 9*(6), 97-100.

Leininger, M. (1997). Transcultural nursing research to transform nursing education and practice: 40 years. *Image, 29*(4), 341-347.

Rosenbaum, J. N. (1995). Teaching cultural sensitivity. *Journal of Nursing Education, 34*(4), 188-189.

U.S. Census Bureau. (2004). *Hispanic and Asian Americans increasing faster than overall population.* Washington, DC: U.S. Census Bureau, U.S. Department of Commerce. Retrieved May 19, 2005, from *www.census.gov/Press-Release/www/releases/archives/race/001839.html*

U.S. Department of Health and Human Services. (1996). *The registered nurse population.* Rockville, MD: U.S. Department of Health and Human Services.

SUPPLEMENTAL READINGS

Alexis, O. (2005). Managing change: cultural diversity in the NHS workforce. *Nursing Management, 11*(10), 28-30.

Chennault, R. E. (2005). A vicarious learning activity for university sophomores in a multiculturalism course, *Multicultural Education, 12*(3), 45-50.

Freeman, H. P. (1997). Concerns of special populations in the national cancer program: The real impact of the reduction in cancer mortality research. In *President's Cancer Panel: Meeting Summary.* Bethesda, MD: National Cancer Institute, National Institutes of Health. Retrieved October 10, 2005, from *www.nci.nih.gov/*

Nagar, B. (2005). Reflecting on cultural considerations for team development in major urban settings. *Organizational Development Journal, 23*(1), 17-25.

Nokes, K. M., Nickitas, D. M., Keida, R., & Neville, S. (2005). Does service-learning increase cultural competency, critical thinking, and civic engagement? *Journal of Nursing Education, 44*(2), 65-71.

Searight, H. R., & Gafford, J. (2005). Cultural diversity at the end of life: Issues and guidelines for family physicians. *American Family Physician, 71*(3), 515-522.

Chapter 19: Patient and Family Cultural Values (pp. 383-406)

1. Why is cultural competence important for nursing?

Cultural competence is an ongoing process that involves expanding one's understanding of different cultures. As client advocates, nurses must be able to recognize, respect, and incorporate the values of other cultures to deliver care effectively. Knowing, respecting, and integrating the values and perspectives of others in care provision and organizational operations are needed to improve health services and to enhance the nursing profession.

2. What are the components of cultural awareness?

Cultural awareness is the result of a purposeful, cognitive process involving a critical analysis of one's own cultural values and biases. Through deep reflection, one can become aware of and sensitive to other cultures without imposing one's own cultural expectations, attitudes, and behaviors. Without self-awareness and sensitivity, cultural competence cannot be achieved.

3. How do you perform a cultural assessment?

Performing a cultural assessment provides an opportunity for the nurse to identify a client's perceptions, beliefs, and practices. According to Davidhizar et al. (1998), six cultural components to assess include communication, interpersonal space, social organization, sense of time, environmental control, and biologic variation. Other elements to assess include health care beliefs and practices, illness beliefs and customs, spiritual practices, and social structure features, including one's worldview. Nurses can use existing cultural assessment tools to assist in conducting a holistic data collection process.

4. How does the nurse apply cultural competence in the workplace?

Nurses can use cultural competence to provide care to diverse clientele, to lead and manage workgroups effectively, and to enhance the nursing profession. Providing culturally competent care results in client and staff satisfaction, and facilitates the success of the organization to recruit and maintain a culturally sensitive workforce. Nurses apply culturally competent strategies such as respect for differences, exploring beyond the comfort zone, withholding judgments of others, emphasizing the positive, and practicing good communication techniques to lead and manage workgroups successfully. A nursing profession that understands and respects other cultures will attract individuals to become members of its discipline, ultimately increasing the diversity and perspectives of the nurses providing care to the society.

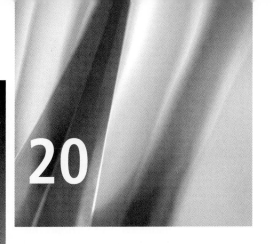

Communication, Persuasion, and Negotiation

20

STUDY FOCUS

A significant component of leadership is the ability to influence individuals to accomplish goals. The three basic *competencies of influencing* are diagnosing, adapting, and communicating. The skill of communication is being able to put forth a message that is easily understood and is accepted by others. Leaders are able to influence others through *personal power* and *positional power*. Personal power is the ability to establish rapport by communicating so that those who are influenced feel comfortable and have trust and confidence in their leader (Hersey et al., 2001). Positional power is having the authority and accountability to perform a specific job based on one's formal title in the organization.

Communication is an essential element in organizing, coordinating, and directing the care of clients. Nurse managers are challenged to create clear communication pathways to facilitate task accomplishment in organizations. *Communication* is the ability to transmit information to another clearly. *Organizational communication* is the ability of an agency to transmit information to and from its members expediently and expeditiously. *Verbal communication* is verbal or written information. *Nonverbal communication* is unspoken and is composed of affective or expressive behaviors. The four *distinctions in communication* are those between the (1) formal/informal, (2) vertical/horizontal, (3) personal/impersonal, and (4) instrumental/expressive types. *Formal communication* is the official information sent by designated officials in an agency, and *informal communication* is information passed via the grapevine. *Vertical communication* is boss to employee, and *horizontal communication* is peer to peer. *Personal communication* is when mutual influence occurs, and *impersonal communication* is one-sided. *Instrumental communication* is transmitting data essential to complete work, and *expressive communication* is transmitting data that are tangential to the work that is done.

Persuasion is the ability to influence others to change their behavior based on argument or reasoning. An individual skillful at persuasion will leave the listener with some perception of choice. Persuaders have a variety of motives for their approach, with the most typical being self-preservation, money, romance, or recognition. Effective communication is essential when attempting to persuade others. A *persuader* is a person who tries to convince others to do what they want them to do. In the course of persuasion, timing, strategy, and credibility are important in the attempt to lower listeners' defenses, as well as in complimenting and supporting them. Commitment, imagination, and trust are three elements crucial to successful persuasion.

Communication is an art and a skill in which a sender and a receiver engage in the transmission of ideas or information. Communication models described in the literature include the sender-receiver, human needs, and transactional analysis models. The sender-receiver model describes communication as messages or signals passed between the sender and receiver. The *steps in communication* whereby information is exchanged include the following: First, there is message formulation where the sender formulates the ideas; second, the message is encoded and the sender formulates the idea into verbal or nonverbal components; third, the message is transmitted and the sender imparts the message; fourth, the receiver acquires the transmission and the message is received by the selected method; and finally, the process is completed when the message is decoded and the receiver interprets the data (Grant, 1994).

Characteristics of successful communication include simplicity, clarity, appropriate timing, relevance, adaptation to circumstances, and credibility. Harmful communication behaviors include offering inappropriate reassurance, rejecting the other, agreeing uncritically, stereotyping, belittling, or being egocentric. The use of communication models focusing on interpersonal skills or transactional analysis emphasize therapeutic communication techniques. These include

135

active listening, attending, questioning, paraphrasing, reflecting feelings, assertion, challenging, confrontation, and interviewing skills (Thies & Williams-Burgess, 1992). In communication, there is always the potential for barriers because of the perception and filtration of information by the sender and receiver. Individuals have their own unique worldview, which colors or changes the message to fit their model of the world. Therefore it is important to keep messages clear, simple, and relevant to the receiver.

Group communication is even more complex than individual communication because of the number of individuals involved. Five *common communication networks* are used: the wheel, the chain, the Y, the all-channel, and the circle. In centralized organizations the wheel, the Y, and the chain are used. In democratic organizations the circle and the all-channel networks are used most often.

Personal communication effectiveness is important aspect of human therapeutic relationships. Communication processes are based on interpersonal, social cognitive, and message competency. *Interpersonal competence* is the understanding of complex cognitive, behavioral, and cultural factors that influence communication efforts. *Social cognitive competency* refers to the ability to interpret message content from each participant's point of view. *Message competency* refers to the ability to use language and nonverbal behaviors in a strategic way to achieve goals (Boggs, 1999). Effective communication requires preparation and determination of the message structure, delivery style, and mode of communication for each interaction. Effective communication relies in part on timing, choice of channel, and personal contact or appeal. The use of words also may significantly influence the acceptance of the message delivered. Individuals respond to certain red flags or emotionally charged words. Examples are superlatives and racist or sexist language. An essential component of communication is assessing whether the receiver understood the message.

Feedback and constructive criticism are important communication activities. Feedback is tied to delegation. After choosing what to delegate (right task), matching the task to the delegate's competence (right person), and making the effective assignment (the right communication), then sharing of the evaluation occurs (the right feedback). Clear, timely, and tactful communication is important when providing feedback and constructive criticism. *Constructive criticism* is an essential aspect of leadership and should not focus on blame or on personal characteristics; it is focused on an analysis of a problem. If feedback in the form of constructive criticism is to be communicated, choose an appropriate time and place to deliver the message,

use communication techniques in terms of outcomes desired, and avoid blanket statements. Feedback is more likely to be accepted when the feedback giver is felt to be reliable and has good intentions; the feedback process is fair, consistent and considerate of facts and opinions; and the feedback communication process is fair, respectful, and supportive.

Communication effectiveness is influenced by the message, the way it is delivered, and the method used to communicate. Persons tend to respond more positively when they are contacted individually. Discrimination or exclusion raises sensitivities and distracts from the message. One must determine whether the receiver understands the message. Feedback is an important managerial tool and enhances subordinates' performance. Clear, immediate, honest input is required for effective outcomes.

Because they work in complex, technologically advanced environments with persons who are not well, nurses typically have been targets of criticism from clients, physicians, and other health care workers. Strategies for dealing with critical individuals include agreeing with the criticism, seeking further information, and guiding the criticism toward problem solving (Deering, 1993). At times, managers must use constructive criticism to improve subordinates' performance. In these cases, blame should not be the focus; instead the focus should be on analysis of the problems and a formulation of goals to be achieved in order to solve the problems. Constructive feedback should be given in an appropriate environment and time. Specific behavioral statements should be used to describe the problem behavior.

Nurses also must remember that image is important in communicating professionalism to the public. Dress and appearance significantly affect the public perception of the nurse's image. Nurses can use language to articulate clearly their values and the nature of their work with clients. Research has demonstrated that 55% of audience interpretations for speaker messages are determined by the speaker's nonverbal communication, such as facial expressions and body language; 38% by the speaker's vocal quality, including tone, pitch, volume, and variation; and 7% by the literal words. Audiences remember concepts and emotional expressions more than the content (Yepsen, 1988). This is true in job interviews as well, where in the first 30 seconds the employer has made a decision. The decision often is based on facial expression, clothing, body posture, and hair. This *30-second hurdle* is based on the *halo effect*, meaning the person's first impression. *External prestige* is the societal view of nursing and *internal prestige* is the nursing values and beliefs. Choice of clothing is important as it relates to professionalism, status and power, infection control, identity, modesty, symbolism, and occupational health and safety (Pearson et al., 2001).

The five basic internal organizational communication systems are (1) downward, (2) upward, (3) horizontal, (4) grapevine, and (5) network. Formal communication channels include downward, upward, and horizontal modes. *Informal communication* channels include the grapevine and network. *Networks* include a group of persons who come together to socialize or work on a team. Communication styles that facilitate communication include affirming, listening, nonaggressive, confident, and indirect approaches. Effective aspects of business communication include brief, simple, and straightforward communications that are receiver-centered (Katz & Green, 1997). Collaboration is important in the act of working together. Effective collaboration occurs when there is a recognition of differences in perspectives and orientation and all parties feel free to speak their minds. Characteristics of effective business communication include all communication must be receiver-centered, communication should be brief, and communication needs to be simple and straightforward rather than complex. The use of committees and task forces to accomplish work is effective in linking and facilitating work flow and problem solving across organizational boundaries. In flat, lean, and customer-oriented organizations, committee structures provide a route for communication and collaborative work.

Conflict is inevitable. Nurses must learn effective strategies to resolve conflict and enhance collaborative efforts among interdisciplinary team members. Two powerful tools that may resolve conflicts are (1) persuasion and (2) negotiation. Individuals use persuasion to get what they want when they believe coercion is unethical. Bargaining and negotiation are also useful in resolving a conflict.

Negotiation is the give-and-take exchange among individuals who want to resolve conflict in a way acceptable to all parties involved. *Bargaining* is related closely to negotiation and is the exchange of favors among individuals. *Collective bargaining* is a type of negotiation governed by specific laws and rules. Individuals engage in negotiation to prevent win-lose situations. To classify an interaction as a negotiation, the following three criteria must be present: the issue must be negotiable, the negotiators must be willing to give and take, and the individuals must trust each other and the process. Four elements in the negotiation process are the (1) goals, (2) values, (3) mutual victory, and (4) incomplete information.

The five reasons for exerting influence are to obtain assistance, to get others to do their jobs, to obtain personal benefits, to initiate change, and to improve job performance (Kipnis & Schmidt, 1980). Assertiveness, ingratiation, rationality, sanctions, exchange, upward appeal, blocking, and coalitions are influence tactics. In effective persuasion, two tactics are used frequently: emphasizing certain points and downplaying other points. Important persuasive techniques are using repetition, avoiding miscommunication, and providing rational explanations while avoiding threats and fear tactics.

The criteria for true negotiations include the following (Smeltzer, 1991):

- The issue must be negotiable.
- The negotiators must be interested in giving and taking.
- The parties must trust each other and the negotiation process.

The four elements of negotiation are the following (Laser, 1981):

1. Goals that are conflicting and nonconflicting
2. Values that vary as to urgency and priority as information is exchanged
3. Mutual victory when both sides realize satisfaction and feel something has been won
4. Incomplete information because parties never reveal all information and thereby shift the negotiating power

The *negotiation process* has 10 steps. The first step is preparing for the negotiation. The second step is communicating a general overview of what is to be accomplished in the negotiation. Third is review of the reasons why each party feels the negotiation is necessary. Fourth, the parties should redefine and clarify the issue(s). Fifth, the parties should agree on the agenda and select when in the course of meeting the issues will be addressed. In the sixth step, discussion should be encouraged and facilitated throughout the negotiation process. During discussions, the seventh step, both parties should explore possible compromise positions. Eighth, during the settlement stage, each party should agree in principle to the solution or possible solutions for the issue. Ninth, a thorough review and summarizing of the agreement should take place. Finally, a process should be established and implemented to monitor the parties' compliance and progress with the final agreement. Tips for successful negotiations include separating the persons from the problem; focusing on interests, not positions; inventing options for mutual gain; and insisting on using objective criteria (Fisher & Ury, 1991). Dimensions of deal-making include tactics, deal design, and setup (Lax & Sebenius, 2003). *Tactics* include individual and process issues such as interpersonal, poor communication, and hardball tactics. *Deal*

137

design is the value and substance, the how-to of crafting agreements, and *setup* is the scope and sequence or the ordering and actions taken to structure the discussions.

Formal negotiations have a specialized language that individuals use to convey the activities that occur throughout the process. Terms such as *issues, deadlock* or *stalemate, impasse, concessions, power, flinch, dead-line,* and *nibble* are used. Issues refer to negotiable items or to those conflicts that need to be resolved. An *impasse* is a point in time when issues cannot be resolved. Impasses lead to deadlocks or stalemates in which individuals are unable to reach agreement. *Concessions* refer to favors given or positions changed in order to continue negotiations or to provide a satisfactory settlement to all parties. They are those items that are of little or no value to you but are important to others and can be used strategically to influence the negotiation process. *Power* is the ability to influence others. A *flinch* is to express displeasure with the initial proposal in order to begin the negotiation process. A *deadline* is an end date on a schedule used to keep both parties on target and progressing in the negotiation process. A *nibble* is a small concession after the agreement has been settled.

Preparation for negotiations is essential for success. The ability to determine the parameters for negotiation helps control the issues and areas of discussion. Dressing professionally and being aware of verbal and nonverbal messages are important in resolving issues and tipping off the opposing party. Good listening skills and a positive communication tone are essential for effective negotiation. Maintaining a flexible position is also important in a successful negotiation.

Nurses have unionized for a variety of reasons. Some of the more recent issues sparking unionization efforts include layoffs, the reduction of hours, elimination of incentives, the cessation of pay increases, and the denial of benefits. The use of unlicensed assistive personnel in place of registered nurses and the increasing number of employees a clinical nurse must supervise have sparked concerns about unsafe client care and inadequate staffing levels. To verbalize the concerns of nurses to management, nurses occasionally have turned to unionization as a method of strengthening their voice and demanding accountability for unilateral administrative decisions influencing client care.

Effective leaders will use communication to strengthen teams and build a positive work culture. They will use communication techniques such as clarity, intention, engagement, medium, language, and alignment to motivate nurses and staff to engender a culture of practice excellence. Visionary leaders will be mindful of the language they use and maintain consistency and congruency in the messages they send.

They will be social entrepreneurs, who create new ways to approach old problems and move the organization and community toward a healthier and enjoyable climate. They will, by example, create a culture and climate in their organization that will foster professional development, encourage innovation, facilitate conflict resolution, and focus on client care and outcomes.

LEARNING TOOLS

Group Activity: Exploring Verbal and Nonverbal Communication

Purpose

To identify the impact of verbal and nonverbal communication when interacting with others. In light of the fact that approximately 55% of a speaker's message is the result of facial and body language (the majority is facial); 38% the vocal quality; and only 7% the actual words used, this activity is designed to help you assess your communication style with others.

Directions

1. Divide yourselves into groups of three. One person will be sending a message; one person will be receiving the message; and one person will observe the interaction and then provide feedback.

2. First, have one person describe the most important thing that has happened to him or her within the past year. Three minutes should be allowed for the interaction.

3. Then reverse the procedure until everyone has had an opportunity to observe, send, and receive a message. Observers should jot down comments about verbal and nonverbal communication. The following observer checklist may be used.

4. Second, have each person describe the worst thing that has happened to him or her in the last year. Again, use the observer checklist to record comments.

Afterward, everyone should share his or her observer comments with the group. Talk with each other about the impact verbal and nonverbal communication has on the content of the message. Receivers should discuss the verbal or nonverbal activity that they focused on the most. Discuss how mannerisms or nonverbal behaviors can distract or support a message.

Observer Checklist

For each of the categories, prompts are provided. Write down the major and minor verbal and nonverbal characteristics that you noted for the sender and receiver.

138

Facial Expression   Sender   Receiver
_____

1. Note the eyes and mouth for expressiveness. Is the sender
   relating happiness? Sadness? Anger?

2. How is the receiver responding?
_____

Body Language   Sender   Receiver
_____

1. Note the arms, hands, legs, shoulders, and hips. How is
   the sender illustrating his or her messsage?

2. How is the receiver acknowledging the message?

3. Is the sender's message supportive, disinterested, or boring?

4. What impact is the sender's message having on the receiver?
   Is the sender changing the content of the message based on
   the receiver's feedback?
_____

Vocal Quality   Sender   Receiver
_____

1. Are the tone, pitch, and volume consistent with the message?

2. Is the sender's message spoken in a monotone? Is there
   variation in tone to make an impact on the receiver?

3. Is the sender forceful? Weak? Bored? Interested? Animated?
   Eager?

4. Does the sender use a strong, soft, reflective, or humorous
   presentation?
_____

Articulated Words   Sender   Receiver
_____

1. What actual verbal message was sent?

2. What words were used to send the message?

3. Were metaphors used? Were red flags or emotionally
   charged words used?
_____

139

Using Persuasion to Influence Others

Character One: Jennifer Smith is the vice president of nursing at a large teaching hospital in Topeka, Kansas. She has decided to organize a team to work on critical pathways and then to implement them in the hospital in an effort to provide cost-effective, high-quality care to clients.

Character Two: Jason Johnson is the chief executive officer of the hospital. He is concerned about rising costs and is tightening up on resources. He plans to hold the line and not distribute money for new projects that cannot guarantee a payoff.

Character Three: Joe James is the vice president of building and maintenance. He is over budget on a new building project and needs additional money to finish the new building. He plans to speak to Mr. Johnson to secure the needed funds.

Character Four: Mary Ann Williams is the chief financial officer. She has crunched some figures and is prepared to speak to Mr. Johnson about the bottom line. She has designed a forecasted projection of the revenue and expenses for the next 6 months, and she is prepared to make recommendations about cost cutting to ensure organizational viability.

Ms. Smith is going to Mr. Johnson's office prepared to share with him a new project (critical pathways) that would improve quality and decrease costs. She knows that there will be an initial outlay of money but is sure that there will be a major payoff for the organization. As she turns the corner toward Mr. Johnson's office, she sees Ms. Williams and Mr. James talking. Mr. Johnson opens his door and sees his executive team waiting to speak to him.

Role-Play Questions

1. What should Ms. Smith do? Should she take the lead and jump right in with her new idea? If so, what should she say? How should she introduce the topic?

2. What persuasive techniques should Ms. Smith use to elicit support for her project?

3. How could she persuade others to support her project and yet support them with their plans?

CASE STUDIES

Case Study 1: Managing Feedback

Martha Boyd is the nurse manager of an operating room in Lake Worth, Florida. Jill Jansen is a registered nurse who has worked in the operating room for 3 years. Lately, Nurse Jansen has been having problems completing the documentation that she is required to do, has been taking long breaks, and is refusing to scrub for several physicians. Nurse Boyd is informed that staffing is short and that they will need her to cover cases just to get through the day. Nurse Boyd enjoys scrubbing and is willing to help out to facilitate a smooth progression of clients through the operating room. After Nurse Boyd has finished her second case, the charge nurse informs her that they are one case behind. Nurse Boyd asks if there was an emergency or a late case. The charge nurse says no, but that Nurse Jansen took a 45-minute break and refused to scrub for a physician. Nurse Boyd walks into the conference room where Nurse Jansen is reading a book. Nurse Boyd angrily reprimands Nurse Jansen in front of two staff members and tells her to scrub for the physician or go home.

Case Study 1 Questions

1. Did Nurse Boyd respond in an appropriate fashion?

2. What other strategies could Nurse Boyd have used to manage this situation?

3. What are characteristics of constructive feedback?

Case Study 2: Communication, Persuasion, and Negotiation

Jennifer Lanze is a nurse manager of an ambulatory care clinic in a large teaching hospital. The ambulatory care clinic is successful and is a good revenue source for the hospital. Recently, the physicians and nurse practitioners in the ambulatory care clinic negotiated a contract with a large employer in the community to provide primary care for all of their employees. The contract was negotiated at a discounted rate. The physicians and nurse practitioners have held a team conference to look at expenses, workload, and equipment usage. They have asked Nurse Lanze to figure out a way to use the registered nurses more effectively and, if necessary, to hire medical assistants. Nurse Lanze knows that the nurses will resist. She also knows that the registered nurses could be used more effectively in client teaching activities, immunizations, and triage.

Case Study 2 Questions

1. What should Nurse Lanze do? Should she be autocratic and demand that the registered nurses comply? Should she use persuasion to get them to do what she wants? Should she negotiate with them?

2. If Nurse Lanze chooses to use persuasion, should she listen to their concerns?

3. If Nurse Lanze chooses to use negotiation and a settlement is agreed upon, who is responsible for evaluating and monitoring progress?

LEARNING RESOURCES

Discussion Questions

1. What is essential for effective communication to occur?

2. What types of communication networks are there? What types of communication networks are used in decentralized and centralized organizations?

3. What are the steps in information exchange?

4. Why are nurses targeted for criticism? What strategies can nurses use to handle criticism?

5. What are the current issues in health care organizations today that might lead to nurses choosing to unionize in order to have a strong collective voice?

6. Describe the process of negotiation that nurses could use to address pressing issues in client care with administrative personnel.

7. Are persuasion, negotiation, and bargaining useful in personal and professional interactions? If so, provide an example of each for a personal and a professional situation.

8. What is the difference between coercion and persuasion? Should both be used? If so, why? If not, why not?

Study Questions

True or False: Circle the correct answer.

T F 1. Verbal communication includes affective and expressive behaviors.

T F 2. Positive communication techniques include agreeing uncritically and reassuringly.

T F 3. Individual communication is more complex than group communication because it is so intensive.

T F 4. Horizontally decentralized organizations are more efficient than centralized organizations.

T F 5. Feedback should be used carefully and only when absolutely necessary because it inhibits effective communication.

T F 6. To respond effectively to communication, place blame on others.

T F 7. The major part of any communication is the words we say to others.

T F 8. Effective communication is clear, direct, and straightforward.

T F 9. Metaphors and political language can be used by nurse leaders to influence governmental officials.

T F 10. Nurses are often targets of verbal abuse.

T F 11. Complex work completed by professionals tends to have organizational structures that are decentralized.

T F 12. Any hint of discrimination or exclusion may raise sensitivities.

T F 13. Nurses are targets of criticism because they are assertive and are client advocates.

Matching: Write the letter of the correct response in front of each term.

_____ 14. Negotiation

_____ 15. Bargaining

_____ 16. Persuasion

_____ 17. Collective bargaining

_____ 18. Flinch

_____ 19. Nibble

_____ 20. Concessions

_____ 21. Deadline

_____ 22. Impasse

_____ 23. Issues

A. A small extra item that is obtained after the settlement

B. Items of little value to one party

C. A point in time when issues cannot be resolved to mutual satisfaction

D. Items to be resolved

E. Activities governed by law and rules

F. Influencing another to modify behaviors

G. Timeframes for negotiations

H. To draw back at an initial proposal

I. Give-and-take exchange aimed at resolving conflicts

J. The exchange of favors

Chapter **20 Communication, Persuasion, and Negotiation**

References

Boggs, K. U. (1999). Communication styles. In E. Arnold & K. U. Boggs (Eds.), *Interpersonal relationships: Professional communication skills for nurses* (3rd ed., pp. 195-208). Philadelphia: W. B. Saunders.

Deering, C. (1993). Giving and taking criticism. *American Journal of Nursing, 93*(12), 56-61.

Fisher, R., & Ury, W. (1991). *Getting to yes: Negotiating agreement without giving in.* New York: Penguin Books.

Grant, A. (1994). *The Professional Nurse: Issues and Actions.* Springhouse, PA: Springhouse.

Hersey, P., Blanchard, K. H., & Johnson, D. E. (2001). *Management of organizational behavior: Leading human resources* (8th ed.). Upper Saddle River, NJ: Prentice-Hall.

Katz, I. M. & Green, E. (1997). *Managing quality: A guide to system-wide performance management in health care* (2nd ed.). St. Louis: Mosby.

Kipnis, D., & Schmidt, S. (1980). Intraorganizational influence tactics: Explorations in getting one's way. *Journal of Applied Psychology, 65*(4), 440-452.

Laser, R. (1981). I win-you win negotiating. *Journal of Nursing Administration, 11*(11/12), 24-29.

Lax, D. A., & Sebenius, J. K. (2003). 3-D negotiation: Playing the whole game. *Harvard Business Review, 81*(11), 64-74.

Pearson, A., Baker, H., Walsh, K., & Fitzgerald, M. (2001). Contemporary nurses' uniforms: History and traditions. *Journal of Nursing Management, 9*(3), 147-152.

Smeltzer, C. (1991). The art of negotiation: An everyday experience. *Journal of Nursing Administration, 21*(7/8), 26-30.

Thies, K., & Williams-Burgess, C. (1992). Communication as a progressive curriculum concept. *Nurse Educator, 17*(2), 39-41.

Yepsen, D. (1988, October 5). Molding a candidate for the media. *The Des Moines Register,* p. 7A.

Supplemental Readings

Dolan, J. P. (2004). Overcome the myths of negotiation for a positive selling experience. *The Secured Lender, 60*(6), 66-70.

Manallack, S. (2002, June). Mastering the art of persuasion. *The National Public Accountant,* pp. 21-22.

Shelton, L. K. (2004). *Communication for nurses: Talking with patients.* Thorofare, NJ: Slack.

Ulijn, J. M., O Duill, M., & Robertson, S. A. (2004). Teaching business plan negotiation: Fostering entrepreneurship among business and engineering students. *Business Communication Quarterly, 67*(1), 41-47.

Warren, B. J., Donaldson, R., & Whaley, M. (2005). Service learning: An adjunct to therapeutic communication and critical thinking skills for baccalaureate nursing students. *Journal of Nursing Education, 44*(3), 147.

Chapter 20: Communication, Persuasion, and Negotiation (pp. 407-438)

1. What are the essential components of the communication process?

The communication process consists of verbal and nonverbal communication. Verbal communication is written and spoken. Nonverbal communication is unspoken and is composed of affective or expressive behaviors. The four distinctions of communication are formal and informal, vertical and horizontal, personal and impersonal, and instrumental and expressive.

2. What are the barriers to effective communication in organizations?

Barriers to effective communication in organizations include political and interpersonal subtleties and the complexity of communicating with multiple individuals. Organizations use various systems for communication such as hierarchical or democratic networks. Barriers in the hierarchical network may be associated with decreased opportunity for individuals to interact with their peers or others on other levels in the hierarchy. Barriers in the democratic network may be associated with communication inaccuracy and the development of subhierarchies.

3. What problems of communication occur frequently in nursing?

Verbal and nonverbal communication problems occur in nursing. These problems frequently center on issues of competency, responsibility, and professionalism and may be related to being on the front lines, being the focus for displaced criticism, working with persons who have health problems, and working in high-stress environments. Nonverbal communication problems exist when the media portrays an unprofessional image of nursing.

4. Are employer-employee communication problems more common than peer-to-peer difficulties?

Communication problems in employer-employee and peer-to-peer relationships are equally common experiences. Problems associated with employer-employee communications may result from intimidation, mistrust, insufficient feedback, or the inability to articulate needs. Similarly, peer-to-peer miscommunications may result from lack of trust or a difficulty with needs expression but also may encompass an inability to give and receive constructive criticism and turf issues.

5. What solutions tend to help communication effectiveness?

Planning the message structure, delivery style, mode of communication, and method for feedback can enhance communication effectiveness. Planning the message involves structuring it so that it will be received positively and will engender the desired response. The selection of delivery style includes careful selection of words to maximize the desired impact. The mode of communication involves decisions about the timing and the optimal vehicle for transmission. The method for feedback includes a plan for determining whether the delivered message was understood. Solutions for responding effectively to criticism include soliciting additional input, clarifying the issues, agreeing with the critic, and using listening skills to enhance understanding.

6. What is the relationship of communication skill to leadership effectiveness?

Communication skill is a key element of leadership effectiveness. Communication skill is a critical and important tool for engaging, motivating, and empowering individuals to accomplish organizational goals. The skill of communication is essential in sharing the vision, in shaping the organizational culture, and in implementing change.

7. What is the leader's role in helping others improve written and oral communication?

The leader plays an important role in mentoring others to improve their communication skills. Mentoring can be accomplished through a variety of methods, such as role modeling, soliciting and providing constructive criticism, and role-playing. It is critical for the leader to model a communication style that is clear, direct, honest, respectful, empathetic, and timely.

8. How important is written communication skill in influencing an individual's image?

Written communication skill is an important professional element that affects an individual's image. Organizations commonly transmit information in the form of fliers, memos, letters, faxes, e-mail, and newsletters. Skill is required to structure a clear and concise written message that will be received positively. Unclear written messages may present ambiguous information that increases the likelihood for misunderstanding.

9. **How do you personally communicate, verbally and nonverbally?**

One's personal communication style may incorporate verbal and nonverbal components. Individuals communicate to others through their appearance, dress, body language, diction, language, mannerism, tone, volume, and word selection. Awareness of your communication strengths and weaknesses and how others receive your intended message is important.

10. **How might you choose some other message or some other channel to increase your personal effectiveness?**

Consider your message structure. Are you consciously thinking about whether it will be received positively and whether it will elicit the desired response? Are your words clear and free from red flags, inflammatory language, and jargon? Are you aware of the nonverbal communications that you portray? Before selecting a communication channel, think about the advantages and disadvantages associated with written and spoken communication.

11. **Do nurses, from the staff nurse to the chief nurse executive, present an image of nursing with which you agree or disagree?**

Think about the image of nursing that you value. Is there consensus or discord among others regarding the image? Do your peers and colleagues agree with the image? How about health care consumers? Do you hold a different image of nursing for the staff nurse and the chief nurse executive? Should you?

12. **What does the ideal nurse's uniform look like? Analyze your response.**

The ideal nurse's uniform is one that conveys a professional appearance and allows the nurse to carry out her or his duties and responsibilities. Although there is consensus that a nurse's uniform should be comfortable and identifiable, disagreement continues over the color and style of the garment. Research has shown that health care consumers prefer white uniforms, in contrast to nurses, who prefer scrubs outfits. How would you blend the two perspectives to meet the needs of both groups? Are they mutually exclusive? Are the preferences of one group more important than the other?

13. **Why do nurses need to look professional?**

Physical appearance and choice of clothing are forms of nonverbal communication that others use to formulate judgments. A professional appearance enhances the image of nursing, influencing the amount of trust, confidence, and prestige that consumers, colleagues, and corporations afford them.

14. **What persuades an individual to become a nurse?**

A variety of factors may influence an individual's decision to become a nurse. For example, some may be drawn to nursing for altruistic reasons or for the excitement of working in a fast-paced health care environment. Still others are drawn to nursing for job security, professional advancement and challenge, and research opportunities.

15. **What feelings are associated with an interview for a nursing position?**

An interview for a nursing position is a process in which applicants seeking employment attempt to persuade the interviewer that they are the best candidates for the position. Applicants may experience feelings of anxiousness, nervousness, excitement, or apprehension during the interview process.

16. **What was the last issue you negotiated?**

Analyze your negotiation process. What was the central issue in the negotiation? What were your objectives or goals? What were the goals of the other person? How did the goals vary with respect to urgency and priority as the negotiation efforts continued? Was it a win-win, win-lose, or lose-lose result? What information was withheld to maintain a sense of negotiating power?

17. **What behaviors contribute to cooperative and productive negotiation?**

Cooperative and productive negotiation can occur only if the issue is negotiable, the negotiators are interested in compromising, and if there is mutual trust and cooperation. In a supportive environment, negotiation is problem focused and sincere. Successful negotiation depends on the participants being well prepared, their use of effective communication skills, and a willingness to take calculated risks and to work toward a mutually supported solution.

18. **What words or actions indicate competitive negotiation?**

A competitive negotiation process may have a defensive milieu in which there are feelings of superiority and domination. Indications of competitive negotiation include ineffective communication, stressful reactions, personal agendas, and unrevealed information. Information may be altered, filtered, given selectively, or withheld as a power-gaining strategy. Questions may be framed to lead the other party to the competitor's point of view rather than genuinely to seek understanding.

19. **What approaches or strategies of negotiation are most effective for nursing?**

Although there are numerous negotiation strategies available for use by nurses, the most effective are those that are planned deliberately and actualized. Laser (1981) identified four significant strategies for negotiation: the flinch, the deadline, the nibble, and the concession. The flinch strategy involves wincing at the initial proposition by the other party in an effort to open the negotiation dialogue. The deadline strategy produces results, is advisable in every negotiation, and must be negotiated among interested parties. The nibble strategy is a small, extra settlement that is reached after a larger decision has been attained. The concession strategy involves giving the other party concessions that are valuable to them but are of little or no value to you. Concessions should be identified, used strategically, and recorded. Other recommended strategies for successful negotiation include separating the persons from the problem; focusing on interests, not positions; inventing options for mutual agreement; and using objective criteria. An awareness of available strategies enhances the negotiator's ability to choose alternative approaches, augment effectiveness, and achieve desirable outcomes.

20. **What factors are facilitators or barriers to collaboration among professionals?**

Facilitators to collaboration among professionals include willingness to compromise, cooperate, and a willingness to work toward a solution that everyone can support. Client-centered goals can be achieved through mutual trust, respect, and acknowledgment of the contribution of each discipline. Barriers to collaboration include turf protection, power issues, arrogance, ineffective communication, and defensiveness.

21. **Does collective bargaining increase professionalism in nursing?**

Some believe that collective bargaining increases professionalism in nursing by ensuring that nursing has a voice in decisions related to client care, working conditions, wages, benefits, and professional practice. Collective bargaining exists to limit employers' ability to take unilateral action. Others believe that collective bargaining limits professionalism by creating a defensive environment between nurses and employers.

22. **What organizational factors are associated with unionization?**

Organizational factors associated with unionization include unilateral decisions made by employers to reduce costs by downsizing, merging, restructuring, and reengineering the workforce. Threats to long-term job security and benefits, reduction in income, increased workload, and concerns over quality care have created an increase in unionization activities.

23. **Is positional power eroding in nursing? With what forms of negotiation can nurses replace positional power?**

Positional power, or legitimate power, relates to the role or position held by nurses in organizations. When organizations make unilateral decisions about issues affecting professional practice without the input of nurses, the nurses' professional power is diminished. Nurses may need to strengthen their expert and referent power to ensure that client advocacy occurs. Nurses may seek and use power to influence professional practice, ethical issues, and national health care policies. Nurses can use negotiation to determine how nursing care is practiced and delivered in organizations by establishing a collaborative environment in which the goals of all parties are respected and valued.

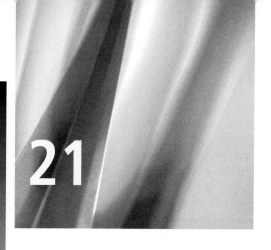

21

All-Hazards Disaster Preparedness

STUDY FOCUS

The tragic September 11, 2001, twin tower catastrophe in New York City changed the world and Americans' perception of their "safe" home environment. This sentinel event triggered a major movement of disaster and bioterrorism preparedness. Significant work has been done on assessing the many possible terrorism acts, including biological mishaps, chemical spills, radiological exposures, nuclear accidents, conventional bombings, agricultural contamination, and cyber viruses. Community members' preparation for bioterrorism includes gathering information from a variety of resources, reevaluating personal perspectives about preparing for an inevitable disaster, and planning what they will do in the event of one (Ashcroft, 2001; Myers, 2001; Ritcher, 2004; Vecchio, 2000). Each health care agency across the country is establishing an all-hazards preparedness program to comply with requirements set forth by the Health Insurance Portability and Accountability Act and the Joint Commission on Accreditation of Healthcare Organizations.

A comprehensive all-hazards preparedness plan assists in establishing an organized hospital-based plan for internal and external disasters, an interhospital plan for effective collaboration among health care organizations, an integrated community plan, and a national health plan. *Disasters* are unforeseen and often sudden events that cause great damage, destruction, and human suffering. Disasters can be internal or external. An *internal disaster* is a catastrophic event that occurs within a single facility and usually is handled by that facility, whereas an *external disaster* is a catastrophic event that is broader and affects the community as a whole. The following definitions are important to know to be prepared for a potential disaster:

- *All-hazards* refers to all types of natural and human terrorist events.
- *All-hazards disaster preparedness* refers to the internal and external disaster preparedness that establishes action plans for every type of disaster or combination of disaster events.
- *Biological disaster* is an incident involving a natural or deliberate outbreak of a pathogen affecting large numbers of individuals (Inova Health System, 2001a).
- *Chemical disaster* is the exposure to hazardous chemically toxic materials (Inova Health System, 2001b)
- *Conventional disaster* is a catastrophic event caused by the use of weapons such as bombs or guns.
- *Cyber disaster* is a catastrophic event affecting large numbers of persons and lasting more than a few hours that affects the ability to use information technology.
- *Radiological/nuclear disaster* is a radiological or nuclear emergency occurring that may be internal or external to the facility.

It is important to design an all-hazards preparedness program. The first step is to establish an interdisciplinary task force to design the plan. The leadership should be filled by a senior executive administrator who is able to communicate preparedness as a priority. In addition, external ad hoc members are important for communication and plan implementation. The development process uses consensus building and standardization to design a dynamic and prepared team process. Internal task force members and external representatives (examples include police, public schools system, church, community physicians, and essential vendors) work together to design an effective all-hazards plan. A *gap analysis* often is performed to uncover any problems, weaknesses, or deficiencies in the plan. These problems and other issues then can be corrected.

Common issues to be addressed in all-hazards plan include the following:

- Establish a common nomenclature, structure, and role definition for writing an all-hazards preparedness plan. Safety and security personnel should have assigned oversight for facility security, quick lockdown, and management of persons moving in and out of the health care facility.

147

- Help staff to overcome fear associated with disaster and all-hazards preparedness. The first rule is to keep the staff and their family members as safe as possible.
- Create procedural addendums for all-hazards preparedness plans. Define procedures of what to do in a variety of potential disasters. Design closely linked and integrated systems with police, fire, and rescue. Design clear algorithms for designing, intervening, and notifying appropriate authorities.
- Create an all-hazards planning subgroup, and develop a command center. Be ready to triage and isolate patients, obtain protective equipment, lock down departments, identify patient contacts, and notify infection control and epidemiological networks.
- Develop processes in the command center; establish the role of the hospital in the community, and test the all-hazards preparedness plans and command center.

A key element of any all-hazards plan is to establish the command center, which serves as the nerve center or command and control center for the entire disaster period. A strong center will provide clear direction and coordination of multiple constituents during a disaster. Essential elements of a command center include the following:

- Setting up the command room: A backup command center in another location is essential to establish to ensure continuation of communication in case of a threat or problem at the main command and control center. Each room is equipped with multiple telephone lines, computer access, fax, copying, radio technology, television access, and other essential supplies.
- Developing processes in the command center: A step-by-step document (1 to 2 pages) describing operational and closedown procedures for the command center is created. In addition, a communication tree and identifiers for staff may be used for coordination of essential services.
- Establishing the role of the hospital in the community: Discussion on the role of the hospital and other agencies is important for proper coordination of services in a disaster. Many health care agencies are using the hospital emergency incident command center for a standardized nomenclature for disasters.
- Testing the all-hazards preparedness plans and command centers: Another important aspect of bioterrorism preparedness is testing the disaster system. Internal and external drills can be conducted in communities. By conducting a test, gaps or problems can be identified and processes improved.

An important leadership and management implication is leadership by the nurse executive in providing direction in all-hazards preparedness. One strategy to provide direction and leadership in bioterrorism preparedness is to establish standards for educational content for staff and develop internal and external networks and partnerships. Nurse leaders not only must plan, implement, and evaluate the all-hazards plans but also must have strong emotional competencies to lead groups effectively. Emotional competencies include good interpersonal skills, excellent and clear communication skills, and calm, controlled delegation (Fahlgren & Drenkard, 2002). These skills are critical in leading groups during periods of uncertainty, challenging circumstances, and unforeseen problems. Current issues in all-hazards preparedness include establishing the level of alertness (low = green; guarded = blue; elevated = yellow; high = orange, and severe = red), developing and using benchmarks for preparedness, establishing the role of long-term care facilities in disaster preparedness, developing disaster preparedness alliances, and creating a national-level incident reporting system.

LEARNING TOOLS

Activity: Analysis of an All-Hazards Preparedness Plan

Purpose
To analyze an all-hazards preparedness plan for an acute care facility in order to understand the complexity, communication networks, and readiness of the organization to implement the disaster plan on a moment's notice.

Directions
1. Obtain an all-hazards preparedness plan from a health care organization to analyze.
2. Conduct a gap analysis survey to identify any potential areas for improvement in the all-hazards preparedness plan. This analysis will illustrate the complexity of disaster preparedness.
3. Use the sample questions to conduct a gap-analysis survey.
4. Review your assessment of the all-hazards survey results that you completed and identify the gaps in the plan. Note the complexity of the all-hazards plan, and share the results of your assessment with your peers and clinical preceptor.

Gap Analysis Survey*

General Questions

- Does your hospital have an internal disaster plan addressing what to do if an emergency occurs only in your facility?
- Does your hospital have an external disaster plan addressing what to do if an emergency occurs in the community and you need to be prepared to respond?
- Do directors know where to find facility internal and external disaster plans?
- Do the directors know who is in charge of the command center in a disaster?
- Does your department staff know the chain of command in an emergency?
- Does your department know its role in a disaster?
- Does your hospital know its role in the community in an emergency situation?
- Are those in charge identified by a vest or have some sort of distinction?
- Are there specific plans for biological, chemical, nuclear, and conventional emergencies? Do all staff members in your department know their role in each emergency?
- Is there a bed and staffing plan for surge capacity for 50 patients? 100 patients? 250 patients? Are there portable cots contracted for use in a surge situation?
- Does your facility have an operational command center to coordinate the response of the hospital in the event of a disaster?
- Is there a central command center telephone number to use in the event of a disaster?

Human Resources

- Do your department staff members know how to prepare themselves, their significant others, and pets in the event of a disaster?
- Is there a credentialing plan for health care professionals who come to the nearest facility in a disaster to volunteer their services?

Safety and Security

Does your facility have the following:

- A lockdown plan in case of an emergency?
- A plan for allowing staff to get to work and allowed entry to hospital during an emergency?

- A plan for facility traffic flow during an emergency?
- A multilanguage signage to direct persons as to where to go during an emergency?

Communication

- Does your hospital have emergency-powered telephones in case of a disaster?
- Does your facility have a backup radio system and volunteer staff to operate it?
- Does your facility have a tiered paging system that can reach multiple staff members simultaneously?
- Does your department know the central command center telephone number (if there is one)?
- Is there a procedure for notifying the administrator on call and opening the command center in the event of a disaster?
- Are there established linkages to the external community (e.g., other hospitals in the region, fire department, police, emergency medical system, public schools, and public health department)?
- Do the telephone operators know how to link patients and families in your facility and in the community should a disaster occur?
- Is there an on-call list for administrative coverage of the command center? If so, do the telephone operators know how to contact the administrator on call for the command center?
- Is there a plan for contacting essential employees and administrators in a disaster?

Logistics

- Does your facility have the following:
  - Backup emergency supplies, pharmaceuticals, and equipment? The ability to release and send pharmaceuticals, medical supplies, and equipment such as respirators to the areas in need in the event of a chemical or biological emergency?
  - Prearrangement plans with physicians, ambulances, nearby churches, and nursing homes to clear beds in an emergency? (What site can take patients?)
  - Contracts with vendors to bring in items such as food, ice, and oxygen?
- Is there an established written psychosocial role for those in social work, chaplaincy, psychiatry, employee health, and case management in the event of a disaster?
- Are there contingency plans for 3 to 5 days for no power, no water, no computers, and/or no food?
- Are there contingency plans for staff to report to the nearest facility to work?

*Courtesy Inova Health System. From Drenkard, K., & Rigotti, G. (2002). Inova Health System Survey 2001. Falls Church, VA: Inova Health System.

- Are there contingency plans for child care during an emergency so parents can work?
- Is there common nomenclature used during an emergency so that everyone understands what is happening and who has what responsibility?

Clinical Operations

- Does your facility have the following:
  - Procedures established to maximize staff safety in the event of a disaster?
  - Procedures for fit testing of respiratory mask for staff?
  - Procedures and training for using protective equipment?
  - The ability to track patients until discharge, admission, or death using Health Insurance Portability and Accountability Act guidelines?
  - Clearly established policies and procedures to respond to biological, chemical, nuclear, and conventional emergencies?
  - A decontamination area and detailed step-by-step procedures on how to work in this area?
  - A backup staff to assist with persons/patients arriving at the hospital?
- Procedures for how to do the following:
  - Open and operate the command center
  - Track available beds
  - Track staff working and direct them to designated area
  - Track volunteer staff and direct them to a designated area
  - Track arriving patients and direct them to a designated area
  - Operate every department of the hospital during an emergency
  - Track discharged patients and direct them to a designated area
  - Handle surge capacity situations
  - Handle operating room cases in the event of an emergency
  - Track biological, chemical, or nuclear events and report them to authorities

Financial

- Is there an established plan to tracking costs during an emergency?
- Is there an established plan for submitting for disaster reimbursement?

Messages/Media

- Is there an established communication plan in case of an emergency?
- Is there an established communication script in the event of an emergency?
- Is there an alternative communication plan if power, telephones, and radios are not working?

CASE STUDY

Jo Ellen Peckesir is the nurse executive at Marion Porter Hospital, a 1,200-bed facility in Greenview, Arizona. She has worked with the community to prepare an all-hazards preparedness plan for the hospital. All stakeholders in the community were included in the development of the all-hazards preparedness plan for the hospital. The plan has integrated all community facilities and is comprehensive. The plan was shared with all employees, who immediately became concerned for their families because the plan requires that staff and health care workers designated as "priority" to respond immediately following a local disaster. Many of the "priority" staff and health care workers are single parents and are concerned for the safety of their families.

Case Study Questions

1. What are the key issues for staff and health care providers with this plan?
2. How should the staff and health care workers alert administration to their concern with this all-hazards preparedness plan? What solutions could they offer to strengthen this plan?
3. What positive characteristics does the all-hazards preparedness plan include?
4. What are the common issues to address in all-hazards preparedness plans?
5. What are the essential elements of a command center?
6. What is a gap analysis? What is its purpose?

LEARNING RESOURCES

Discussion Questions

1. Describe the process of developing an all-hazards preparedness plan. Discuss the type of individuals in the organization that should be included in plan development.
2. Define the following terms: disaster, all-hazards, biological disaster, chemical disaster, conventional disaster, cyber disaster, radiological/nuclear disaster, and gap analysis.

3. Discuss the concept of gap analysis, and describe a situation in which this would be useful and what information it might provide.

4. Identify and discuss common issues that need to be addressed in the development of all-hazards plans. Discuss the implications of each issue.

5. Discuss the development of a command center for an acute care organization or community and describe the importance and function of the center.

Study Questions

True or False: Circle the correct answer.

T   F   1. Individuals in communities are gathering information on all-hazards preparedness, developing community-based plans, and conducting disaster drills.

T   F   2. The Health Insurance Portability and Accountability Act and the Joint Commission on Accreditation of Healthcare Organizations require an all-hazards preparedness plan.

T   F   3. A disaster is an unforeseen and often sudden event that causes great damage, destruction, and human suffering.

T   F   4. Acute care facilities only need to be prepared and have a plan in place only for external disasters.

T   F   5. A biological disaster is a catastrophic event caused by the use of weapons such as guns, bombs, missiles, and grenades.

T   F   6. A chemical disaster is an incident involving a natural or deliberate outbreak of a pathogen affecting large numbers of adults and children.

T   F   7. A cyber disaster is a catastrophic event affecting large numbers of persons and lasting more than a few hours that affects the ability to use information technology.

T   F   8. The first step in establishing an all-hazards preparedness plan is to create an all-hazards preparedness task force.

T   F   9. When designing an all-hazards preparedness plan, membership should include only internal organizational members.

T   F   10. A gap analysis is a punitive tool used when acute care organizations do not meet accreditation criteria for all-hazards preparedness.

T   F   11. The role of gap analysis in all-hazards preparedness is to identify the areas in which there are gaps in the preparedness plan of a facility.

T   F   12. The development of a command center is integral to an all-hazards plan.

T   F   13. The hospital emergency incident command system is a nomenclature for disasters.

T   F   14. It is important to include the public health department, police, and other critical community organizations in a all-hazards community preparedness plan.

References

Ashcroft, T. (2001). Braced for disaster. *Nursing Management, 32*(5), 49-52.

Fahlgren, T., & Drenkard, K. (2002). Health care system disaster preparedness, part 2: Nursing executive role in leadership. *Journal of Nursing Administration, 32*(10), 531-537.

Inova Health System. (2001a). *All-hazards disaster preparedness plan. Annex B.* Falls Church, VA: Inova Health System.

Inova Health System. (2001b). *All-hazards disaster preparedness plan. Annex C.* Falls Church, VA: Inova Health System.

Lindholm, M., & Uden, G. (2001). Nurse managers' management, direction, and role over time. *Nursing Administration Quarterly, 25*(4), 14-29.

Myers III, F. E. (2001). Bioterrorism: Responding to militant microbes. *Nursing 2001, 31*(9), 32hn1-32hn4.

Ritcher, P. (2004). *Hospital disaster preparedness: Meeting a requirement or preparing for the worst?* Chicago: American Society for Health Care Engineering. Retrieved June 9, 2004, from *www.ashe.org/ashe/codes/jcaho/ec/emergency/hospdisasterprepare.html*

Vecchio, A. (2000). Plan for the worst before disaster strikes. *Health Management Technology, 21*(6), 28-30.

Supplemental Readings

Foldy, S. L., Biedrzycki, P. A., Baker, V. K., Swain, G. R., Howe, D. S., Gleryn D., et al. (2004). The public health dashboard: A surveillance model for bioterrorism preparedness. *Journal of Public Health Management and Practice, 10*(3), 234-240.

Hilton, C., & Allison, V. (2004). Disaster preparedness: An indictment for action by nursing educators. *The Journal of Continuing Education in Nursing, 35*(2), 59-65.

Saliba, D., Buchanan, J., & Kington, R. S. (2004). Function and response of nursing facilities during community disaster. *American Journal of Public Health, 94*(8), 1436-1441.

Sebastian, S. V., Styron, S., Reize, S. N., Houston, S., Luquire, R., & Hickey, J. V. (2003). Resiliency of accomplished critical care nurses in a natural disaster. *Critical Care Nurse, 23*(5), 24-36.

Stokes, E., Gilbert-Palmer, D., Skorga, P., Young, C., & Persell, D. (2004). Chemical agents of terrorism: Preparing nurse practitioners. *The Nurse Practitioner, 29*(5), 30-41.

Weber, C. J. (2004). Update on bioterrorism preparedness. *Urologic Nursing, 24*(5), 417-419.

Chapter 21: All-Hazards Disaster Preparedness (pp. 439-460)

1. **How does an all-hazards disaster plan differ from a typical disaster plan?**

   A disaster is an unforeseen and often sudden event that causes great damage, destruction, and human suffering. A typical disaster plan outlines actions to be taken to meet the needs of the community as a result of a disaster caused by event such as hurricanes, building collapse, explosion, and tornados. Since the terrorist attack in the United States on September 11, 2001, disaster plans have been expanded to include bioterrorism preparedness and are deemed all-hazards disaster plans. An all-hazards disaster plan encompasses all types of natural and/or human terrorist events or combination of disaster events. These disasters may include biological, chemical, conventional, cyber, and radiological/nuclear events. A comprehensive all-hazards preparedness plan encompasses the following: (1) an organized hospital-based plan for internal and external disasters at the department/unit level, (2) an interhospital plan for effectively collaborating with other hospitals within a health care system and within the vicinity, (3) a community plan that integrates the hospital plan with other external community plans, and (4) a national plan that guides nurse leaders in accessing financial assistance from federal and state all-hazards preparedness resources.

2. **What is the difference between an internal disaster plan and an external disaster plan?**

   An internal disaster plan outlines actions for a catastrophic event that occurs within a facility and usually is handled within the facility depending on the size of the event. Events that involve the community use an external disaster plan. These events may or may not affect the facility.

3. **What is the role of nursing leadership and the chief nurse officer in creating an effective all-hazards disaster preparedness plan?**

   High-level administrative support and oversight are important in the development of all-hazards preparedness plan. This signifies to others the high priority that this must have within a health system.

A representative chief nurse officer and emergency care physician serving as co-chairs with the senior executive administrator are also key in the success of this endeavor. Nurse leaders have the necessary skills, competencies and experience that serve them well in taking on a primary role in disaster preparedness (Lindholm & Uden, 2001).

4. **Why is it important for each department/unit to define its role and responsibility in a disaster?**

   Each department best understands what contributions it can add to the all-hazards disaster plan. The incorporation of the expertise of each department is essential in developing a well-thought-out program. Each department can outline the detailed step-by-step processes necessary in actualization of the plan. Coordination between departments is also important.

5. **What types of addenda are needed in addition to the basic all-hazards disaster plan? Why are they important?**

   Procedures need to be outlined for specific types of disasters in addition to the basic all-hazards plan. For example, a biological disaster will require specific procedures to follow in the event of an occurrence. These procedures should provide easy-to-follow, step-by-step action plans, fact sheets, and algorithms for identifying, intervening, and notifying the appropriate authorities. With proper planning, hospitals and communities can be prepared to act quickly when such a disaster occurs.

6. **Why is it important to partner with external resources such as local hospitals, fire, police, and public health departments in creating and implementing an all-hazards disaster plan?**

   Partnering with external agencies is essential to define the roles of each in an emergency situation. Clearly defined roles can prevent duplication of efforts and enhance the coordination and orchestration of the all-hazards plan during an actual disaster.

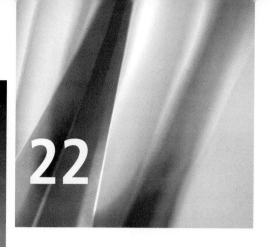

22

Evidence-Based Practice: Strategies for Nursing Leaders

STUDY FOCUS

The use of research in practice in nursing dates back to Florence Nightingale's work. Using the best evidence to guide client care improves client outcomes. *Evidence-based practice* is the integration of research and other best evidence with clinical expertise and client values in health care decision making (Sackett et al., 2000). Evidence-based practice (EBP) uses a similar process to that of utilization research. *Research utilization* is a process of using research findings as a basis for practice. Research utilization is the critique of research studies, synthesis of findings, determination of applicability of findings, review of the application with implementation of scientific findings in practice, and evaluation of practice change. *Translation research* is the scientific investigation of methods and variables that influence rate and extent of adoption of EBPs by individuals and organizations to improve care delivery (Titler & Everett, 2001). Audit and feedback involves ongoing monitoring of critical indicators of practice and periodic reporting of the data/information back to clinicians to improve client care (Davis et al., 1995; Oxman et al., 1995). The goal of *best practice* is to apply "the most recent, relevant and helpful nursing interventions in clinical practice" (John A. Hartford Center for Geriatric Nursing Excellence, 2004, p. 1).

Change champions are clinicians who continually promote EBP in their organization. *Opinion leaders* are informal leaders from the local health care setting who are viewed as important and respected sources of influence among their peer group. Change champions and opinion leaders can partner to "sell" the practice change to colleagues. The *organizational context,* the health system environment in which the proposed EBP is implemented, is an important component for implementation of EBP. The core elements that help describe the organizational context include the prevailing culture of the system, the nature of human relationships in the system and the leadership styles, and the approach of the organization to routine monitoring of

performance of systems (Kitson et al., 1998). *Outreach* or *academic detailing* is using a market strategy in which a trained individual meets one-on-one with practitioners in their setting to provide information about EBP. *Performance gap assessment* is a strategy of demonstrating an opportunity for improvement at baseline, outlining current practice related to specific indicators (Oxman et al., 1995; Schoenbaum et al., 1995). *Practice guidelines* are statements designed to assist providers and clients in making decisions about appropriate health care for special clinical circumstances (Sackett et al., 2000). *Systematic review* is a rigorous scientific process used to combine findings from research (usually randomized controlled trials) into a powerful and clinically useful report to guide practice. The *components of a systematic review* include questions being reviewed, search strategies, selection criteria/inclusion or exclusion criteria, review/appraisal methods, study description, synthesis method, results and implications (Titler, 2002a).

The best process to use when addressing clinical issues depends on the issue or problem and the extent of evidence on the topic. The movement toward EBP shows the movement to use the best available evidence to improve client outcomes. One model to guide implementation is the diffusion of innovations model (Rogers, 2003). Rogers defined diffusion of an innovation as a process by which (1) an innovation (2) is communicated through certain channels (3) over time (4) among the members of a social system.

Topic selection is an important first step in the EBP process. When a topic is chosen, clinical issues, the amount of organizational commitment, and adoptability of the practice change should be considered. When determining the appropriate topic, one should consider the following:

- Staff involvement
- Complexity of the intervention
- Interest and commitment to the topic
- Observability of impact of the practice change
- Centrality to the day-to-day work

- Technical/clinical versus administrative focus
- Pervasiveness/extent of change required
- Radicalness or extent the practice differs from the norm
- Uncertainty about outcomes
- Appeal to local power holders
- Additional resources needed

Centrality of the new practice to daily operations improves adaptation. The use of a *bottoms-up approach,* doing what is important to the staff at the bedside, improves implementations and positive outcomes. If there are competing topic areas, developing criteria for topic selection, and then establishing topic priorities can be useful (Titler, 2002a, 2002b). *Localization* is the process of revising a practice guideline to fit the needs of the clients and organization. A strategy to facilitate the use of EBP is to provide practice prompts. *Practice prompts* are just-in-time clinically relevant information to guide practice and are provided to busy clinicians.

Once a topic is selected, critique of evidence is undertaken. Many different evaluation strategies can be used, including quantitative research, qualitative research, systematic reviews, guidelines, and websites. Synthesis of evidence may lead to an organizational policy or procedure. Nationally, evidence summaries may be transmitted in the form of national guidelines. There are many different ways to disseminate the information to clinicians. Strategies to facilitate adoption include interactive education, use of opinion leaders and change champions, core group strategies, outreach or academic detailing, and use of action plans. Rewards, recognition, individual education, and feedback are other useful tools to promote adoption. Developing an action plan for each step in the EBP process, with responsible individuals and clear timelines, facilitates practice change adoption. A *reinfusion plan* or reinforcement of the practice change is also important to maintain the integrated change. Part of the reinfusion plan strategies may include brief memos with updates, sharing success, providing resources, and designing a network for communications.

Support can be garnered for EBP through data analysis and continuous monitoring and audit-feedback. Issues to be addressed in data collection and reporting include having reasonable sample size, identifying key indicators, defining the data sources, identifying the frequency of data collection, and timeframes for reporting. Feedback results facilitate adoption of practice changes through discussions and decisions among participants. Additional strategies to implement practice changes include pilot projects in which the practice change is implemented with a small number of clients and focus group discussions provide clinicians with the opportunity to provide suggestions and give feedback in a facilitated group discussion.

Organizational systems also must change to support EBP. Developing systems to facilitate implementation of EBP includes revising documentation systems, developing policy and procedures to support EBP, incorporating EBP in the quality improvement activities, and educating staff. Celebrating successes in EBP also can be a powerful tool. The celebrations should include formal recognition from high-level organizational leaders, visibility for the project champions, accessibility to practitioners within the organization, and a clear articulation of the benefits of the EBP project. A key component of EBP is building the infrastructure. A building block structure for EBP includes (1) incorporating EBP in the mission, vision, strategic plan, and performance appraisal system; (2) integrating EBP in the governance structure; (3) demonstrating the value of EBP through administrative support; and (4) establishing an EBP culture for nurse leaders who value clinical inquiry (Titler et al., 2002).

Nurse leaders are responsible for creating a culture that supports EBP. The advanced practice nurse partners with project teams and supports and facilitates project development. Development of clear action and reinfusion plans are critical to the success of practice changes. Oftentimes, innovations take 10 to 20 years to be incorporated into practice because the research findings are not disseminated in a way that clinicians can apply them easily, clinicians are not skilled in critique and synthesis of research findings, continuing education methods are ineffective in creating practice changes, clinicians do not have ready access to the research synthesis findings, and time limitations. To promote practice change adoptions, interventions must be multifaceted, interactive, and repetitive and must include positive reinforcement. Nurse leaders are challenged to build infrastructures to support EBP.

LEARNING TOOLS

Activity 1

Purpose

To discuss EBP with a registered nurse on the clinical unit in which you are completing your clinical rotation. Query a registered nurse on what clinical practice change has been implemented as part of the EBP process and the role of the nurse in implementation of the change. Ask the following questions:

- What are the benefits of the practice change?
- What are the barriers you have experienced with implementation of this change?

- Did you and the other registered nurses on the unit have input in selecting the practice change topic?
- Was the practice change a response to a critical problem or issue on the unit?
- Has the practice change made a major impact on client outcomes?
- Do you feel the practice change is important in your daily work?
- Was the change implemented incrementally or suddenly?
- How significant was the change from the routine?
- Were policies or procedures put in place before implementing the change?
- Was their adequate educational and managerial support for the change?
- Were adequate resources available to implement the change?
- Is there ongoing evaluation of the practice change?

Based on your reading of the textbook Chapter 22 on EBP, is there a correlation between administrative support for the practice change and adaptation? Is there a correlation between staff selection of the topic and implementation of the practice change? Who provides support for the staff? Were their celebrations based on successful adaptation. Is there ongoing reinfusion of the practice change?

Activity 2

Purpose

To become familiar with examples of national practice guidelines.

Introduction

Practice guidelines are statements designed to assist providers and clients in making decisions about appropriate health care for specific clinical circumstances (Sackett et al., 2000). Guidelines are developed systematically, link evidence with health outcomes, and continue to require subjective judgments when making decisions (Woolf & Atkins, 2001).

Directions

Working in a group of three, each of you should access three of the websites from the following list. Share what types of national guidelines you have accessed. Discuss how each of the national guidelines evidence is rated. Discuss how these documents can be used in practice.

Examples of Organizations Publishing Practice Guidelines

American Association of Critical-Care Nurses: *www.aacn.org*

Association of Women's Health, Obstetric and Neonatal Nurses: *www.awhonn.org*

Centers for Disease Control and Prevention: *www.cdc.gov*

Gerontological Nursing Intervention Research Center (at the University of Iowa): *www.nursing.uiowa.edu/centers/gnirc/*

National Guideline Clearinghouse: *www.guideline.gov*

Oncology Nursing Society: *www.ons.org*

Registered Nurses' Association of Ontario: *www.rnao.org*

The Joanna Briggs Institute: *www.joannabriggs.edu.au/about/home.php*

U.S. Preventive Services Task Force, Agency for Healthcare Research and Quality: *www.ahrq.gov/clinic/uspstfix.htm*

CASE STUDY

Alisha Hoanick is a registered nurse on the surgical unit in a 400-bed hospital in Alma, Nebraska. She recently attended a national conference titled the "Surgical Options for Breast Cancer Patients." A breakout session described an interdisciplinary team approach to discussing treatment options for breast care for women who were diagnosed with breast cancer. The team consisted of an oncologist, radiologist, clinical nurse specialist, surgeon, plastic surgeon, and the client. The conference presenter provided several references to studies that compared key outcomes for those women who had participated in the interdisciplinary team conference and those who did not. Results demonstrated positive outcomes for participants of interdisciplinary teams.

Case Study Questions

1. Nurse Hoanick is unsure whether this is an appropriate EBP project, but she has heard the clinical nurse specialist talking about practice changes. Whom should she contact to discuss her idea?

2. What is the process that organizations use to determine priority topics for EBP?

3. What organizational infrastructure should be in place to support EBP?

4. What are strategies to recognize success in adaptation of EBP?

5. What is the building block approach to EBP?

LEARNING RESOURCES

Discussion Questions

1. Describe the four building blocks of integrating evidence-based practice into an organization.

2. Define evidence-based practice and research utilization. Describe how these two terms are different.

3. What is a change champion and an opinion leader? What is their role in facilitating adaptation of evidence-based practice?

4. How does an organization determine what topic to select for the evidence-based practice project/process?

5. Describe several strategies that could be used to communicate the practice change?

Study Questions

Matching: Write the correct response in front of each term.

_____ 1. Evidence-based practice

_____ 2. Research utilization

_____ 3. Translation research

_____ 4. Audit and feedback

_____ 5. Best practice

_____ 6. Change champions

_____ 7. Opinion leaders

_____ 8. Organizational context

_____ 9. Outreach or academic detailing

_____ 10. Performance gap assessment

_____ 11. Practice guideline

_____ 12. Systematic review

A. A process of using research findings as a basis for practice

B. Integration of research and other best evidence with clinical expertise and client values in health care decision making

C. Applying the most recent, relevant nursing interventions in clinical practice

D. The scientific investigation of methods and variables that influence rate and extent of adoption of EBP by individuals and organizations to improve clinical services

E. Informal leaders from the local health care setting who are viewed as important and respected sources of influence among their peer group

F. Statement designed to assist provider and client in making decisions about appropriate health care for specific clinical circumstances

G. Health system environment in which the proposed EBP is to be implemented

H. Practitioners from the local peer group who continually promote the EBP

I. A strategy of demonstrating an opportunity for improvement at baseline outlining current practice related to specific indicators

J. Ongoing monitoring of critical indicators of practice and providing periodic reporting of the data/information back to the clinicians responsible for client care

K. A rigorous scientific process used to combine findings from research into a powerful and clinically useful report to guide practice

L. The use of a marketing strategy in which a trained individual meets one-on-one with practitioners in their setting to provide information about the EBP

REFERENCES

Davis, D. A., Thomson, M. A., Oxman, A. D., & Haynes, R. B. (1995). Changing physician performance: A systematic review of the effect of continuing medical education strategies. *Journal of the American Medical Association, 274*(9), 700-705.

John A. Hartford Center for Geriatric Nursing Excellence. (2004). *Best practices.* Iowa City: The University of Iowa College of Nursing. Retrieved March 2, 2004, from *www.nursing.uiowa.edu/hartford/nurse/bestrpractice/best_practice.htm*

Kitson, A., Harvey, G., & McCormack, B. (1998). Enabling the implementation of evidence based practice: A conceptual framework. *Quality in Health Care, 7*(3), 149-158.

Oxman, A. D., Thomson, M. A., Davis, D. A. & Haynes, R. B. (1995). No magic bullets: A systematic review of 102 trials of interventions to improve professional practice. *Canadian Medical Association Journal, 153*(10), 1423-1431.

Rogers, E. (2003). *Diffusion of innovation* (5th ed.). New York: Free Press.

Sackett, D. L., Straus, S. E., Richardson, W. S., Rosenberg, W., & Haynes, R. B.(2000). *Evidence-based medicine: How to practice and teach EBM.* London: Churchill Livingstone.

Schoenbaum, S. C., Sundwall, D. N. Bergman, D., Buckle, J. M., Chernov, A., George, J. H. C., et al. (1995). *Using clinical practice guidelines to evaluate quality of care. Volume 2: Methods.* Rockville, MD: U.S. Department of Health and Human Services, Public Health Service, Agency for Health Care Research and Quality.

Titler, M. G. (2002a). Use of research in practice. In G. LoBiondo-Wood & J. Haber (Eds.), *Nursing research* (5th ed.). St Louis: Mosby.

Titler, M. G. (2002b). *Toolkit for promoting evidence-based practice.* Iowa City: Research, Quality and Outcomes Management, Department of Nursing Service and Patient Care, The University of Iowa Hospitals and Clinics.

Titler, M. G., Cullen, L., & Ardery, G. (2002). Evidence-based practice: An administrative perspective. *Reflections on Nursing Leadership, 28*(2), 26-27, 46.

Titler, M. G., & Everett, L. Q. (2001). Translating research into practice: Considerations for critical care investigators. *Critical Care Nursing Clinics of North American, 13*(4), 587-604.

Woolf, S. H., & Atkins, D. (2001). The evolving role of prevention in health care. Contributions of the U.S. Preventive Services Task Force. *American Journal of Preventive Medicine, 20*(3, Suppl. 1), 13-20.

SUPPLEMENTAL READINGS

Busby, A. (2004). Creating nursing research opportunities in rural healthcare facilities. *Journal of Nursing Care Quality, 19*(2), 162-168.

Maramba, P. J., Richards, S., & Larrabee, J. H. (2004). Discharge planning process: Applying a model for evidence-based practice. *Journal of Nursing Care Quality, 19*(2), 123-129.

Melnyk, B. M. (2004). Integrating levels of evidence into clinical decision making. *Pediatric Nursing, 30*(4) 323-325.

Olade, R. A. (2004). Evidence-based practice and research utilization activities among rural nurses. *Journal of Nursing Scholarship, 36*(3), 220-225.

Rycroft-Malone, J. (2004). The PARIHS framework: A framework for guiding the implementation of evidence-based practice. *Journal of Nursing Care Quality, 19*(4), 297-304.

Chapter 22: Evidence-Based Practice: Strategies for Nursing Leaders (pp. 461-478)

1. **What process is used to identify topics for development of an evidence-based practice project?**

   Clinical interest or issues, the amount of organizational commitment, and the adoptability of the practice changes are important aspects to consider when choosing topics. Several processes may be used to identify topics for development such as quality/performance improvement or conducting research.

2. **What implementation strategies are effective in supporting adoption of a practice change?**

   Implementation strategies that support successful practice changes include the following:

   - Staff involvement in topic selection
   - Minimal complexity of the intervention
   - Staff buy-in
   - Practices that show a direct impact on client care
   - Centrality to the day-to-day work
   - "Bottoms-up" staff approach
   - Small extent of change required
   - Extent that the practice differs from the norm
   - Certain/clear expected outcomes
   - Appeal to local power holders
   - Additional sources needed

3. **What are the four building blocks used to develop the organizational structures supporting an evidence-based practice environment? How can nurses put these in place?**

   Titler and colleagues (2002) outline four building blocks for the development of organizational structures supporting an evidence-based practice environment, as follows:

   1. Incorporation of evidence-based practice terminology into the mission, vision, strategic plan, and performance appraisals of staff
   2. Integration of the work of evidence-based practice into the governance structure of nursing departments and the health care system
   3. Demonstration of the values of evidence-based practice through administrative behaviors of the chief nurse executive
   4. Establishment of explicit expectations about evidence-based practice for nursing leaders who create a culture that values clinical inquiry

4. **What is the role of the nurse manager in developing an evidence-based practice culture?**

   The role of the nurse manager is critical to the success of the project and its outcomes. The nurse manager is responsible for developing the unit culture by setting expectations for the unit, discussing the importance of the work of evidence-based practice with unit nurses and other disciplines, supporting the team with time to work on the project, being a project cheerleader, tracking progress, and facilitating the movement of the project through appropriate committees, along with allocation of resources as needed.

5. **What current nursing issues can be addressed through translation research?**

   Current nursing issues such as the nursing shortage, the effects of collaborative practice on client outcomes, and level of education for entry into practice are some issues that may be addressed through translation research. Each of these issues possibly could have an impact on the promotion of adoption of evidence-based practices.

6. **How is evidence-based practice used in a multidisciplinary team?**

   Evidence-based practices may be used within a multidisciplinary team to make clinical and operational decisions. Other tools such as clinical pathways, preprinted orders, and other clinical aides can be developed from these practices.

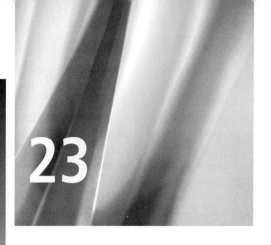

23 Motivation

STUDY FOCUS

Motivation is central to the energy or drive needed to accomplish a task. Motivation is the ability to get individuals to do what you want them to do, when and how you want it done. Motivation is a sense of energy, enthusiasm, and goal directedness. *Motivation* describes factors that energize human behavior, describes the mechanism of how and where the behavior will occur, and encompasses insights on how the behavior is sustained over time.

Motivation is a complex process requiring strong leadership and management skills to enhance employee productivity creatively. Nurse managers of health care organizations are faced with trying to increase employee productivity while maintaining or decreasing labor costs. An *activity* is the basic unit of behavior or a discrete plan. Individuals perform activities based on their *motives* or *needs,* what they desire or want, their drives or impulses. Nurse managers are challenged to motivate employees to work in a way that achieves organizational goals expeditiously. Energizing, facilitating, and maintaining high levels of employee productivity can be problematic. *Motivation to work* is the degree to which members of an organization are willing to work.

Traditionally, managers of bureaucratic organizations used direct supervision to control employees; whereas managers using a human relations approach in decentralized organizations use the methods of participation and cooperation. Many motivational models have been developed to help guide managers in motivating employees to maximum productivity. Many schemes exist to categorize the plethora of motivational theories. A common method is to categorize motivational theories as a content theory or a process theory. A *content theory* describes behavior and factors that exist within the individual, whereas a *process theory* describes behaviors as a function of decision making and includes environmental factors that motivate individuals (Porter et al., 2003). Motivation can be viewed as follows:

$$Performance = Ability \times Motivation$$

The *needs satisfaction model* states that there is a felt need followed by an activity or behavioral response. Then a process results to decrease frustration and meet individual needs. Individual needs arise from internal and external motivating forces. *Internal motivation* is a personal desire to achieve and accomplish. *External motivation* is a stimulus external to an individual that generates an incentive to complete an activity.

Maslow's hierarchy of needs theory is based on levels of human needs starting with basic needs and ending with self-actualization. Maslow's hierarchy has five levels, beginning with physiological drives, progressing to safety and security needs, to belonging needs, to esteem and ego needs, and to self-actualization. Maslow's work was refined by Alderfer, who collapsed the five levels to three: existence, relatedness, and growth needs.

Herzberg's motivation-hygiene theory describes two categories of needs, hygiene or maintenance factors and motivators. *Hygiene* or *maintenance factors* are security, status, money, working conditions, interpersonal relations, supervision, and policies and administration. *Motivators* include the need for growth and development, advancement, increased responsibility, challenging work, recognition, and achievement. Motivators encourage superior performance, whereas hygiene factors maintain satisfaction. This is considered a "job enrichment" theory.

McClelland's theory describes three basic needs: achievement, power, and affiliation. McClelland's theory lends itself to self-assessment. Nursing leaders were found to have a leadership motive pattern with no need to moderately high levels of need for power, low levels of affiliation needs, high levels of self-control needs, and minimal achievement motivation.

159

Operant conditioning is a classic approach to motivation focusing on how behavior and motivation are shaped by the external environment. Individuals respond to stimuli they perceive as rewarding and avoid stimuli that they perceive as undesirable. This theoretical perspective emphasizes the process of shaping behavior through environmental stimuli such as rewards.

Expectancy theories, including Vroom's, examine the attractiveness of an outcome, a valence, and the likelihood that the outcome will occur. In these theories, employees assess the value of an outcome and the degree to which individuals perceive that they can attain the reward. Then they decide whether they will expend the energy to perform the activity.

The most prominent motivational theory today is the *goal-setting theory.* The basic premise is that goals serve as targets for human behavior. Difficult, specific goals motivate the individual to search for strategies for effective performance. Self-efficacy, a person's confidence, and sense of capability in accomplishing goals are enhanced by the goals set before an individual.

Job characteristics theory examines the core dimension of any job, the psychological state of the individual, and personal work outcomes. Core job dimensions of the theory include task identity, task significance, skill variety, and autonomy and feedback. The core job dimensions interact with three critical psychological states: the meaningfulness of the work, responsibility for outcomes, and the actual result of the work. The outcomes may improve productivity, enhance quality, decrease turnover and absenteeism, and improve personal and professional job satisfaction.

McGregor published *theory X* and *theory Y.* The basic assumptions of theory X are that employees are lazy and nonproductive and require close supervision. The theory portrays employees as resistant to autonomy and unable to assume responsibility. In contrast, the basic assumptions of theory Y are that employees enjoy autonomy and need only guidance as opposed to supervision. Employees are depicted as creative, self-directed individuals who embrace responsibility and autonomy.

The classic *Hawthorne studies* were conducted in 1924 at the Hawthorne plant of Western Electric, outside of Chicago. The studies examined the motivation and productivity of assembly line workers. Several variables—including improving lighting, scheduling breaks, providing lunches, and shortening work hours—were studied with control and experimental groups. To the researchers' surprise, all the variables had a significant positive impact on employee productivity. Even after all the variables were withdrawn, productivity climbed. Study outcomes showed that interpersonal relationships were also a significant factor in motivating employees.

Involving workers in planning, organizing, and controlling their work increased workers' positive cooperation. To create circumstances in which individuals are more likely to become self-motivated is important. In creating a positive work culture, employers can incorporate the following list of needs that employees expect of their employers (McConnell, 1998):

- Capable
- Respected leadership
- Decent and safe surroundings
- Acceptance as a member of a group
- Recognition and other feedback
- Fair treatment
- A reasonable sense of job security
- Knowledge of the results of individual effort
- Knowledge of the organizational policies, rules, and regulations
- Recognition for special effort
- Respect for individual beliefs; assurance that others are doing their fair share of the work
- Fair monetary compensation

Organizational commitment is the intensity of an individual's identification with and involvement in the employing organization. Employee involvement is the participation in decision making. Employees are key assets in the work environment. Managers must use creative strategies to maximize the human talents and achieve high levels of productivity in their organizations.

Interpersonal relationships with colleagues are ranked as the most important factor related to motivation. Critical motivating factors include recognition at work, the amount of responsibility, and the nature of the work, the quality of the work environment, rewards, part of the decision making, and feelings of being valued. Work experiences are a strong predictor of affective feeling about work. Magnet hospitals are one strategy to create a positive work environment that supports professional practice, increases positive working environments, increases employee commitment, improves employer retention, and enhances client care (McClure & Hinshaw, 2002).

Managers who use the art of leading and managing groups of professionals use creative, interesting, and continuous improvement strategies to make individuals feel good about what they do. Generalizations from motivational theory include the following:

- The complexities of human behavior likely will never be explained by one simple theory.
- Nurses are aware of individual differences as they work with clients.

- Goals are important regardless of the task at hand.
- Incentives and rewards are always important.
- Equity is important.

Current issues and trends include increasing use of information technologies and the rapid diversification in society.

LEARNING TOOLS

Role Play: Motivating Subordinates to Improve Productivity

Character One: Jo Ellen Mae is the nurse manager of a neurorespiratory unit of a medium-sized hospital in Beaumont, Texas. Nurse Mae believes in rewarding staff for superior performance and tailors rewards based on individual accomplishments.

Character Two: Bob Segar is a registered nurse who was hired 10 years ago and has been doing an adequate, but not exemplary, job.

Character Three: Jon Nemy is a registered nurse who was hired 5 years ago and who consistently exhibits superior performance in client care.

Character Four: Jane James is a registered nurse who was hired 1 year ago and consistently performs well.

Nurse Mae is preparing annual reviews (performance appraisals) on all of her employees. She knows that Nurses Segar, Nemy, and James are best friends and share information with one another. Nurse Mae wants to reward Nurses Nemy and James for their exemplary performance but does not want Nurse Segar to be disgruntled. She decides to give special merit pay to Nurse Nemy and award him the neurological nurse of the year because he consistently performs outstandingly. She puts Nurse James' name in for the hospital's professional nurse of the year award and sends her to a national neurosurgical nursing convention in California. One morning, Nurse Mae enters the neurorespiratory unit to see Nurses James, Segar, and Nemy arguing loudly in the conference room. Upon entering the conference room, Nurse Segar aggressively approaches Nurse Mae and demands an explanation for her poor choices as a manager. He demands to know why his 10 years of loyal service were not recognized. What should Nurse Mae do?

Role-Play Questions

1. What should Nurse Mae say? Should she give Nurse Segar a reward?

2. What strategies can be used to motivate Nurse Segar to work harder?

3. How can Nurse Mae manage the situation to empower all three individuals?

Role-Play Worksheet

Characters	Student Assigned
Jo Ellen Mae, the nurse manager	_____
Bob Segar, registered nurse of 10 years	_____
Jon Nemy, registered nurse of 5 years	_____
Jane James, registered nurse of 1 year	_____

Which character have you been assigned?

What are your character's goals in this situation?

How can the other characters assist you in achieving your goals?

What might the other characters do to hinder you in achieving your goals?

What strategies and probes do you plan to use in this situation?

CASE STUDY

Jackie Burdock is a charge nurse on the 11 AM to 7 PM shift at Middleville Hospital in Little Rock, Arkansas. Her leadership style includes directing employees to accomplish tasks. She feels that the nurse's aides, licensed practical nurses, and orderlies are lazy and do only what they are required to do. Nurse Burdock requires them to report to her any client changes, large or small, because she feels that they cannot handle responsibility. She has developed detailed, step-by-step procedures for her staff to follow to prevent mistakes.

Case Study Questions

1. From which motivational theory is Nurse Burdock practicing?

2. What are the characteristics of this theory?

3. Is this an effective theory to practice leadership behaviors?

4. What motivational theory might you use when assigned the job of charge nurse?

LEARNING RESOURCES

Discussion Questions

1. What types of rewards motivate nurses to improve productivity?

2. What did the Hawthorne studies show? Why were the results of the Hawthorne studies important to managers?

3. What is the difference between internal and external motivation? How can a nurse manager capitalize on these?

4. What is the difference between the needs satisfaction model and Vroom's theory?

5. How can you apply Maslow's hierarchy of needs theory to nursing management?

6. In an information age, what is the nature of the work needed in health care organizations? How does the nature of work differ from the industrial age to the information age?

Study Questions

Matching: Write the letter of the correct response in front of each term.

_____ 1. Motivation

_____ 2. Motives

_____ 3. External motivation

_____ 4. Activity

_____ 5. Internal motivation

_____ 6. Vroom's theory

_____ 7. McClelland's theory

A. A unit of human behavior

B. Identifies individual's basic needs

C. Represents valence, instrumentality, and expectancy

D. Energizing and eliciting human activity

E. Wants, desires, and drives

F. Individuals who provide incentives for activity

G. Accomplishments arising from within the individual

True or False: Circle the correct answer.

T   F   8. Organizational commitment is a strong involvement and identification with the employing organization.

T   F   9. The reward that has been found to be most effective in increasing employee productivity is pay.

T   F   10. Herzberg's motivation-hygiene theory describes three basic needs: achievement, power, and affiliation.

T   F   11. Motives are the wants, desires, and drives of individuals.

T   F   12. Traditional bureaucratic organizations use participation to enhance employee morale.

REFERENCES

McClure, M. L., & Hinshaw, A. S. (2002). *Magnet hospitals revisited: Attraction and retention of professional nurses.* Washington, DC: American Nurses Publishing.

McConnell, C. R. (1998). Employee involvement: motivation or manipulation? *Health Care Supervisor, 16*(3), 69-85.

Porter, L., Bigley, G. A., & Steers, R. M. (Eds.). (2003). *Motivation and work behaviour* (7th ed.). Boston: McGraw-Hill/Irwin.

SUPPLEMENTAL READINGS

Asselin, M. E., Baker, B. J., Bullinger, R., & Perry, D. (2003). Motivating LPNs. *Nursing Management, 34*(8), 40-45.

Cohen, S. (2003). Motivation: Your key IC ingredient. *Nursing Management, 34*(6), 10.

Greggs-McQuilkin, D. (2004). The power of self-motivation. *Medsurg Nursing, 13*(2), 73.

Joshua-Amadi, M. (2003). Recruitment and retention in the NHS: A study of motivation. *Nursing Management, 9*(9), 14-19.

Ossman, S. S. (2004). Motivational interviewing: A process to encourage behavioural change. *Nephrology Nursing Journal, 31*(3), 346-347.

Chapter 23: Motivation (pp. 479-500)

1. **How do you stay motivated to love nursing for the rest of your life?**

   It is important for nurses to be cognizant of the factors that provide them internal and external motivation. Ask yourself, which values, beliefs, and assumptions motivate you to love nursing. How have they changed? Will the same factors motivate you in the future? What impact will career advancement, increased responsibility, and work challenges have on your motivation?

2. **Does loving nursing guarantee quality care?**

   Although loving nursing cannot guarantee quality care, the nurse's motivation is a powerful influence on the provision of quality care. The love of nursing may serve as an internal force that motivates nurses to provide excellent care, which in turn may generate external reinforcement from positive client outcomes and professional satisfaction.

3. **What is the motivation to enter nursing as a career? Is this changing?**

   Individuals enter nursing for a variety of reasons. Some individuals are motivated by the need for recognition, acknowledgment, status, or economic compensation, whereas others are motivated by the need for autonomy, a sense of doing important work, helping others, the need for competence, or self-actualization. Motivation to enter nursing as a career may change depending on expanded roles, educational requirements, professional recognition, societal contribution, and competitive salaries.

4. **How does real-world nursing practice compare with what motivation theories say?**

   Many motivation theories can be applied to real-world nursing practice. For example, nurses use the need satisfaction model in the provision of care, and they use Maslow's hierarchy of needs theory to formulate effective teaching strategies. Herzberg's motivation-hygiene theory fits well in describing job satisfaction and dissatisfaction.

   Real-world nursing practice is affected by challenging work, collegial relationships, and professional/societal recognition. To ascend the self-actualization hierarchy, nurses must perceive safe working conditions, administrative support, and financial security.

5. **What positive incentives are most important to nurses? To you personally?**

   Positive incentives vary depending on the needs of the individual nurse. The love of the work itself is often a significant motivator for nurses. Positive incentives may include providing quality client care, client advocacy, professional acknowledgment, and a challenging work environment. What professional, personal, and financial incentives are important to you?

6. **What are the elements of a motivating environment?**

   Rantz and colleagues (1996) found that interpersonal relationship with peers at work was important to nurses. Recognition at work, the amount of responsibility, and the nature of the work itself also were identified as critical motivating factors. Tzeng (2002) discovered that nurses who felt rewarded had positions where they were involved in decision making and felt valued by the hospital. Elements of a motivating environment include explicit goals, clear expectations, direct feedback and reinforcement, elimination of threats, individual responsibility, rewards, and trust. The nurse leader's job is to create an environment that fosters motivation by identifying what nurses need to succeed, to be satisfied, and to feel what they do is an important service to clients.

7. **Is it manipulative or Machiavellian deliberately to plan and implement rewards and incentives to get others to perform? Do you ever do this?**

The art of leading and managing groups of professional nurses requires creative, interesting, and innovative ways to make individuals feel good about what they are doing. Although the rewards and incentives can be viewed as manipulative, the relationship is mutually beneficial in which recognition is provided in exchange for quality performance. Showing nurses that the work and input they provide are valued is key. Personal, professional, and economic rewards have been shown to be powerful motivators in nursing.

8. **Under cost-containment pressures, what is the effect on nurses of relying on recognition as the organizational motivation strategy?**

Cost-containment pressures may create dissatisfaction in nurses who rely on economic rewards as an entitlement or as a motivator to perform. Productivity may decrease while perceptions of betrayal and cynicism increase. Nurse leaders may need to develop and implement personal and professional recognition programs to compensate for the loss of economic rewards.

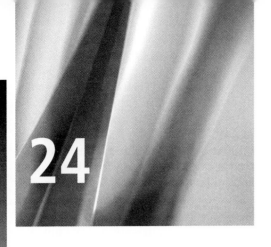

24

Power and Conflict

STUDY FOCUS

Nurses often view power with a negative connotation. With a fragmented health care delivery system, nurses must feel comfortable with using power to influence health care decisions. This is especially important when $1.6 trillion were spent on health care in 2002, which was 14.9% of the gross domestic product (Centers for Medicare & Medicaid Services, 2004). Nursing is the largest health care profession and could use this power to influence and facilitate positive change in the health care system. *Power* is the ability to influence another's actions in order to attain a scarce resource. The *three formal dimensions of power* are relational, dependence, and sanctioning aspects (Bacharach & Lawler, 1980). *Relational aspect* of power describes power as a property of a social relationship; *dependency aspect* describes power residing in the other's dependency (mutual dependence); and *sanctioning aspect* describes power relationships in relation to direct manipulation of other's outcomes. *Reciprocal interdependence* is where the output of operation X is the input of operation Y, and the output of operation Y is the input to operation X. *Empowerment* is giving responsibility and accountability to individuals to complete tasks. The two meanings to empowerment are (1) the transfer of actual power and (2) the inspiring of self-confidence. Empowerment initiatives take two forms: the *relational approach*, improving performance by decentralizing and delegating power, authority, and decision making; and the *motivational approach*, facilitating open communication and inspirational goal setting.

Two major content dimensions of power are authority and influence (Bacharach & Lawler, 1980). The *eight forms of influence behavior* are assertiveness, ingratiation, rationality, sanctions, exchange, upward appeal, blocking, and coalitions. *Assertiveness* is standing up for your rights without infringing on others' rights. *Ingratiation* is praising someone for a job well done in hopes of gaining recognition for your support.

Rationality is the logical presentation of ideas. *Sanctions* include the use of threats and negative activities to gain a desired response. *Exchanges* are trades for services or goods in which both parties receive something desired. *Upward appeals* involve the act of seeking opinion of a higher authority about a decision. *Blocking* is stopping someone's activities or progress by threatening them, ignoring them, or physically interfering with their progress. *Coalitions* are the banding together of individuals for the purpose of presenting a single voice.

French and Raven (1959) identify *five sources of power. Reward power* is the use of praise, pay, promotions, or advancements. *Coercive power* is the use of force such as threatening to fire an individual or to discipline the individual. *Expert power* is based on knowledge, competence, and skill. *Referent power* is based on a person's interpersonal appeal, charisma, and image. *Legitimate power* is based on the job title or position a person holds. *Other sources of power* include *connection,* a network of powerful persons or information sources; *informational power,* the control of special information, and *group decision-making power,* the creative synergy and force when groups work in a united front. *Persuasive power* is the skill in making rational appeals. Position power consists of legitimate, reward, coercive, and information power; whereas personal power consists of expert, referent, and persuasive power (Yukl & Falbe, 1991). Kanter (1977) developed the structural theory of organizational behavior, which asserts that with sufficient power, organizational tasks and goals will be realized. Recognition is the visibility of an employee's accomplishments among peers and supervisors. Relationships with individuals at higher hierarchical levels confers approval and prestige, whereas peer networks provide reputation and "grapevine" information (Kanter, 1977). Higher levels of structural empowerment are associated with higher levels of organizational commitment (Laschinger et al., 1997), increased job autonomy (Sabiston & Laschinger, 1995), and increased job

165

satisfaction (Laschinger & Havens, 1997). Basic methods of acquiring and maintaining power include gaining control of resources, obtaining and controlling information, and establishing favorable relationships. Keys to gaining power are being sensitive to power, taking calculated risks, recognizing that any and all actions affect power, avoiding actions that decrease power, and trying to move up in the organizational hierarchy. Structural determinants of power within organizations are derived from providing resources, dependence, coping with uncertainty, being irreplaceable, ability to affect the decision process, and shared consensus within the organizational subunit (Pfeffer, 1981).

The strategic contingencies theory of intraorganizational power describes the conditions for the differentiation of power among organizational subunits (Hickson et al., 1971). The main difference between power and leadership is goal compatibility. Power requires dependence and focuses on intimidation but does not require goal compatibility, whereas leadership requires congruence between the goals of the leader and followers and focuses on downward influence. Leadership focuses on answers, whereas power focuses on gaining compliance. Leaders who are effective are able to manage uncertainty. Areas of uncertainty in health care include improving quality of care and client safety, expanding of the aging population, advancing technology, increasing number of chronic illnesses, emerging diseases, increasing cost and limited access to health care, and being central and controlling substitutability of nurses.

Conflict is natural and can be a useful growth experience for individuals. *Conflict* arises between two or more individuals from a perceived threat to their wants, needs, feelings, behaviors, or attitudes. *Organizational conflict* arises from competition for the limited available resources in an organization. *Job conflict* is the struggle between individual and organizational goals. *Social conflict* is struggle between individuals or groups over values and claims to scarce resources, status, or power (Coser, 1956). Factors that underlie conflict are interdependence, differences in goals, and differences in perception. *Interpersonal conflict* is interference with goal attainment and negative emotional reactions to perceived disagreements between interdependent parties (Barki & Hartwick, 2001). *Competitive conflict* is where rules are followed with the goal of winning, whereas *disruptive conflict* is engaging in activities to attack, defeat, or eliminate an opponent. Conflict occurs because of discord between one individual's values, philosophies, and beliefs and

those of other individuals. When conflict is handled positively, there can be personal or professional growth; improved relationships; and increased productivity, creativity, and satisfaction. When it is handled poorly, fear, retaliation, anger, and hostility are the result.

Conflict can be categorized three ways: intrapersonal, interpersonal, and intergroup. *Intrapersonal conflict* arises within an individual from two competing demands or ideas. *Interpersonal conflict* is the battle between two or more individuals arising from miscommunication or differences in values. *Intergroup conflict* is the result of struggles between two or more groups. The *three broad types of conflict* are *relationship* (awareness of interpersonal incompatibilities), *task* (awareness of differences in viewpoints), and *process* (awareness of controversies about task accomplishments).

Pondy (1967) has identified *four stages of conflict.* The first stage is *latent (antecedent conditions),* in which are the conditions that begin stirring the pot of discontent. Examples could include the competition for resources, differing goals, or a lack of individual responsibility. The second stage, *perception and feeling,* is where perceived conflict emerges and emotions become charged. During the third stage, *behavior manifestation (manifest),* an individual has a felt conflict and expresses these emotions. The individual initiates behavior to correct or alleviate the felt conflict by negatively talking about the other individuals, by initiating actions to correct the situation, or by removing himself or herself from the uncomfortable environment. Manifest behavior occurs when the individual acts and resolves or suppresses the conflict. The fourth and final stage, *aftermath* to the conflict, occurs when there is an effect, either resolution to the conflict or a cyclic process in which increasing antecedent behaviors take place.

Many conflict models can be found in the literature. Filley's (1975) conflict model is composed of six stages: antecedent conditions, perceived conflict, felt conflict, manifest behavior, resolution or suppression, and conflict aftermath. The Thomas (1976) process model has five major concepts: frustration, conceptualization, behavior, other's reaction (interaction), and outcome. The Robbins (2003) model is composed of five stages: potential opposition, cognition and personalization, intentions, behavior, and functional or dysfunctional outcomes. Common elements of these conflict models are (1) causes that occur before the conflict, (2) perception of conflict followed by an affective state, and (3) outcomes such as resolution or aftermath consequences. The underlying sources of organizational conflict include competition for scarce resources, drives for autonomy, and divergence of subunit goals. The potential sources of conflict in nursing include unclear roles, conflicts of interest, communication barriers, dependence on one another, relationship differences, response to regulation, unresolved prior conflict, and unique health care conflicts. Three general dimensions are thought to underlie conflict: disagreement, interference, and negative emotions (Barki & Hartwick, 2001).

Positive outcomes of conflict resolution in nursing include better client care and satisfaction, improved relationships and communication, personal and professional growth, efficient use of resources, increased staff satisfaction, and improved collaboration. *Negative outcomes* include hostility, gossip, burnout, lack of professional growth, increased turnover, lack of professional collaboration, and less efficient use of resources. Two conflict scales are available to measure conflict: the Rahim Organizational Conflict Inventory—I and the Perceived Conflict Scale. These tools can be used to conduct a conflict assessment.

Effectively managing conflict is essential for positive work groups. The *three frameworks for resolving conflict* are defensive, compromise, and creative. The *defensive mode* leaves individuals feeling losses and wins. Strategies for defensively addressing conflict are separating the competing parties, suppressing conflict, restricting the conflict, smoothing over the conflict through change, and avoiding the conflict. A *compromise mode* solves conflict through negotiation until a mutually acceptable solution is reached in which each party receives something and forfeits something. The creative *problem-solving mode* is the best possible scenario, in which all parties gain and do not feel a loss. In *creative conflict resolution, a five-step process* is used: initiating discussion at a set time in private, understanding and respecting differences, empathizing with each party, engaging in an assertive discussion, and agreeing on a solution.

Conflict resolution techniques include *avoiding* (avoiding conflict at all cost), *withholding* (opting out of participation), *smoothing over* (maintaining surface harmony), *accommodating* (preserving harmony), *forcing* (voting on it), *competing* (winning at all cost), *compromising* (splitting the difference), *confronting* (using "I" and "you" messages), *collaborating* (working together), *bargaining* (working together to benefit everyone), and *problem solving* (finding a workable solution for all). Outcomes for conflict resolution include win-win, win-lose, and lose-lose. *Win-lose* is when one party wins without concern about the other. *Win-win* occurs when both parties are satisfied with the outcome, and *lose-lose* is when neither party gets

what he or she wants. Nurse managers are challenged to build positive interdisciplinary work teams, and the process usually requires conflict management and resolution. One group strategy nurses have used to manage conflict is collective bargaining, which is aimed at preventing total control by employers over work conditions, skill mix, and compensation.

Face negotiation theory explains differences in responses to conflict using cultural backgrounds (Ting-Toomey, 1988; Ting-Toomey & Kurogi, 1998). The dimension of self-construal (self-image) is central to this theory in terms of independent and interdependent self. In high-power distance cultures, differences in treatment based on status are accepted; whereas in low-power distance cultures, differences in treatment based on status are less accepted.

Negotiation is an important concept in conflict resolution. *Negotiation includes three mechanisms: bargaining power* (another person's inducement to agree to terms), *distributive bargaining* (what side gains at the others expense), *integrative bargaining* (problem solving to reach a mutually acceptable solution), and *mediation* (each party acknowledges injury to the other but are also dependence on each other). Distributive bargaining tends to be more competitive, whereas integrative bargaining is more cooperative. *Principled negotiation* is a process in which negotators use five fundamental principles to negotiate in a collaborative fashion. *These principles are* separating the person from the problem; negotiating about interests, not positions; inventing options for mutual gain; insisting on objective decision criteria; and knowing the best alternative to a negotiated agreement. *Five styles of handling interpersonal conflict* are (1) avoiding, (2) obliging, (3) compromising, (4) integrating, and (5) dominating. Studies have shown that avoiding and compromising were the most frequently used conflict-handling intentions in nursing.

Organizational conflict is interpersonal conflict generated by styles of management, rules, procedures and communication channels. Organizational conflict can be assessed by looking at the big picture using four factors: (1) examining behavioral predisposition of individuals, (2) assessing social pressure in the environment, (3) reviewing the incentive structure of the organization, and (4) evaluating the rules and procedures. *Three strategies can be used to resolve organizational conflicts:* (1) bargaining; (2) using rules, procedures, and administrative control; and (3) using a system integrator. The *sources of conflict* in organizations include power, communication, goals, values, resources, roles, and personalities. Nurses can experience conflict in the form of *role overload,* in which they are required to do the work of other health care disciplines; in role ambiguity, in which the nurses' responsibilities and duties expand without a job description change; or role stress, in which a nurse's boss has one idea about the job and the nurse has a different perception. *Burnout* is often a result of role overload. *Successful strategies to manage conflict* includes reversing the negative emotion associated with the conflict; choosing an appropriate approach to manage the situation; and using good communication skills. *The six types of power* exercised by nurses are (1) *transformational power* (assisting individuals to transform their self-image), (2) *integrative power* (helping clients to return to normal lives), (3) *advocacy power* (removing obstacles), (4) *healing power* (creating a healing climate and relationship), (5) *participative/affirmative power* (drawing strength from caring interactions), and (6) *problem-solving power* (being sensitive to cues and searching for solutions).

In organizations, formal power is attained through position. Nurse managers must use power to be effective in leading the staff in care delivery. To be powerful, one must be able to access support, information, and resources and must be aware of opportunities to seize advancement or achievements. Those who use power positively resolve conflicts with creativity, innovation, and novelty, whereas those who use power ineffectively create barriers, decrease efficiency, and encourage distrust and uncomfortable work environments. Strategies to gain and maintain power include gaining access to information, controlling resources, accessing key decision makers, and networking with powerful individuals. Empowering others promotes excellence and motivates others. Empowerment—a method to improve productivity, lower costs, and raise customer satisfaction—is an important strategy for organizational productivity.

LEARNING TOOLS

Self-Assessment: Power

Power Inventory
Power is an important aspect of our personal and professional lives. Understanding your own level of comfort with power will help you gain support and resources in your work environment.

Directions

1. Write a brief response to the statement under each item.
2. Circle a number on the continuum that best corresponds with how you view yourself. (1 = Strongly agree; 2 = Moderately agree; 3 = Agree; 4 = Somewhat agree; 5 = Disagree)

1. I am sensitive to where power   1   2   3   4   5
exists in organizations.

_____

_____

_____

2. I feel that power can be used   1   2   3   4   5
effectively without disadvantaging individuals.

_____

_____

_____

3. I feel comfortable taking risks.   1   2   3   4   5

_____

_____

_____

4. I try to obtain additional   1   2   3   4   5
resources in my work setting.

_____

_____

_____

5. I engage in activities to strengthen my power base.

1 2 3 4 5

_____

_____

_____

6. I avoid activities that will decrease my power.

1 2 3 4 5

_____

_____

_____

7. I feel I have a base of colleagues on whom I can count to support my ideas or projects.

1 2 3 4 5

_____

_____

_____

8. I enjoy taking charge of situations or projects to accomplish goals.

1 2 3 4 5

_____

_____

_____

9. I enjoy speaking in front of groups, meeting new people, and being the center of attention.

1 2 3 4 5

_____

_____

_____

10. I enjoy competing for resources with others.

1 2 3 4 5

_____

_____

_____

Scoring: Review the scoring of each of the 10 questions. Count the number of items that you ranked high (3, 4, or 5). Were the majority of your rankings high? Examine the items that you scored high. If you scored many items high, you probably do not feel comfortable gaining and using power. Focus on one or two items where you would like to gain confidence in gaining power. Identify activities in which you can engage to empower yourself in personal and professional interactions.

Self-Assessment: Conflict

Conflict management is an important skill for nurses to acquire in order to build teams, to work in complex client care situations, and to obtain scarce resources. By evaluating your conflict management style, you can gain insight into what strategies have been effective methods for resolving conflict. Huber's Perceived Conflict Scale measures the conflict among hospital nurses.

The Perceived Conflict Scale

Purpose

To become aware of job conflict levels. If you do not work in a health care organization, rate the following assessment from the perspective of a student working in the clinical agency.

Directions

Read each question (see p. 170) and circle the number that most accurately represents your feelings. Select option 3 if conflict exists but you are unable to identify its strength. Each item has a 5-point Likert-type scale: 1 = strongly disagree; 2 = disagree; 3 = neutral; 4 = agree; 5 = strongly agree.

	Strongly Disagree	Disagree	Neutral	Agree	Strongly Agree
1. Other nurses often disagree with each other on how work on this unit should be handled.	1	2	3	4	5
2. I usually agree with the way other nurses think things should be done on this unit.	1	2	3	4	5
3. My supervisor and I usually agree about what my job is and the requirements I must fulfill.	1	2	3	4	5
4. I usually agree with the decisions my head nurse and supervisor make.	1	2	3	4	5
5. Clients often demand that I do things I simply cannot do.	1	2	3	4	5
6. When I do something that satisfies one person or group, other people are frequently upset with what I have done.	1	2	3	4	5
7. The employees that I see who are from other areas of the hospital are often difficult to deal with.	1	2	3	4	5
8. The various departments that I deal with in my hospital are usually helpful and make it easy for me to do my job.	1	2	3	4	5
9. I frequently encounter problems when I transfer my clients to other units or departments	1	2	3	4	5
10. Support services (e.g., dietary and maintenance) are readily available when I need them.	1	2	3	4	5
11. Many times, the things that support services are supposed to do are not adequately done, and I either have to argue with another unit or do someone else's job.	1	2	3	4	5
12. I am unable to provide adequate care because of the time that I spend dealing with hospital rules and red tape.	1	2	3	4	5
13. I often cannot get equipment, supplies, or medications when I need them.	1	2	3	4	5
14. My clients often make requests or need care that I feel I should provide but cannot because I lack the time or energy.	1	2	3	4	5
15. My obligations to my work frequently conflict with my obligations to family, friends, or myself (outside the job).	1	2	3	4	5
16. I often have too many things to do at one time.	1	2	3	4	5

Reverse Score Items: For items 2, 3, 4, 8, and 10 reverse the 1-to-5 Likert scale to score them. For example, if you scored 5, change it to 1; if you scored 1, change it to 5; if you scored 4, change it to 2; and if you scored 2, change it to 4.

Subscales: Name	Items
1. Intrapersonal conflict	5, 14, 15, 16

*Conflict that arises within the individual from two competing demands.

2. Interpersonal conflict	1, 2, 3, 4

*Conflict between two or more individuals arising from miscommunication or differences in values.

3. Intergroup/support conflict	10, 11, 12, 13

*Conflict between two or more groups that are supportive in work or personal lives. Differences in competition for resources, power, or status may occur.

4. Intergroup/other departments	6, 7, 8, 9

*Conflict between two or more groups for resources or services. The conflict may be competitive or disruptive and may center around resources or control.

CASE STUDIES

Case Study 1: Power

Sandy Bandergest, a staff nurse on a 66-bed medical-surgical unit in Sagers, Hawaii, decides to establish a strong power base for herself. She has read a book about power mechanisms and decides to experiment with them. Nurse Bandergest arrives on the unit and notices that her assignment is heavy. She decides to address the charge nurse by stating the facts about the number of clients she has and their condition severity levels. She requests that the assignment be adjusted in light of the data presented. The charge nurse refuses the request and walks away. Nurse Bandergest decides to approach the nurse manager and again presents all the facts. The nurse manager intervenes and modifies the assignment. Nurse Bandergest meets Ruth Ann Marion, a clinical nurse specialist, in the hall and praises her for the new client care delivery model she developed. Finally, Nurse Bandergest begins care delivery and realizes she cannot handle the turning and positioning alone. She seeks assistance from Judy Jackson and says she will return the favor. Nurse Jackson agrees to help.

Case Study 1 Questions

1. What power mechanisms did Nurse Bandergest use?
2. Is Nurse Bandergest empowering herself by using these power mechanisms?
3. What else can Nurse Bandergest do to garner power?

Case Study 2: Conflict

Jennifer Radsovick is a nurse manager on a neuroscience unit in Chicago, Illinois. She has been trying to get funding for renovating the neuroscience unit. Jonathan Joseph is a nurse manager on the orthopedic unit in the same hospital. The vice president of nursing has announced that there is enough money to renovate only one unit in the hospital and that she would like proposals from Nurses Radsovick and Joseph because their units are those in the most need for repair. Nurse Radsovick calls Nurse Joseph after the meeting and asks if they could meet and discuss the renovation issue. He eagerly accepts the invitation because he has wanted to work with Nurse Radsovick to resolve this conflict of interest.

The nurse managers meet to develop a detailed work plan of desired renovations for each of their units. They have costs for the projects and agree that they do not want to compete for the renovation because morale will suffer greatly on the unit that loses. The two units adjoin, and they freely share staff back and forth as the census demands. Nurses Radsovick and Joseph brainstorm and come up with several options, such as rebidding the work based on two units that are adjacent (perhaps they could get a discount); renovating the units in phases, part one this year and part two the next; or perhaps if this were not possible, renovating one unit this year and purchasing new equipment for the other unit and then reversing the process. The nurse managers make a joint appointment to speak with the vice president of nursing.

Case Study 2 Questions

1. What type of conflict outcome were Nurses Radsovick and Joseph attempting to elicit?
2. What types of conflict strategies were these nurse managers using?
3. What type of framework for conflict strategy were these nurse managers using to get their desired outcome?

---

* *Scoring: The higher the mean score, the greater the level of conflict.*

171

Copyright © 2006, 2000, 1996 by Elsevier Inc. All rights reserved.

Chapter **24 Power and Conflict**

LEARNING RESOURCES

Discussion Questions

1. What are the five power bases described by French and Raven (1959)?

2. What is the difference between personal power-oriented individuals and institutionalized power-oriented individuals?

3. How can a nurse manager empower the staff? What effect does empowerment have on care delivery?

4. What are effective strategies for staff nurses to use to empower themselves and their colleagues?

5. What are the differences between fight, negotiation, and collaboration? Identify a situation in which each might be appropriate.

6. Describe and discuss the three conflict resolution outcomes in terms of team building and long-term positive relationships among individuals competing for resources.

7. Discuss the use of conflict resolution strategies, and identify the outcome possible when using each of the strategies.

8. How can nurses as a group work together to have significant impact on legislative issues affecting nursing practice?

9. What are sources of conflict in nursing, and what can nurses do to resolve this conflict and promote growth?

Study Questions

Matching: Write the correct letter of the correct response in front of each term.

_____ 1. Power

_____ 2. Empower-ment

_____ 3. Reward power

_____ 4. Coercive power

_____ 5. Expert power

_____ 6. Referent power

_____ 7. Legitimate power

_____ 8. Ingratiation

_____ 9. Upward appeal

_____ 10. Coalitions

A. Power based on charisma and interpersonal appeal

B. The authority to act based on position

C. Providing the opportunity for others to take responsibility and accountability for their work

D. Influencing an individual or group in order to gain a scarce resource

E. Lavishing praise on another in order to gain favor

F. Formation of a group for the purpose of a single voice in order to affect change

G. Taking concern to a higher authority

H. The use of threats, discipline, or negative consequences

I. Individuals who possess special skills or talents

J. Providing a pay raise, promotion, or advancement

True or False: Circle the correct answer.

T   F   11. Conflict arises because job descriptions are clear, policies and procedures are written, and growth is fostered in an organization.

T   F   12. Organizational conflict arises from the competition for scarce resources.

T   F   13. To build effective interdisciplinary teams, conflict must be present, and managers must not interfere with conflict resolution.

T   F   14. Role ambiguity is the expectation that nurses take on duties from other disciplines.

T F 15. Individuals are most comfortable around those who are like them.

T F 16. A defensive framework for conflict resolution includes winning some resources and losing others.

T F 17. Using the conflict strategy of withdrawing provides the participant with the time to calm down or avoid confrontation.

T F 18. In a win-lose situation, both parties end up losing because nobody is 100% satisfied.

T F 19. Negotiation and collaboration are strategies used to promote cooperation in power moments.

T F 20. Role stress occurs when the nurse's responsibilities expand faster than the formal job description.

T F 21. Ingratiation is an attempt to make another feel good or important.

T F 22. Referent power is based on the individual's position in an organization.

References

Bacharach, S. B., & Lawler, E. J. (1980). *Power and politics in organizations.* San Francisco: Jossey-Bass.

Barki, H., & Hartwick, J. (2001). Interpersonal conflict and its management in information system development. *MIS Quarterly, 25,* 195-228.

Centers for Medicare & Medicaid Services. (2004, January 8). Health care spending reaches $1.6 trillion in 2002. Baltimore: Author. Retrieved May 15, 2004, from *www.cms.hhs.gov/media/press/release.asp?Counter=935*

Coser, L. A. (1956). *The functions of social conflict.* Glencoe, IL: Free Press.

Filley, A. C. (1975). *Interpersonal conflict resolution.* Glenview, IL: Scott Foresman.

French, J., & Raven, B. (1959). The bases of social power. In D. Cartwright (Ed.), *Studies in social power* (pp. 150-167). Ann Arbor: University of Michigan, Institute for Social Research.

Hickson, D. J., Hinings, C. R., Lee, C. A., Schneck, R. E., & Pennings, J. M. (1971). A strategic contingencies theory of intraorganizational power. *Administrative Science Quarterly, 16,* 216-229.

Kanter, R. M. (1977). *Men and women of the corporation.* New York: Basic Books.

Laschinger, H. K., & Havens, D. S. (1997). The effect of workplace empowerment on staff nurses' occupational mental health and work effectiveness. *Journal of Nursing Administration, 27*(6), 4-50.

Laschinger, H. K., Sabiston, J. A., & Kutszcher, L. (1997). Empowerment and staff nurse decision involvement in nursing work environments: Testing Kanter's theory of structural power in organizations. *Research in Nursing and Health, 20,* 341-352.

Pfeffer, J. (1981). *Power in organizations.* Boston: Pitman Books.

Pondy, L. (1967). Organizational conflict: Concepts and models. *Administrative Science Quarterly, 12,* 296-320.

Robbins, S. P. (2003). *Organizational behavior* (10th ed.). Englewood Cliffs, NJ: Prentice-Hall.

Sabiston, J. A., & Laschinger, H. K. (1995). Staff nurse empowerment and perceived autonomy: Testing Kanter's theory of structural power in organizations. *Journal of Nursing Administration, 25*(9), 42-50.

Thomas, K. W. (1976). Conflict and conflict management. In M. D. Dunnette (Ed.), *The handbook of industrial and organizational psychology* (pp. 889-935). Chicago: Rand McNally.

Ting-Toomey, S. (1988). Intercultural conflict styles: A face-negotiation theory. In Y. Y. Kim, & W. Gudykunst (Eds.), *Theories in intercultural communication* (pp. 213-235). Newbury Park, CA: Sage.

Ting-Toomey, S., & Kurogi, A. (1998). Facework competence in intercultural conflict: An updated face-negotiation theory. *International Journal of Intercultural Relations, 22,* 187-225.

Yukl, G., & Falbe, C. M. (1991). Importance of different power sources in downward and lateral relations. *Journal of Applied Psychology, 76*(3), 416-423.

Supplemental Readings

Cox, K. B. (2003). The effects of intrapersonal, intragroup, and intergroup conflict on team performance effectiveness and work satisfaction, *Nursing Administration Quarterly, 24*(2), 153-163.

Jones, M., & Malone, B. (2004). Nursing skills in the corridors of power. *Nursing Standard, 18*(51), 16-17.

Kozub, M. L., & Kozub, F. M. (2004). Dealing with power. *Journal of Psychosocial Nursing & Mental Health Services, 42*(2), 22-31.

Larson, L. (2004). Restoring the relationship: The key to nurse and patient satisfaction. *ABI/INFORM Global, 57*(9), 8-14.

Leifer, D. (2004). Nurse power. *Nursing Standard, 18*(50), 14-15.

Chapter 24: Power and Conflict (pp. 501-542)

Power

1. Think of a manager who has had the most influence over you. Why was that individual influential?

Persons can be influential for a variety of reasons. What strategies did they enlist to exert their influence? Did they use assertiveness, ingratiation, rationality, sanctions, exchange, upward appeal, blocking, or coalitions? Were they influential because you felt guilty, motivated, encouraged, or defeated? Or did this manager empower you?

2. With what types of power are you most comfortable? With which types would you consider it difficult to cope?

There are many sources of power. Are you more comfortable with reward power, coercive power, expert power, referent power, legitimate power, connection power, information power, group decision-making power, and persuasive power? In what situation might you use each? Which sources of power are you least comfortable exercising? Which are you the most comfortable exercising? Why do you think you feel that way?

3. Think about yourself as acting with strength and power and feeling the most satisfied about it. What kinds of things would you be doing?

Analysis of what gives you a sense of power is important. Nurses may be inclined to avoid an acknowledgment or analysis of power. However, to lead and manage, nurses need to acquire, possess, and use power effectively. Nurses may use power to improve client outcomes, to advance the nursing profession, and to improve the organizational climate.

4. How do you react in situations in which you feel powerless? Why do you respond in this way?

Individuals may react differently when facing situations in which they feel powerless. A loss of control may precipitate emotions such as fear, anxiety, and anger. They also may exhibit behaviors such as withdrawal and aggression. How do you react when you feel powerless? Do you withdraw, fight, negotiate, or collaborate? Do you develop behaviors that are counterproductive to the organization? How do you regain a sense of power?

5. Does a lack of power affect the way that you feel about situations?

A lack of power may negatively affect the way one feels about a given situation. Situations in which one feels powerless may result in passive participation, work dissatisfaction, and diminished productivity. Prolonged feelings of powerlessness may lead to demoralization and depression. How do you perceive your attitude in powerless situations? How could you modify your outlook to regain a sense of power?

6. When you are trying to control a situation, what makes you feel comfortable or uncomfortable?

Attempting to control a situation may cause an individual to use power to control others, rather than to empower others to improve the situation. How a person responds to a power conflict is related to personality, experience, position, perspective, and the problem. Which approach do you take when faced with power conflicts?

7. How can power principles be structured to advance nursing professional goals?

Nurses can use power principles to establish a foundation that will enlist support to advance the image, power, and prestige of nursing. Each nurse has the power to project enthusiasm, self-confidence, and self-esteem. Professional introductions and the display of academic credentials are two ways that nurses can reinforce their image. Power also is derived from the art and science of nursing practice. Nurses can use expertise, information, and nursing research data to render cost-effective client care.

8. What are your sources of power? What other sources of power can you develop?

Benner (1984) describes six types of power in nursing practice: transformational, participative/affirmative, integrative, advocacy, healing, and problem-solving. What are your sources of power, and what ones might you consider developing?

Conflict

1. What types of conflict are most common among nursing staff?

Nurses may experience intrapersonal, interpersonal, or intergroup conflicts. Intrapersonal conflict may result as a nurse wants to spend more time comforting a client's grieving spouse, but another client is nearing an arrest situation and needs immediate attention. An interpersonal conflict may erupt between a nurse and unlicensed assistive personnel over uncompleted tasks or miscommunication. An intergroup conflict may occur between nurses and the pharmacy department regarding the timeliness of medication delivery.

2. What sources of conflict are most common in nursing practice?

Nurses may experience conflict because of the need to work collaboratively with individuals with different values, beliefs, and perspectives. Conflicts may arise from differences in communication styles, goals, expectations, resources, and roles. Power distribution for nurses employed in a hierarchical system may lead to conflicts as they attempt to meet the needs of their clients and advocate for scarce resources to provide the care.

3. Does the way your immediate superior handles conflict help or hinder you?

Think about the conflict resolution outcomes achieved by your immediate supervisor. Are they win-lose, lose-lose, or win-win? How is the conflict framed? Is conflict viewed constructively from the perspective of increasing group cohesion and morale, promoting creativity, producing change and growth, improving work relationships, promoting effective problem solving, and motivating group members? Or is conflict viewed as a destructive force that interferes with stability and harmony?

4. Is there one best way to handle the conflicts most common to nursing practice? Why or why not?

A variety of strategies can be used to handle conflicts in nursing. An assessment of the conflict situation is important in order to identify the parameters of the conflict, areas of agreement and disagreement, and a person's perspective and goals. The factors that limit the possibilities of managing the conflict constructively must be communicated, explicated, and resolved.

5. What is the difference between functional and dysfunctional conflict? What determines functionality?

Functional conflict improves the quality of decisions, stimulates creativity and innovation, encourages interest and curiosity, provides a medium through which problems can be aired and tensions released, and fosters an environment of self-evaluation and change. Dysfunctional conflict occurs with poor communication, reduction in group cohesiveness, and subordination of group goals to the primacy of infighting between members (Robbins, 2003). An extremely high or low level of conflict can hinder performance.

6. What are the components of the conflict process model? From your own experience, give an example of how a conflict episode proceeded through the stages.

Several conflict process models are available for use (Filley, 1975; Pondy, 1967; Robbins, 1994, 2003; and Thomas, 1976). The following are commonalities found in all of these models:

- Causes that are conditions that occur before the conflict
- Core processes including the perception that conflict exists followed by some kind of affective state or emotional response
- Conflict behaviors including a variety of behaviors from subtle to violent
- Effect that includes outcomes such as resolution or aftermath consequences

How did your conflict proceed through the stages of one of the foregoing models?

7. What are the largest obstacles to effective conflict resolution?

Conflict resolution may be slowed or halted if the group's performance is hindered through interference with communication, reductions in group cohesiveness, and subordination of group goals to the primacy of infighting.

8. Identify two specific situations that you are facing currently that involve conflict. Apply the steps in the chapter to the conflict you identify.

A variety of strategies can be used to handle conflicts in nursing. An assessment of the conflict situation is important in order to identify the parameters of the conflict, areas of agreement and disagreement, and person's perspective and goals. The factors that limit the possibilities of managing the conflict constructively must be communicated, explicated, and resolved.

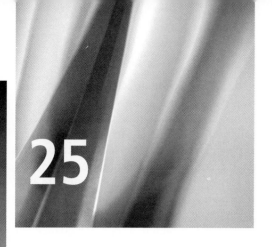

25

Delegation

STUDY FOCUS

The complexity and cost-constrained nature of the health care delivery system necessitates a multidisciplinary, multilevel approach to the provision of client care. Nurses must learn to delegate effectively to coordinate multidisciplinary teams and to manage complex client cases to provide quality care. *Delegation* is the ability to accomplish tasks through other persons while maintaining accountability. A *delegator* is an individual who assigns or delegates the task to another. A *delegatee* is an individual who accepts the delegated task. To delegate effectively, the delegator must supervise the work by providing direction for task accomplishment, periodically checking on the progress, and then evaluating the outcome. *Supervision* is the process of directing, guiding, and influencing the outcome of an individual's performance of a task. Unlicensed assistance personnel function in assitive roles under the direction of a registered professional nurse to provide client care. Nurse extenders are ancillary personnel trained to perform basic care (clinical) or supportive (nonclinical) tasks (Gardner, 1991; Hall, 1997).

Delegation is not dumping unpleasant work on others, being bossy, or abdicating responsibility and accountability. Managers should *not delegate* personal accountability, the disciplining of employees, or the recognition and praise of good work to others or morale issues. Delegation is used to improve others' skills, assign new tasks, build teams, and complete tasks that you do not have time to do. As a nurse, you will delegate nursing activities (the tasks essential to provide client care) and nonnursing activities (the tasks necessary to support client care). Nonnursing tasks include cleaning, running errands, clerical, stocking, and maintenance not involving client contact (American Association of Critical-Care Nurses [AACN], 1995). The National Council of State Boards of Nursing (NCSBN) describes delegation as a dynamic decision-making process and has formulated

practice guidelines for delegation. Questions to ask before delegating include the following (NCSBN, 1998):

- What is the task to be delegated?
- Is the task complex or simple?
- How much intensive decision making is needed to complete the task?

Factors to consider in delegating include the task, the staff available, the client's needs, the potential delegate's competency, and the level of supervision available. The two main *legal responsibilities* of a nurse making assignments are (1) delegating duties appropriately and (2) providing adequate supervision (Barter & Furmidge, 1994).

The NCSBN has developed a tool and a decision-making process for delegation. The tool assists with assessing critical elements in delegation decisions. The seven *critical elements in delegation decisions* are (1) the level of the client's condition, (2) level of unlicensed assistive personnel competence, (3) level of licensed nurse competence, (4) potential for harm, (5) frequency, (6) level of decision making, and (7) ability of client for self-care (NCSBN, 1997).

The decision-making process of delegation requires expert judgment. The delegation process is designed to give a directive, set a timeframe, and provide periodic review. An effective method of delegation is to provide a verbal directive with written instructions. When trying to decide which tasks are appropriate to delegate, the nurse should consider the following factors: the potential for harm, the complexity of the activity, the degree of problem solving and innovation required, the predictability of the outcome, and the extent of interaction necessary with clients (AACN, 1995). Carefully analyzing each task and matching it to an appropriate individual will assist in positive task accomplishment. The NCSBN delegation decision-making process is based on the nursing process and is in the assessment, planning, implementing, and evaluating format. The *NCSBN model* includes the following (NCSBN, 1995):

- Reviewing the delegation criteria
- Assessing the situation
- Planning for specific tasks to be delegated
- Ensuring appropriate accountability
- Supervising performance of the task
- Evaluating the entire delegation process
- Reassessing and adjusting the overall plan of care as needed

The *five rights of delegation* can help the nurse in making delegation decisions. The nurse must determine the *right task* to delegate within the guidelines established by the policies and procedures of the employing organization, the American Nurses Association Code of Ethics, and legal regulations of practice. The nurse must determine the *right circumstance* in which to perform the task with the necessary resources and supervision. The nurse must choose the *right person* who has the education and competency to complete the task. The nurse must provide the *right direction/communication* for the delegatee to complete the task. Finally, the nurse must provide the *right supervision* to complete the task. Often questions arise about whether the delegator needs to be present when the delegatee completes the task. Delegation (indirect) is providing direction through written and verbal communication (Association of Operating Room Nurses, 2004). Tasks can be delegated that reflect the ability, experience, and education of the delegatee; however, the ultimate responsibility and accountability rests with the delegator.

Many managers *choose not to delegate because of fears* that include the following: the need to control situations, fear of the incompetence of their subordinates, an attitude of superiority, worry about the risk of overdelegating, concern about a delegatee surpassing them in ability or prestige, fearful of potential harm to a client, perception of their failure to accomplish work personally, or are concern about poor outcomes (Poteet, 1989). *Subordinates also may be fearful of delegation* because they fear criticism for mistakes, lack information and resources to complete the work, have an overwhelming workload, lack self-confidence, fear criticism and overwork, have no incentives to complete new tasks, are discouraged by the delegator's personality and preferences, and like the convenience of having the boss solve the problems. Once a task is delegated, the delegator is still accountable for the outcome. Nurses must become familiar with the Nurse Practice Act for their state to understand the rules that govern nursing practice and provide direction on delegation. The American Nurses Association Code of Ethics is a handy guide for ethical problems. Nurses must understand the liability that is inherent in delegating activities so that they can avoid any *negligence* through a failure to act in accordance with established standards.

Delegating involves assigning the appropriate task to the right person who can complete the task in an established timeframe and clearly identifying who will undertake the task. Registered nurses are challenged with the delegation of tasks to unlicensed assistive personnel. Evaluating individuals, their job description, skill level, task, and the required level of supervision they need is essential for effective delegation. Guidelines for delegating to unlicensed assistive personnel include assigning tasks that are routine and standard with outcomes that are relatively predictable and where the illness and hospitalization is not life threatening. *Malpractice* refers to improper performance of professional duties resulting in a failure to meet the standard of care that results in harming a person (Zerwekh & Claborn, 2003). *Accountability* is the obligation to answer for one's actions, including the act of supervision. *Legal issues associated with delegation* include the following:

- The registered nurse remains legally responsible for the activities delegated.
- The registered nurse is accountable for the appropriateness of the delegated task and its accurate completion.
- The organization is liable for negligence or malpractice.
- Unlicensed assistive personnel cannot supervise other unlicensed assistive personnel.
- Unlicensed assistive personnel cannot redelegate to another unlicensed assistive person or student.
- Unlicensed assistive personnel cannot complete a pain assessment.
- Licensed practical nurses cannot complete discharge teaching.

Leaders usually adopt a problem-solving style of an *adaptor* who generates ideas to solve problems or an *innovator* who is detached from the problem, critically thinks about it, and searches for a solution. Coaching activities often are used to guide individuals in completing tasks effectively. Effective use of delegation builds teams, improves an individual's skills, and enhances quality care. Nurse leaders are challenged to evaluate the staff-mix configurations in relation to cost, quality, and outcomes in client care and to provide effective staffing to improve client outcomes and quality and safety of care.

LEARNING TOOLS

Role-Play: Delegating Tasks and Exploring Roles

Character One: Jessica Meyer is a nurse manager of a 45-bed surgical unit. Nurse Meyer is supportive of her staff and facilitates their growth and development.

Character Two: Barb Leve is a registered nurse (RN) on the surgical unit. She has worked for 3 years as an RN and is well respected by the staff. She leads a team that includes Julie Smanski and Anna Barrett, who are nurse's aides.

Character Three: Julie Smanski is an experienced nurse's aide on the surgical unit. She enjoys client care and works well with Nurse Leve. She is hesitant to offer any additional assistance to Nurse Leve, even though she knows the RN is busy. Ms. Smanski is afraid that if she offers additional assistance, it will become expected of her, and she wants to leave the hospital exactly at 3:30 PM so that she can pick up her son from school to avoid the additional expense of day care.

Character Four: Anna Barrett is a nurse's aide who was hired 3 months ago and has no previous experience beyond the training she has received at the hospital. Ms. Barrett also feels that RNs should do more work than she does because they get paid more.

Nurse Leve is having trouble completing her work before the 7 AM to 3 PM shift ends. She feels that there is not enough time in a shift to complete the required activities for safe client care and becomes frustrated when she notices the nurse's aides sitting down and chatting at the desk while she provides care at an unrelenting pace. She approaches Nurse Meyer, explaining that she is overworked and the nurse's aides are unproductive. She requests to have another registered nurse put on her team and tells Nurse Meyer that she would be willing to give up both nurse's aides for one experienced RN. Nurse Meyer explains to Nurse Leve that there is not enough money in the budget for any more RNs and that she will have to learn to delegate her work to the nurse's aides.

Role-Play Questions

1. What process should Nurse Leve use to determine what tasks she could delegate to the aides?
2. What should she say to the aides when she delegates tasks to them? How do you think Ms. Smanski and Ms. Barrett will respond?
3. Can the nurse's aides refuse to take on additional work?
4. Would both nurse's aides be able to take on the same tasks?
5. How can Nurse Leve manage the situation without becoming frustrated and burned out?

Directions

Role-play this scenario showing how Nurse Meyer can help Nurse Leve become comfortable with delegating. Practice delegating tasks to the nurse's aides.

Role-Play Worksheet

Character	Student Assigned
Jessica Meyer, the nurse manager	_____
Barb Leve, the RN	_____
Julie Smanski, the experienced nurse's aide	_____
Anna Barrett, the new nurse's aide	_____

Which character have you been assigned?

What are your character's goals in this situation?

How can the other characters assist you in achieving your goals?

What might the other characters do to hinder you in achieving your goals?

What strategies and probes do you plan to use in this situation?

CASE STUDY

Jon Burnard is an RN on the 3-to-11 PM shift for a medical unit. The nurse manager just announced that because of budget cuts, unlicensed assistive personnel are going to be hired to assist RNs. Nurse Burnard is assigned to a pod that consists of himself and two unlicensed assistive persons to care for 18 clients. He realizes that he cannot complete the work himself, so he requests a description of the experience, skill level, and familiarity with the hospital of the two unlicensed assistive persons.

After the nurse manager provides him with this information, Nurse Burnard goes home and identifies all the tasks that he must complete in an 8-hour shift. Based on the nurse manager's description of the unlicensed assistive persons' experience and skills, he assigns tasks to himself and to them. Finally, he develops a written mini-job description for himself and the unlicensed assistive persons. The next day Nurse Burnard asks the nurse manager to review the job descriptions he has developed and asks for input. She is thrilled with the job descriptions and feels they are appropriate. He then asks her to provide at least 2 hours of scheduled time for his team to get to know one another and to establish guidelines. Nurse Burnard also requests one 8-hour shift when he and the two nurse's aides can have half of a normal assignment to try the new job descriptions, work out any bugs, and become comfortable with each others' expectations.

Case Study Questions

1. Is Nurse Burnard using an appropriate delegation process to solve an immediate problem?

2. What are the advantages and disadvantages of the plan Nurse Burnard has described?

3. What factors should Nurse Burnard consider when he determines what is appropriate for delegation?

LEARNING RESOURCES

Discussion Questions

1. What are some advantages and disadvantages of delegation?

2. What is the National Council of State Boards of Nursing delegation decision-making process? How can this process be useful in practice?

3. What legal and ethical considerations do nurses who delegate tasks need to consider?

4. When a task is delegated, who then has the authority, responsibility, and accountability for the task?

5. Can all unlicensed assistive personnel perform the same tasks? Provide a rationale for your answer.

6. Are there any tasks that managers should not delegate to their subordinates? If so, what are they, and why should they not be delegated?

Study Questions

Matching: Write the correct response in front of each term.

_____ 1. Delegator

_____ 2. Delegatee

_____ 3. Supervision

_____ 4. Nursing activities

_____ 5. Nonnursing activities

_____ 6. Negligence

_____ 7. Nurse practice act

_____ 8. Board of nursing

_____ 9. American Nurses Association Code of Ethics

_____ 10. Adaptors

A. To generate new solutions to problems

B. Failure to act in accordance with established standards

C. A source useful in exploring ethical problems

D. A set of rules that governs nursing practice

E. To function to interpret and enforce the law

F. Tasks necessary to support client care

G. Tasks necessary to provide care to clients

H. Guidance to accomplish a specific task or activity

I. The individual who accepts a new task

J. The individual who assigns a task to another

True or False: Circle the correct answer.

T   F   11. Staffing patterns and methods of care delivery should be evaluated on client outcomes and basic safety.

T   F   12. The National Council of State Boards of Nursing is opposed to delegation to unlicensed assistive personnel.

T   F   13. A key element in delegation is to assess the competency level of the staff.

T   F   14. When a registered nurse delegates a task, he or she is responsible for supervision but is not accountable for the outcome.

T   F   15. The state Nurse Practice Act consists of rules that govern nursing practice and provide guidance on delegation.

REFERENCES

American Association of Critical-Care Nurses. (1995). *Delegation: A tool for success in the changing workplace.* Aliso Viejo, CA: Author.

Association of Operating Room Nurses. (2004). *Official statement on unlicensed assistive personnel.* Denver, CO: Author.

Barter, M., & Furmidge, M. (1994). Unlicensed assistive personnel: Issues relating to delegation and supervision. *Journal of Nursing Administration, 24*(4), 36-40.

Gardner, D. (1991). Issues related to the use of nurse extenders. *Journal of Nursing Administration, 21*(10), 40-45.

Hall, L. M. (1997). Staff mix models: Complementary or substitution roles for nurses. *Nursing Administration Quarterly, 21*(2), 31-39.

National Council of State Boards of Nursing. (1995). *Delegation: Concepts and decision-making process.* Chicago: Author. Retrieved September 17, 2004, from *www.ncsbn.org/regulation/uap_delegation_documents_delegation.asp*

National Council of State Boards of Nursing. (1997). *Delegating decision-making grid.* Chicago: Author.

National Council of State Boards of Nursing. (1998). *The continuum of care: A regulatory perspective.* Chicago: NCSBN.

Poteet, G. (1989). Nursing administrators and delegation. *Nursing Administration Quarterly, 13*(3), 23-32.

Zerwekh, J., & Claborn, J. C. (2003). *Nursing today: Transitions and trends* (4th ed.). Philadelphia: W. B. Saunders.

SUPPLEMENTAL READINGS

Anthony, M. K., Standing, T. S., & Hertz, J. (2001). Nurses' beliefs about their abilities to delegate within changing models of care. *The Journal of Continuing Education in Nursing, 32*(5), 210-215.

Curtis, E., & Nicholl, H. (2004). Delegation: A key function of nursing. *Nursing Management, 11*(4), 26-31.

Fisher, M. (2000). Do you have delegation savvy? *Nursing 2000, 30*(12), 58-59.

Nagelkerk, J., & Henry, B. (1992-1993). Power delegating. *Graduating Nurse,* 56-57.

Chapter 25: Delegation (pp. 543-560)

1. **What does your Nurse Practice Act in your state say about delegation and supervision?**

   Although similarities exist, the Nurse Practice Act in each state has unique information concerning delegation and supervision. As a result, it is important to know the specific requisites for delegating legally and effectively in your state. You may obtain a copy of the Nurse Practice Act from your State Board of Nursing.

2. **Should a nursing student delegate nursing activities?**

   Nursing students must learn and practice delegation skills. Because these skills require critical thinking and advanced clinical judgment, principles of effective delegation are integrated into the final semesters of the curriculum to afford students the opportunity to practice delegation under the auspices of a supervised clinical experience.

3. **How often is delegating to unlicensed assistive personnel performed in your work setting?**

   In addition to thinking about how often delegation is used, you also should consider which tasks are delegated and in which situations delegation occurs. Do you feel that the delegation was appropriate? To evaluate this, the nurse should assess the following before delegation (American Association of Critical-Care Nurses, 1995):

   - Potential for harm
   - Complexity of task
   - Problem solving and innovation required
   - Unpredictability of the outcome
   - Level of client interaction

4. **How comfortable do you feel with delegation?**

   You may be hesitant or uncomfortable delegating tasks to others. The basis for your discomfort may be related to a belief that you could do it better or quicker yourself, a lack of confidence in your staff, a fear of taking a risk, a need to feel indispensable, inability to direct others, a fear of losing authority, or anxiety about experiencing decreases in personal satisfaction.

5. **How can the nurse delegate to assist others to develop further?**

   Delegation should be viewed as a learning opportunity. Delegating increasingly complex tasks after providing a foundation of knowledge and skills is an excellent way for delegatees to grow. Providing responsible incremental growth experiences with adequate supervision will enhance job satisfaction and build team relationships.

6. **What criteria can be used to assess co-workers' competency?**

   The criteria used to assess competency must be preestablished and measurable and must be completed within an established timeframe. Before delegating a task, the nurse should know the job description, including the type of education and training required to function in that role. The evaluation process should include whether the task was completed correctly, completely, and within the designated timeframe. Supervision and evaluation should be an ongoing process with periodic review and feedback.

7. **How do competency criteria differ for registered nurses, licensed practical nurses/licensed vocational nurses, unlicensed assistive personnel, and nursing students?**

   Competencies for registered nurses differ from those for unlicensed assistive personnel. Registered nurses are skilled in clinical judgment and complex decision making, necessitating cognitive, affective, and psychomotor competency validation. Nursing students are evaluated by the same criteria as the registered nurse, taking into consideration their evolving level of skill and knowledge. Unlicensed assistive personnel are evaluated according to the job description and policies of the health care agency that dictate their level of education and skill.

8. **What routine tasks can registered nurses delegate to others?**

Registered nurses can delegate tasks and procedures that are routine, such as specimen collection, vital signs, bathing, and assisting with procedures. However, the nurse must remember that just because it was right to delegate a task in one instance, it may not be right the next time. A thorough assessment of the client, task, and the abilities of the delegate should be completed before any delegation process. Also, the nurse should never delegate components of professional nursing practice including nursing process, nursing diagnoses, clinical judgment, or interventions that require the specialized knowledge or skill of a registered nurse.

9. **When you delegate your work, what type of work do you then perform?**

The goal of delegation is to have others assist you in completing certain tasks or activities. A registered nurse remains accountable and responsible and must supervise all those to whom nursing activities are delegated. The level of supervision will depend on the experience and the expertise of the delegate. The nurse should make sure that the delegate is aware of the resources that are available to assist him or her and any parameters for reporting back to you. If the individual has never completed the task before, use it as an opportunity to teach.

10. **What is a safe or minimum nurse/client ratio? Does this differ across care settings?**

A safe or minimum nurse-to-client ratio depends on the setting, shift, skill mix, client condition severity, and care context. It can vary from 1:1 in a perioperative or critical care setting to 1:10 or more in a nonacute care setting. The primary determinant of an appropriate staffing ratio is that nurses must be able to provide safe care and adequate supervision for care delivery. Staffing guidelines often are established by specialty nursing organizations and the Joint Commission on Accreditation of Healthcare Organizations.

11. **When and what is a nurse responsible for during client care and delivery coordination?**

The registered nurse (RN) retains the responsibility and accountability for the provision of care to an assigned group of clients. The RN has the responsibility of completing the nursing process. The RN may delegate aspects of care for clients after assessing the potential for harm, the complexity of the task, the degree of problem solving needed, the predictability of the outcome, and the competency of the delegate. As the coordinator of care, the RN delegates appropriate aspects of care but remains accountable for care delivery.

12. **What type of relationships have you observed among registered nurses, licensed practical nurses/licensed vocational nurses, and unlicensed assistive personnel? Were they positive? If not, what changes could be implemented to help the relationships?**

Registered nurses, licensed practical nurses, and unlicensed assistive personnel can work well together if each provides care according to the policies and procedures of the agency, the American Nurses Association Code of Ethics, and legal regulations for practice. For example, the unlicensed assistive person only does tasks that are supported by policy and after having achieved a level of competency in that task. Mutual respect and trust is important in a team. Registered nurses need to be able to trust those to whom they delegate, and licensed practical nurses and unlicensed assistive personnel need to be able to trust the registered nurse's judgment. What situations have you experienced? What changes could be implemented to help the relationships?

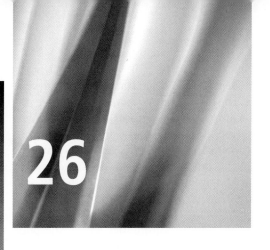

26

Team Building and Working with Effective Groups

STUDY FOCUS

Nursing leaders must be skilled in group facilitation to accomplish organizational objectives because a significant portion of the work requires collective efforts. Reasons why teamwork is a new imperative includes changing reimbursement, managed care organizations, increasing complexity, technological advances, rapid information dissemination, and shift to a knowledge worker–based service society. The emergence of teamwork in health care organizations is imperative for the building of knowledge work teams. *Knowledge work teams* are small numbers of persons working together who have complementary knowledge to achieve a desired goal for which they hold themselves mutually accountable (Sorrells-Jones & Weaver, 1999). Knowledge work teams provide a competitive edge and boost productivity under conditions of constrained resources. Such teams capitalize on improved productivity, better decisions, and process innovations. Health care delivery systems are becoming more complex, requiring interdisciplinary work teams to tackle difficult systems problems in a cost-controlled manner. In most health care environments, nursing is at the core of client care, providing around-the-clock access to health care services. As central players in the delivery of client care, nurses are expected to assume the role of team leaders, case managers, and coordinators of care. Many of the care-coordinating roles entail interdisciplinary consultation and intense group work.

A *group* is a collection of interrelated individuals working toward a goal. Groups are important because of the informal network dynamics and the formation and functioning of formal committees and teams. A *committee* is a stable and formally composed group with a mechanism for maintaining and selecting members. Committee members have official status and sanction within organizations. *Team building* is a process of creating and unifying a group to accomplish specific goals (Farley & Stoner, 1989). A *team* is a small number of persons with similar skill sets committed to

a common purpose and goal set for which they are mutually accountable (Katzenbach & Smith, 1993). A *work group* is a collection of individuals who are led by a strong, focused leader. A team engages in collective work, whereas in a work group each individual may feel accountability, but there is no collective accountability. In a true team, individuals rotate leadership and share roles, there are collective work products, there is group and individual accountability, the whole team is responsible for solving the problems, and all members assist their fellow team members to meet quality goals. A pseudo-team is a group of persons who believe they are a team, but which exhibits confusion over the purpose, unhealthy or toxic interpersonal issues and communication patterns, individual needs that are put above group needs, hierarchical rituals, unclear goals, and lack of evaluation criteria.

Group interactions are composed of five elements: process, standards, decision making, communication, and roles (Book & Galvin, 1975). *Process* is the way the group works together to accomplish goals. *Standards* are values and norms that the group uses to process information. *Decision making* is the method the group uses to solve problems. Communication includes verbal and nonverbal interactions within and external to the group. *Roles* describe each individual's part in the group. Creative techniques used by groups to enhance group process and improve outcomes include brainstorming, nominal group technique, tri-council, and the Delphi survey. Characteristics of highly effective groups include having a common purpose, agreeing on performance goals, recruiting competent members, working together, developing a collaborative climate, being mutually accountable, and setting standards of excellence.

Groups progress through a series of four stages: orientation, adaptation, emergence, and working (Farley & Stoner, 1989). The *orientation stage* occurs at the beginning of the group's formation and involves trust and boundary issues. During *adaptation*, a team identity is formed and individual roles are differentiated. In the *emergence* (control) phase, issues arise and are resolved. The *working* phase is the productive stage when decision making and task accomplishment take place. These stages of the group process are not necessarily sequential and may be iterative.

Individuals join groups for a variety of reasons. Often, individuals seek group participation to fulfill affiliation and achievement needs. When individuals work in groups, they gain the advantage of a greater depth and breadth of knowledge and information. In nursing the formation of groups occurs primarily to provide a personal or professional socialization and exchange forum and to provide a mechanism for work accomplishment. Reasons why groups are established in organizations include creating a sense of status and esteem, testing and establishing reality, getting a job done, and utilizing the complexity of knowledge and skill. Five major advantages of group problem solving over individual problem solving are (1) greater knowledge and information, (2) increased acceptance of solutions, (3) more approaches to a problem, (4) individual expression, and (5) lower economic costs. Members of groups tend to accept and endorse group solutions to problems because of their commitment and investment in the decision-making process. Complex problems are more manageable within groups because they tend to have an increased knowledge base and a varied approach to problem solving. In groups, individuals are provided with the outlet for expression of ideas.

The disadvantages of groups can include premature decision making, individual domination and control, and disruptive conflicts. Individuals will belong to groups as long as their needs are being met. Once the costs of membership become greater than the benefits, termination likely will occur. Work group disruption leads to negative outcomes (Leppa, 1996). Group decision-making power occurs on a continuum. On one end of the continuum is an *autocratic decision* procedure in which the leader makes the decision. In this type of committee the leader controls the power and the committee exists for the sake of appearance. A *consultative decision* procedure occurs when decisions involve employee participation, but the final decision is made by the leader. In *joint decision* making, the entire group decides. Employees have as much influence as the leader, and the leader can use persuasion. Finally, a *delegated decision* procedure is when the committee chairperson allows the participants to make the decision and does not override the followers' decision. A leadership or conflict moment may occur when a group assumes that delegation is the decision procedure rule in effect.

High-performance teams are essential for organizational efficiency and effectiveness. Work teams are forming in health care organizations as a survival mechanism. The *three types of health care teams* are primary work teams (client care teams), executive leadership teams (top executive team), and ad hoc teams (specific problem-solving teams). All teams have the potential to become *self-directed work teams* that accept increasingly higher levels of authority and responsibility. *Key steps to designing highly effective health care teams* include defining the work of the team, differentiating responsibilities within the pool, narrowing the options to those most attractive, and identifying the best design to implement. Issues in designing interdisciplinary teams include a lack of a common vocabulary and understanding about other disciplines' practice, confusion about the work, lack of real authority, lack of team building, dysfunctional behavior, and lack of coaching (Manion et al., 1996). Trust and communication are critical elements of building effective work teams. A key characteristic of an emotionally intelligent team is the establishment of norms that guide team behavior (Cherniss & Goleman, 2001). The process of developing norms is often leader initiated. Topics for behavioral norms include communication, treatment of members, support, decision-making process, and conflict resolution. Norms also may be referred to as *team operating agreements, code of conduct,* or *articulated expectations.* Points on a team performance curve include a working group, a pseudo-team with no common goals, a potential team, a real team, and a high-performance team (Katzenbach & Smith, 1993). A framework to understand team development is group process (Farley & Stoner, 1989). Four essential components of high-performing teams are roles, activities, relationships, and the environment (Sovie, 1992). Skill categories useful in completing team tasks include functional expertise, decision-making skills, and interpersonal skills. The six basic elements of teams are small size, complementary skills, a meaningful purpose, specific goal(s), clear work approach, and mutual accountability (Katzenbach & Smith, 1993). Characteristics of highly effective teams include a common goal, performance goals, competent members, common approach to work, unified commitment, complementary skills, collaborative climate, mutual accountability, standards of excellence, external support and recognition, and principled leadership (Katzenbach & Smith, 1993; Manion et al., 1996).

Committees are formally designated groups. Committees meet at scheduled times and have an identified purpose. Committee structures are preferable when each member's input is needed to attain a goal and when situations in which diverse representation facilitates implementation of proposed activities. The types

186

of committees include standing committees (ongoing part of an organizational mission), task forces (project or ad hoc committee is used for an emergent need and then disbands), councils (membership based on organizational position), and multidisciplinary committees (multiple specialties). Efficient and effective committees have appropriate representation and authority for decision making (Wilson et al., 1999). For committees to remain vital, they must be evaluated, restructured, and revitalized periodically.

Much of group work is organized and completed through meetings. Meetings typically are held to disseminate information, seek opinions, and solve problems. The important components of a successful meeting are distribution of an agenda, careful selection of members, attention to starting times and seating positions, and facilitation of discussion of the topic. The ideal size of a group is 4 to 7 persons, but groups can be managed effectively with 12 persons. It is important to draw out silent members, avoid stomping out creative ideas, protect junior members, control compulsive talkers, and provide recognition and encouragement (Jay, 1982). The chairperson should take responsibility for comfort and convenience for group members. Questions to ask when preparing an agenda include the following:

- Where are we?

- What needs to be done?

- What supporting materials might help the committee?

- Who should be invited?

A continuum of authority in group decision making includes the autocratic, the consultative, the joint, and the delegated styles. The leader's style of facilitating the group's decision making affects the power of the group. The leader's role is pivotal in facilitating positive work groups to accomplish organizational goals. Three categories of group members are (1) facilitator, (2) recorder, (3) group member. Roles that build the group include initiator, encourager, opinion giver, clarifier, listener, and summarizer. Roles that maintain groups include tension reliever, compromiser, gatekeeper, and harmonizer. Facilitators provide everyone the opportunity to speak, maintain the meeting focus, and ensure a positive environment. The group recorder takes minutes and facilitates group process. The leader must redirect disruptive group members such as compulsive talkers (thank them and then ask to hear from others), nontalkers (encourage them to submit their ideas or share them verbally), interrupters (control and redirect), squashers (encourage openness to all ideas or provide an equal time for positive and then negative input), and busybodies (give them a concrete assignment with accountability) (Jacobs & Rosenthal, 1984). Team building is an essential component of the group leader's role. Methods to generate creative ideas or solutions include brainstorming (encouraging multiple diverse ideas without limitations of feasibility or practicality), Delphi survey technique (sequential questionnaires with expert consensus to prioritize), and nominal group technique (writing ideas with round-robin feedback and individual voting on priority ideas).

The leader's role is to prepare the materials, setting, and the group for the work required to fulfill the mission and goals of the organization. Coaching, the transfer of responsibility with guidance and support, is an important aspect of a leader's role. The coaching of group leaders, interdisciplinary teams, and future leaders is critical in health care today. Strong leaders who are skilled at leading groups, accomplishing work, and providing innovative solutions to thorny health care problems are essential to direct the provision of quality, cost-effective health care services. Current issues and trends with which health care leaders must grapple include workforce shortages in health care, designing cohesive interdisciplinary care teams, designing new methods of compensation, encouraging innovative groups, and speaking in a unified voice (multiple nursing organizations). The success of health care organizations in developing effective and productive knowledge-based work teams will provide strategic advantages in a highly competitive, turbulent environment.

LEARNING TOOLS

Individual Activity: Effective Meeting Checklist for Leaders*

Purpose
To review and understand the elements that are important to consider and act upon to conduct an effective meeting.

Instructions
1. Review the information in the textbook Chapter 26 on conducting effective meetings.

2. Review the following Effective Meetings Checklist for Leaders.

*Data from Jay, A. (1982). How to run a meeting. Journal of Nursing Administration, 12(1)22-28.

3. Attend a meeting of your choice, and use the checklist to determine how well the leader was prepared for the meeting and how you ranked the leader on the Effective Meeting Checklist for Leaders.

4. Did your overall impression of the effectiveness of the meeting correlate with the score you gave it? By reviewing your evaluation of this meeting, you can identify areas in which the leader could improve key elements to make a more effective and efficient meeting. This information is useful for you as you prepare to lead meetings.

Effective Meetings Checklist for Leaders

Directions

Check each numbered Meeting Element according to the following scale:

O = Outstanding
G = Good
S = Satisfactory
P = Poor
U = Unsatisfactory

Meeting Element	O	G	S	P	U
1. Identify the purpose of the meeting.					
• Information dissemination					
• Opinion seeking					
• Problem solving					
2. Prepare an agenda and related materials.					
3. Identify the category of each agenda item.					
• For information					
• For development					
• For implementation					
• For change in the system					
4. Set the size at four to seven people.					
5. Carefully select members (based on skill and expertise).					
6. Distribute agenda well in advance of meeting.					
7. Start on time.					
8. Listen carefully.					
9. Process the interactions.					
10. Control the flow of interactions.					
11. Keep the meeting directed toward accomplishing objectives.					

Scoring: Add the number of check marks in each of the columns. If the majority of check marks are in the Outstanding and Good columns, the leader is skilled in preparing and conducting effective meetings. If the checks are scattered in the Outstanding, Good, and Satisfactory columns, the leader has been effective in conducting the meeting. If the check marks are in the columns of Poor or Unsatisfactory, this leader and meeting were not effective. This tool can be used to identify areas in which leaders or meeting facilitators can strengthen their skills in conducting effective meetings.

Group Activity: Winter Survival Decision Exercise*

Purpose

To compare autocratic, consultative, joint, and delegated group decision-making authority.

---

* *Modified from Johnson, D. W., & Johnson, F. P. (1986).* Joining together: Group theory and group skills *(3rd ed.). Upper Saddle River, NJ: Allyn & Bacon/Pearson Education.*

Instructions

1. Divide the study group into four small groups of 7 to 12. One member of each small group will be the designated leader, one member will be the designated observer, and all other members will be participants in the small group during this exercise. Group 1 should be assigned autocratic group decision authority, Group 2 should be assigned consultative group decision authority, Group 3 should be assigned joint group decision authority, and Group 4 should be assigned delegated group decision-making authority.

2. The observer should be attuned to the process by which the groups make decisions. Crucial issues are how well the group uses the resources of its members, how much commitment to implement the decision is mustered, how the future decision-making ability of the group is affected, and how members feel about and react to what is taking place. The observer should address the following issues: Who does and does not participate in discussion? Who participates most? Who participates least? Who influences the decision? Who does not influence the decision? How is influence determined (expertise, loudness)? What are the dominant group feelings? What resources are used to make a decision?

3. Give each group the following exercise and the Winter Survival Decision Form.

4. Provide 45 minutes for each group to work through this exercise; then ask them to score their answers.

5. Have the observer brief the small groups with his or her observations. This is a good time to discuss effective group decision-making techniques. Provide 15 minutes for this activity.

6. Get the whole class back together and have the leader of each group share group scores, the type of group decision-making authority that the group role-played, and key observations made by the observers of the small groups.

You have crash-landed into a lake in the northern Minnesota woods. It is 11:32 AM in mid-January. The pilot and copilot were killed. Shortly after the crash, the plane sinks completely into the lake with the pilot's and copilot's bodies inside. None of you is seriously injured, and you are all dry.

The crash came suddenly, before the pilot had time to radio for help or inform anyone of your position. Because your pilot was trying to avoid a storm, you know the plane was considerably off course. The pilot announced shortly before the crash that you were 20 miles northwest of a small town that is the nearest known habitation.

You are in a wilderness area made up of thick woods broken by many lakes and streams. The snow depth varies from above the ankles in windswept areas to knee-deep where it has drifted. The last weather report indicated that the temperature would reach −25° F in the daytime and −40° F at night. Plenty of dead wood and twigs are in the immediate area. You are dressed in winter clothing appropriate for city wear: suits, pantsuits, street shoes, and overcoats.

While escaping from the plane, several members of your group salvaged 12 items. Your task is to rank these items according to their importance to your survival. You may assume that the number of passengers is the same as the number of persons in your group and that the group has agreed to stick together.

Winter Survival Decision Form

Directions

Rank the following items according to their importance to your survival, starting with 1 for the least important item and proceeding to 12 for the most important item.

_____ Ball of steel wool

_____ Newspapers (one per person)

_____ Compass

_____ Hand ax

_____ Cigarette lighter (without fluid)

_____ Loaded .45-caliber pistol

_____ Sectional air map made of plastic

_____ 20- by 20-foot piece of heavy-duty canvas

_____ Extra shirts and pants for each survivor

_____ Can of shortening

_____ Quart of 100-proof whiskey

_____ Family-size chocolate bars (one per person)

Scoring: Score the net difference between the participants' answers and the correct answer. For example, if a participant's answer is 9 and the correct answer is 12, the net difference is 3. Disregard all plus or minus signs. Find only the net difference for each item. Total all the item scores. The lower the score the more accurate the ranking.

Winter Survival Exercise: Answer Key

Item	Expert Ranking	Your Rank	Difference Score
Ball of steel wool	2		
Newspaper (one per person)	8		
Compass	12		
Hand ax	6		
Cigarette lighter (without fluid)	1		
Loaded .45-caliber pistol	9		
Sectional air map made of plastic	11		
20 × 20 foot piece of heavy-duty canvas	5		
Extra shirt and pants for each survivor	3		
Can of shortening	4		
Quart of 100-proof whiskey	10		
Family-size chocolate bar (one per person)	7		
TOTAL			

CASE STUDY

Jackie Hanson, a nurse practitioner who works in a primary care setting, feels isolated from other nurse practitioners because there are only physician assistants and physicians where she is employed. Nurse Hanson organizes a nurse practitioner group, invites other nurse practitioners to attend, and arranges the meeting place. The first meeting is a formal organizational gathering where nurses introduce themselves, socialize, and become familiar with one another and the purpose for the group. Goals are set and roles are assigned at the second, third, and fourth meetings. During the next several meetings, a number of individuals try to control the issues that are to be addressed. Once the issues are determined and the group agrees to be responsible for tasks, the work progresses quickly, and the group feels a sense of accomplishment.

Case Study Questions

1. Through what stages did this group work?
2. What are the four stages of group progress, and what do they include?
3. Do groups progress sequentially through the stages?

LEARNING RESOURCES

Discussion Questions

1. What is the continuum of authority for group decision making? How does the leader's style of facilitating the group affect group decision-making authority?

2. What are the types of disruptive group members, and what are strategies to redirect their energy toward group work and goal accomplishment?
3. What are the possible roles for clinical nurses in an interdisciplinary team?
4. What is the difference between a team, a committee, and a task force?
5. What are the stages of group development? Provide leader strategies to facilitate the group process for each stage.
6. What are the advantages and disadvantages of group work?
7. Describe the leader's role in planning and conducting a meeting.
8. Why are knowledge-based work teams important to the success and viability of a health care organization?

Study Questions

True or False: Circle the correct answer.

T F 1. Interdisciplinary work teams are necessary for complex situations.

T F 2. Groups sequentially go through the stages of orientation, adaptation, emergence, and working.

T F 3. The major reason individuals join groups is to gain information.

T F 4. Group decision making is cost-effective in all situations.

T F 5. A group leader must organize and structure a group for success.

190

T   F   6. In all groups, decision making is a joint process with all members participating.

T   F   7. A committee is a formally designated group designed to meet organizational objectives.

T   F   8. A task force is designed to solve long-term problems.

T   F   9. Team building is a complex process that requires leader and group commitment and cooperation.

T   F 10. The ideal number of members in a group is between 10 and 14.

T   F 11. A knowledge work team is a large number of highly skilled individuals with complementary knowledge who come together to accomplish specific goals.

T   F 12. In large health care organizations, interdisciplinary teams are an integral part of the core structure.

T   F 13. Research has linked work group disruption with increased productivity and collaboration.

T   F 14. Two elements that promote efficient and effective committee decision making are appropriate representation and delegation of authority to the committee.

Matching: Write the letter of the correct response in front of each term.

_____ 15. Brainstorming

_____ 16. Delphi survey

_____ 17. NGT

A. Sequential rounds of questionnaires to collect expert opinions on a topic

B. Silently gathered written input, round-robin feedback, and individual voting

C. Generating a large number of ideas through open, noncritical participation

REFERENCES

Book, C., & Galvin, K. (1975). *Instruction in and about small group discussion.* Falls Church, VA: Speech Communication Association.

Cherniss, C., & Goleman, D. (2001). *The emotionally intelligent workplace: How to select for, measure, and improve emotional intelligence in individuals, groups, and organizations.* San Francisco: Jossey-Bass.

Farley, M., & Stoner, M. (1989). The nurse executive and interdisciplinary team building. *Nursing Administration Quarterly, 13*(2), 24-30.

Jacobs, B., & Rosenthal, T. (1984). Managing effective meetings. *Nursing Economic$, 2*(2), 137-141.

Jay, A. (1982). How to run a meeting. *Journal of Nursing Administration, 12*(1), 22-28.

Katzenbach, J., & Smith, D. (1993). *The wisdom of teams: Creating the high-performance organization.* New York: Harper Collins.

Leppa, C. J. (1996). Nurse relationships and work group disruption. *Journal of Nursing Administration, 26*(10), 23-27.

Manion, J., Lorimer, W., & Leander, W. J. (1996). *Team-based health care organizations: Blueprint for success.* Gaithersburg, MD: Aspen.

Sorells-Jones, J., & Weaver, D. (1999). Knowledge workers and knowledge-intense organizations. I. A promise framework for nursing and healthcare. *Journal of Nursing Administration, 29*(7/8), 12-18.

Sovie, M. (1992). Care and service teams: A new imperative. *Nursing Economic$, 10*(2), 94-100.

Wilson, R. D., Mateo, M. A., & Brumm, S. K. (1999). Revitalizing a departmental committee. *Journal of Nursing Administration, 29*(3), 45-48.

SUPPLEMENTAL READINGS

Blount, K., & Nahigian, E. (1998). How to build teams in the midst of change. *Nursing Management, 29*(8), 27-29.

Gaynor, S. E., Reschak, G. L., & Verdin, J. (1994). Evaluating a committee structure. *Journal of Nursing Administration, 24*(7/8), 59-63.

Herman, J. E., & Reichelt, P. A. (1998). Are first-line nurse managers prepared for team building? *Nursing Management, 29*(10), 68-72.

Wheelan, S. A., & Burchill, C. (1999). Take teamwork to new heights. *Nursing Management, 30*(4), 28-82.

Chapter 26: Team Building and Working with Effective Groups (pp. 561-586)

1. Where in nursing are the most appropriate uses for teams? For work groups? For committees?

There are differences in the definitions of a team, a work group, and a committee. A team is a group of individuals working together for a common cause, each member doing the collective work of the team. A true team goes through a developmental process that takes time and the investment of energy to become a true team; otherwise, the team is a workgroup (Katzenbach & Smith, 1993). Institutions benefit from the work of a true synergistic team. Multidisciplinary teams such as client care teams, ad hoc teams, and quality improvement teams are a few examples of teams that can be beneficial in nursing.

A work group is a gathering of individuals who come together to share ideas. They have individual work products for which they are responsible. An example of this is the client care unit in which the secretary, registered nurse, charge nurse, and managers work together but have specific responsibilities to perform, possibly with individual accountability, but no collective accountability. A committee is a specific type of group that meets periodically, has an identified purpose within the institution, and has a mechanism for maintaining and selecting members. An example of a committee is a policy and procedure committee. The work group provides the forum for nurses and other care providers to join together to formulate client care decisions and to improve work processes.

2. What motivates an individual to join a group?

An individual may join a group to satisfy psychological drives and primary needs. The need for socialization, affiliation, and recognition, as well as an opportunity for self-achievement, often motivates group participation.

3. What are the significantly different elements between a work group and a team? What elements are similar? How do you determine whether you need a team?

Since the 1990s, hospitals and other organizations have transformed the traditional hierarchical bureaucratic structure into team-based structures. Knowledge has become so specialized in the health care settings that it is imperative to have all disciplines involved to achieve high-quality outcomes. A team is a group of individuals working together for a common cause with each member doing the collective work of the team. A true team goes through a developmental process that takes time and the investment of energy to become a true team; otherwise, the team is a workgroup (Katzenbach & Smith, 1993). A true team also shares the leadership of the group. A work group is a gathering of individuals who come together to share ideas. They have individual work products for which they are responsible. The boundaries remain separated, and there is little collaboration.

Teamwork and collaboration are essential to achieving high-quality work outcomes and cost control in client care. Ideally, all groups should strive toward becoming a team. Groups that are struggling may benefit from team building.

4. How is leading a group like the nursing process? The management process?

Leading a group parallels the nursing process in that it consists of assessment, diagnosis, planning, intervention, and evaluation. Essential functions of the group leader are to assess the group's role and responsibility and to articulate its purpose. The group leader is responsible for planning functional and operational processes, facilitating group consensus, and evaluating group work. The management process is also useful in leading a group. It involves planning, diagnosing, coordinating, implementing the best solution, and evaluating and tracking outcomes. Additional components of the management process include organizing the physical environment, preparing and motivating participants for action, and facilitating the group accomplishments.

5. What team-building strategies are most useful when one is trying to develop a team?

Interactive leadership, a leadership style prevalent in nursing, facilitates team building. It uses strategies such as participatory management, mutual respect, and generating trust through shared governance models. Building team cohesion and performance can be enhanced by facilitating interdisciplinary collaboration, using conflict resolution skills, forming strong alliances with top decision makers, and enhancing collaboration and coordination skills.

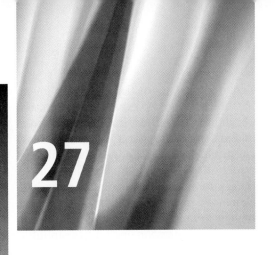

27

Confronting the Nursing Shortage

The nursing shortage is a major national issue influencing the delivery of health care services. The United States has more than 2.3 million licensed registered nurses; however, there is a projected deficit of 275,000 nurses by 2010 (National Center for Health Workforce Analysis, 2002). Furthermore, enrollment in nursing schools is falling at the same time that enrollments in nursing programs must increase by 40% to meet the projected demand for nurses (American Association of Colleges of Nursing, 2003). Further compounding the problem is that the average age of a registered nurse (RN) is 44 years old (National Center for Health Workforce Analysis, 2002) and that between 1980 and 2000 the proportion of RNs under the age of 30 declined from 25% to 9%.

To confront the nursing shortage challenge, the following strategies should be examined and implemented: (1) implementing educational strategies to increase nursing school enrollment; (2) improving work environments to retain staff; and (3) redesigning the health delivery system to reduce the demand for nursing services. A *nursing shortage* is defined as the number of nurses that employers would like to hire in relation to the number of nurses willing to be employed. A nursing shortage is different from *understaffing* in that understaffing is often due to local factors such as tight budgets or working conditions; it is not related to the workforce supply of nurses. Data reported as indicators on the nursing shortage include employer reports, vacancy rates, turnover, recruitment difficulties, staffing levels, RN supply per population or forecasting models. The *span of control* is the number of individuals who report to a single manager (Hattrup & Kleiner, 1993). The smaller the span of control, the more satisfied employees are and the more they are apt to stay in the organization. A *transformational leader* is one who inspires and transforms followers by enhancing their sense of value and importance. The *four components of transformation leadership* are charisma, inspirational motivation, intellectual stimulation, and individualized consideration (Bass, 1998). *Turnover* is termination of membership in an organization.

Cycles of nursing shortages and surpluses have occurred despite the fact that there were 2.3 million nurses in jobs in 2002, with 1 in 5 working part time (Bureau of Labor Statistics, 2004). The following shortage periods occurred: 1915-1920, 1945-1965, 1970-1980, and 1986-1992. The basis of the nursing shortages has been attributed to the nature of the work, low wages, poor working conditions, and hospital administrators' desire to keep nursing costs down and preventing salaries from increasing (Carlson et al., 1992; Grando, 1998; King, 1989). The major reasons cited for a projected increased demand for nurses are increasing incidence of chronic illnesses and an aging population. The nursing shortage is particularly troublesome because research has demonstrated that with a greater RN mix, there are fewer negative care outcomes (Kovner & Gergen, 1998). Not only is there a shortage in all of the states in the United States, but also there are significant shortages in many other countries. Some countries are concerned that their nurses will go to the United States or another country, creating a situation in which their national supply of nurses is even worse.

Many factors contribute to the nursing shortage. These factors include changing demographics of an aging RN workforce; not only are the existing nurses aging, but also there is a higher average age of recent graduating nurses. Also, the number of young women choosing nursing as a career has declined during the past several decades because of the increased career opportunities available to them. *Factors that affect the supply of nurses* include nursing education, work environment, and demographics. For nursing education, there is a shortage of nursing faculty to prepare new nurses. In addition, there are more students electing a baccalaureate degree rather than an associate degree, which requires twice as long to complete and to enter the workplace. Several work environment factors influence turnover, including workload, autonomy, relations with managers, and compensation (Buerhaus et al., 2000; Laschinger et al., 2001; Tri-Council for Nursing, 2004). Nurses with the highest nurse-to-patient ratio were more likely to describe burnout, emotional exhaustion, and job dissatisfaction. Professional autonomy was identified as the strongest predictor of nurses' identification with the organization (Apker et al., 2003). Additional factors influencing job satisfaction include the manager's leadership style and compensation. The majority of employment growth will occur in hospitals (National Center for Health Workforce Analysis, 2002).

Increased demand for nursing and health care services increases with age; those over 65, and particularly those 85 and over, make the greatest use of services. Strategies to confront the nursing shortage include formal recruitment and retention programs, collaboration between education and practice settings to recruit more persons into nursing, sign-on and other types of hiring bonuses, and actions to improve the work environment of nurses (American Hospital Association, 2002). Educational strategies to increase enrollment in nursing programs include additional nursing education funding; encouraging a younger, more diverse population; enhancing the image of nursing; and articulating a clear vision that includes career progression. Making nursing attractive to the next generation with scholarship opportunities, attractive compensation, and employee-friendly work environments can contribute to filling nursing positions. Centers of excellence in leadership and management are important in establishing supportive leadership and management structures, providing nurses with sufficient autonomy, ensuring adequate nursing staffing, and implementing strong compensation and benefit programs. Transformational leaders were more likely to have staff nurses with higher job satisfaction scores (Medley & Larochelle, 1995; Stordeur et al., 2000). Transformational leaders provide support, encouragement, positive feedback, and individual consideration and promote an open environment supporting cooperation and teamwork. Another important environmental factor is the size of the unit and span of managerial control. Research demonstrates that the larger the work unit, the less positive the relationship between the manager and staff (Green et al., 1996; Gittell, 2001). Managers who encourage professional autonomy in practice have more satisfied nurses. These managers encourage promotion and advancement, flexible scheduling, and a culture that promotes respect and collaboration.

Current trends to encourage experienced nurses to work for longer periods include developing clinical ergonomic adaptations to minimize the physical strain in the work environment, to use flexible scheduling, to increase part-time positions, to expand new roles, and to provide economic incentives. Implementing good compensation and benefit packages may entice nurses to work longer. Nurses may choose to specialize in primary prevention and build autonomous practices. Another strategy to affect the nursing shortage is to conduct research on methods of health care delivery, design technology to support nursing care, and develop innovations in care delivery. Nursing leaders can influence the nursing shortage by applying and accepting executive leader positions, designing supportive health care environments, encouraging research and innovations, and mentoring junior nurses.

LEARNING TOOL

Activity: Factors in the Work Environment that Support Nursing Practice

Purpose

To interview an RN to understand better the factors that support nurses in a work environment. These factors often influence the attractiveness of nursing as a profession and influence the retention of nurses.

Instructions

Carve out time before, during, or after your clinical rotation experience to interview an RN on the unit you are assigned. Ask an RN to schedule 10 minutes to answer a few questions about professional nursing practice. Use the following questions to guide the discussion:

- What factors in this work environment support RNs in providing care to patients?

- What characteristics do you appreciate in a nursing leader?

- What do you like most about professional nursing practice?

- Do you feel that there are opportunities for career advancement in the work environment?

- Are professional activities (such as meetings and inservices) a requirement of employment?

By interviewing an RN, you can compare the material that you have been reading on the nursing shortage and determine those factors that attract and retain nurse. You also can begin to formulate ideas of where you may wish to practice based on factors that support nurses in work environments.

CASE STUDY

Jackie Yange is a graduate nurse on the 45-bed women's care unit at University Hospital in Honolulu, Hawaii.

She has been employed in the women's care unit for 6 months and has become discouraged and dissatisfied with her work experience. Nurse Yange has talked to several new nurses about how disorganized, inflexible, and controlling the nurse manager and assistant nurse manager have been with her work requests. She is working on her graduate degree and has requested specific days off to accommodate her school schedule. In return for her work requests, Nurse Yange has agreed to cover all of the major holidays and give up a few "extra" weekend days. To her dismay, the schedule consistently is posted without her input and the days that she has requested are not even granted; instead only the exact shifts during which her classes fall are scheduled. Nurse Yange is disheartened because she has asked for the entire day of her scheduled class be a day off so she can arrive at class relaxed and prepared. To make matters worse, she has been scheduled for every holiday and weekend.

When Nurse Yange approached the assistant head nurse, Andrea Jacobs, she was told to "take it or leave it"; after all, she was getting the time off for her class, which was a major inconvenience for the nursing unit. Nurse Yange also tried to discuss a new "reporting method" because she noticed it took almost 1 hour for a total report to be provided to the on-coming shift. She was told by the head nurse, Nancy Smith, that she should not worry about improving systems, when she should be focusing on increasing her clinical proficiency. When Nurse Yange asked Nurse Smith whether there was a problem with her patient care, Nurse Smith abruptly stated, "No, and let's keep it that way!" Nurse Yange decided that she was unhappy and would quit to move to a more supportive environment. She went to the nurse recruiter in the human resource department and asked to be considered for an open position on a medical-surgical unit. She had heard good things about the nurse manager, Kelly Young, and the supportive environment. The nurse recruiter told her that she was not eligible for a transfer until she had completed 1 year of service. Nurse Yange went home that night and wrote her resignation letter.

Case Study Questions

1. What types of nurse leaders were Nurses Yange and Jacobs? Would you classify them as transformational or transactional leaders?

2. What strategies could Nurses Smith and Jacobs have implemented to provide a more supportive climate for Nurse Yange?

3. Would a smaller span of control on the women's care unit have helped Nurse Yange be supportive to the nursing staff?

4. What types of strategies could be implemented in a nursing unit to build collegiality, support, respect, and flexibility?

5. What impact does professional autonomy have on nursing environments?

LEARNING RESOURCES

Discussion Questions

1. Describe why the nursing shortage is a major national issue in the United States. How does a nursing shortage in other countries around the world affect the nursing shortage in the United States?

2. What is the basis for the nursing shortage problem?

3. Why is the nursing shortage projected to be so intense? Describe the factors contributing to the nursing shortage.

4. What strategies can be implemented to increase the number of nurses in the United States?

5. What work environmental factors have been cited as reasons for increased nursing staff turnover? Describe why these factors contribute to the nurse turnover.

6. Describe the nurse managers role in providing a supportive work environment and the role of professional autonomy in nurse job satisfaction.

Study Questions

True or False: Circle the correct answer.

T F 1. A nursing shortage is the understaffing of nursing units because of tight budgets or poor working conditions.

T F 2. A large span of control is conducive to a supportive work environment and autonomous practice.

T F 3. A transformational leader is one who inspires and transforms followers by increasing their sense of value and importance.

T F 4. The future projected demand for nurses is related to the increase in chronic illnesses and an aging population.

T F 5. The greater the RN mix, the fewer the care outcomes that are negative.

T F 6. Using foreign nurses to fill U.S. vacancies is a useful strategy to improve the nursing shortage and is not problematic because there is a surplus of nurses in many countries.

T F 7. The majority of nursing employment openings will be in primary care in the future.

T   F   8. Infants and toddlers are the highest consumers of health care services.

T   F   9. It is important to enhance the image of nursing and nurses to attract individuals into the profession of nursing.

T   F   10. A manager's role in an organization is important and influences the retention of nurses.

REFERENCES

Aiken, L. H., Clarke, S. P., Sloane, D. M., Sochalski, J., & Silber, J. H. (2002). Hospital nurse staffing and patient mortality, nurse burnout, and job dissatisfaction, *Journal of the American Medical Association, 288*(16), 1987-1993.

American Association of Colleges of Nursing. (2003). *Faculty shortages in baccalaureate and graduate nursing programs: Scope of the problem and strategies for expanding the supply.* Washington, DC: Author. Retrieved May 21, 2004, from *www.aacn.nche.edu/Publications/WhitePapers/Faculty Shortages.htm*

American Hospital Association. (2002). *In our hands: How hospital leaders can build a thriving workforce.* Chicago: Author.

Apker, J., Zabava Ford, W., & Fox, D. (2003). Predicting nurses' organizational and professional identification: The effect of nursing roles, professional autonomy, and supportive communication. *Nursing Economic$, 21*(5), 225-233.

Bass, B. (1998). *Transformational leadership: Industrial, military, and educational impact.* Mahwah, NJ: Lawrence Erlbaum Associates.

Buerhaus, P., Staiger, D., & Auerbach, D. (2000). Implications of an aging registered nurse workforce. *Journal of the American Medical Association, 283*(22), 2948-1954.

Bureau of Labor Statistics. (2004). U.S. *Department of Labor: Occupational outlook handbook—Registered nurses* (2004-2005 ed.). Washington, DC: Author. Retrieved May 21, 2004, from *www.bls.gov/oco/ocos083.htm*

Carlson, S. M., Cowart, M. E., & Speaker, D. L. (1992). Perspectives of nursing personnel in the 1980s. In M. E. Cowart, & W. J. Serow (Eds.), *Nurses in the workplace* (pp. 1-27). Newbury Park, CA: Sage.

Gittell, J. (2001). Supervisory span, relational coordination and flight departure performance: A reassessment of postbureaucracy theory. *Organization Science, 12,* 468-483.

Grando, V. T. (1998). Making do with fewer nurses in the United States, 1945-1965. *Image, 30*(2), 147-149.

Green, S., Anderson, S., & Shivers, S. (1996). Demographic and organizational influences on leader-member exchange and related work related attitudes. *Organizational Behavior and Human Decision Processes, 66,* 203-214.

Hattrup, G., & Kleiner, B. (1993). How to establish the proper span of control for managers. *Industrial Management, 35,* 28-30.

King, M. G. (1989). Nursing shortage, circa 1915. *Image, 21*(3), 124-127.

Kovner, C., & Gergen, P. J. (1998). Nurse staffing levels and adverse events following surgery in U.S. hospitals. *Image, 30*(4), 315-321.

Laschinger, H., Finegan, J., & Shamian, J. (2001). Promoting nurses' health: Effect of empowerment on job strain and work satisfaction. *Nursing Economic$, 19,* 42-52.

Medley, F., & Larochelle, D. (1995). Transformational leadership and job satisfaction. *Nursing Management, 26*(9), 64.

National Center for Health Workforce Analysis. (2002). *Projected supply, demand and shortages of registered nurses: 2000-2020.* Rockville, MD: U.S. Department of Health and Human Services, Health Resources and Services Administration, Bureau of Health Professions. Retrieved May 21, 2004, from *http://bhpr.hrsa.gov/healthworkforce/reports/rnproject/report.htm*

Stordeur, S., Vandenberghe, C., & D'Hoore, W. (2000). Leadership styles across hierarchical levels in nursing departments. *Nursing Research, 49,* 37-43.

Tri-Council for Nursing. (2004). *Tri-Council for Nursing policy statement: Strategies to reverse the new nursing shortage.* New York: National League for Nursing. Retrieved May 24, 2004, from *www.nln.org/aboutnln/news_tricouncil2.htm*

Wieck, K. (2003). Faculty for the millennium: Changes needed to attract the emerging workforce into nursing. *Journal of Nursing Education, 42* (4), 151-159.

SUPPLEMENTAL READINGS

Albaugh, J.A. (2005). Resolving the nursing shortage: Nursing job satisfaction on the rise. *Urological Nursing, 25*(4), 293.

Evans, M. (2005). Losing their faculty. *Modern Healthcare, 35* (24), 24-27.

Lindsay, G. & Kleiner, B. (2005). Nurse residency program: An effective tool for recruitment and retention. *Journal of Health Care Finance, 31*(3), 25-32.

Mikhail, J. (2005). The nursing shortage: Clear and present danger. *Journal of Trauma Nursing, 12*(2), 38-39.

Stuenkel, D. C., Cohen, J. & de la Cuesta, K. (2005). The multigenerational nursing workforce: Essential differences in perception of work environment. *Journal of Nursing Administration, 35*(6), 283.

Chapter 27: Confronting the Nursing Shortage (pp. 587-604)

1. **What creative strategies can the average nurse consider to tackle one or more factors contributing to the nursing shortage?**

   Nurses can encourage young persons to consider the profession of nursing through informal conversations, volunteering to present at high school career days, and role modeling at social events. Nurses also can volunteer to be shadowed by high school students in the work environment while discussing how the nurse is critically thinking, that is, using the nursing process and knowledge of physiology and behavioral sciences to make important decisions. What creative strategies can you think of?

2. **What would make nursing attractive to the next generation of nurses?**

   Several strategies can be helpful in making nursing attractive to the young, such as the establishment of tuition funding and scholarships, enhancing the image in society, developing career paths, increasing compensation to be competitive with other professional roles, and the provision of employee-friendly work environments.

3. **How can mentorship help alleviate the nursing shortage? Who should do this? How?**

   Aiken and colleagues (2002) found that 43% of nurses in their study who experienced high levels of burnout and dissatisfaction intended to leave their jobs within a year. Registered nurses mentoring new nurses to acclimate to the workforce can help decrease the burnout rate. Nursing leaders can initiate a mentoring program in which each nurse new to the institution has a nurturing mentor.

4. **How and in what ways can the image of nursing be enhanced?**

   Wieck (2003) recommends that expanding the image of nursing from caring and caregiver to opportunities and outcomes may affect the image of nursing positively. Younger persons want opportunities to succeed and outcomes by which they can measure their success; for example, the operating room and emergency room are perceived as exciting places to work. Marketing the relationship between better patient outcomes and the role of the professional nurse is another positive image of nursing. Increasing compensation also can enhance the image of nursing because our society values well-compensated professional roles.

5. **How can technology be of use in a nursing shortage?**

   Technology, research, and innovation can reduce the demand on services and enhance the capacity of a reduced nursing workforce. For instance, the use of cellular telephones, palm pilots, and computers can reduce the workload. Cellular telephones may be used in the hospital to contact other health professionals such as physicians, pharmacists, physical therapists, and nutritionists to coordinate care. Rather than walking back to the nurse's station every time the nurse is paged or needs to contact another professional, the nurse can use a readily available cellular telephone.

   Computers with interactive programs designed to decrease charting time can enhance the role of the nurse. Palm pilots can be used as an instant reference for looking up medications, the care of a particular disease process, or the preferred preparation for a radiological test.

6. **Describe how demand affects the health care delivery system and nursing.**

   The demand for nurses may depend on the local health system characteristics. For example, if prevention methods or early diagnosis strategies are not in place, patients may wait too long to receive appropriate care. This delay results in sicker patients needing a higher level of care. This higher condition severity results in a higher demand for critical care nursing services. Critical care nurses care for fewer patients than do nurses on a general medical-surgical floor because of the patient's condition severity, thus resulting in a higher demand for nursing services.

7. **Give examples of policies that would address the nursing shortage at the nursing unit level, hospital level, and national level.**

   Policies that would address factors that contribute to the nursing shortage include establishing appropriate leadership and management structures, providing nurses with sufficient autonomy, ensuring adequate nurse staffing, and implementing appropriate compensation and benefit programs.

8. **What research questions would increase our understanding of the causes and effects of nursing staff shortage?**

A diverse and wide range of research questions are possible when considering research questions that could help increase the understanding of the causes and effects of the nursing staff shortage. "What is the relationship between the level of condition severity and the number of registered nurses caring for patients on a medical surgical unit?" "How do high school seniors perceive the role of the registered nurse?" "What are enticements for college students in choosing careers?" "What is the relationship between higher compensation, job satisfaction, and retention of experienced nurses?" "How do other health care professionals define the role of the registered nurse?" "What is the image of nursing as perceived by physicians?" "Do institutions that support professional nursing autonomy show less preferential treatment to other health care professionals than those who do not support nursing autonomy?"

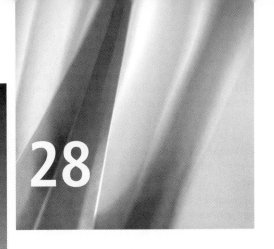

28 Cultural and Generational Workforce Diversity

STUDY FOCUS

Diversity is part of the changing nature of society, and business leaders must be skilled at managing cultural and generational workforce diversity to gain a competitive advantage. The advantages of managing a diverse workforce are providing supportive work environments, improving the retention of the best individuals, fortifying team effectiveness and exploiting rich skill sets, enhancing recruitment from nontraditional environments, having the ability to relate to customer needs, and laying the groundwork and providing the context for future business growth. The five major sociodemographic developments that define American society are (1) emergence of a global economy; (2) technoshrink, the diffusion of information and telecommunication technology; (3) maturation of the Baby Boomer generation; (4) rise of individualism; and (5) deterioration of the principles of economic justice. The growing appreciation for the global community has raised the awareness of cultural differences and of the differing values in subcultures in local communities. For successful delivery of health care services, nurses must recognize the values of other cultures as they relate to health and must take positive steps to recruit persons from diverse cultures to the nursing profession.

The demographic makeup of the U.S. population in the areas of ethnicity and age are radically changing. Of the four major U.S. populations (white, black, Hispanic, and Asian American/Pacific Islander), the Hispanic and Asian-American/Pacific Islander groups are growing at a rapid rate (Freeman, 1997). Latinos now surpass blacks as the largest ethnic minority in the United States. In fact, as of 2001, one in four Americans were nonwhite. The world population is expected to double by 2050, with the majority of growth (85%) occurring in developing countries. In contrast, in industrialized nations the median age is rising and the population is aging. Changes in societal needs will occur as the population ages and becomes more ethnically diverse. With the projected demographic changes there will be an increase in diagnoses of chronic illnesses, rising generational issues, increasing language and cultural challenges, conflicting perspectives on the use of resources, and challenging ethical issues. In the United States, individualism has been a value that has contributed to the fragmentation of the family structures, poor public school systems, and mistrust of the government and businesses. In addition, the distribution of wealth has shifted to the advantage of the affluent. This fact partially supports the statement that this country no longer has a middle class. Individuals are "haves" or "have nots." Older adults experience a better lifestyle than children.

Despite the rapidly changing demographic characteristics of the U.S. population, there is failure to obtain parity in positive health care outcomes for members of minority groups. Nurses are in a pivotal role to enact changes in effectively managing quality health care and managing resources to affect positively the vulnerable populations in communities. Statistics show that 90% of the total registered nurse population is white, which is higher than 72% of the total U.S. population (U.S. Department of Health and Human Services, 1996). Recruitment efforts need to be aimed at attracting a diverse cultural mix of individuals into the nursing profession.

Cultural diversity is the variations among groups of people in habits, values, beliefs, preferences, taboos, and rules of behavior. *Corporate culture* is the way business is conducted in organizations and is comprised of written and unwritten rules. *Culture* is values and beliefs. Culture is the actions in organizations of what receives attention, what is rewarded, what things mean, and what reactions are acceptable and which are not. *Diversity* is differences that make a difference in that which is stripped of its cultural and political baggage. *Racism* is defined as discrimination based on race or color. *Prejudice* is an emotional mode of mental functioning involving rigid prejudgment (stereotypes) and misjudgment of individual activities. *Stereotypes* are clouded viewpoints and perceptions that may occur even though an individual disagrees or does not consciously hold that stereotype. *Cultural relativism* is when individuals do not judge but rather consider actions, beliefs, or traits of their own cultural context in order to better understand them. *Bias* is when an individual's emotional perspective is prejudiced. *Cultural competence* is providing care effectively to persons from a multiplicity of cultures. Competence is a dynamic and evolving process that embodies an evolution of knowing, respecting, and incorporating the values of others. Cultural competence involves recognition of the importance of integrating persons with other values in the process of health care delivery. *Ethnicity* is shared origins and culture. *Transcultural nursing* is a formal area of study and practice that focuses on cultural care, comparison of cultural variations, and the provision of culturally compassionate care.

on all members in one or another way. The following table presents four cohorts and their characteristics.

The *mature generation,* born 1925 to 1945, has strong respect for authority and conforms to the situation. In their generation, children were to be seen but not heard. For *Baby Boomers,* born 1946 to 1964, efficiency, teamwork, quality, and service have been hallmarks of their leadership. They grew up believing they were special, ignored or broke rules, enjoy conveniences and often said "charge it." The *X'ers,* born 1965 to 1980, are the first latchkey kids and have become resourceful. They enjoy a balanced life and do not look for long-term employment agreements. The *Millennial workers,* born 1981 to 1999, are technologically adept, multitask, and have a positive outlook. They bend rules and work to live.

The United States has been a melting pot resulting from waves of immigration. Degrees of cultural

Generational Characteristics

Matures	Baby Boomers	Generation X	Millennials
Hard work	Personal fulfilment	Uncertainty	What's next?
Duty	Optimism	Personal focus	On my terms
Sacrifice	Crusading causes	Live for today	Just show up
Thriftiness	Buy now/pay later	Save, save, save	Earn to spend
Work fast	Work efficiently	Eliminate the task	Do exactly what's asked

Source: Center for Generational Studies, Aurora, Colo.

Common sources of conflict include differences in time orientation, communication patterns, value systems, perceptions of staff responsibilities or nursing roles, and differences in educational preparation. Conflict is common in organizations, with supervisors spending as much as 29% of their time resolving personality and relationship issues. In fact, 85% of persons fired in 2003 were fired because of relationship issues (The Murphy Leadership Institute, 2004). Those who act differently most often are labeled as problems.

A new challenge for nurse leaders is generational workforce diversity. *Generational groups* often are referred to as *call cohorts.* These cohorts are linked together through shared life experiences in their formative years. Each group or cohort is influenced by generational markers, which are events that have an impact

awareness vary in the United States, but the predominant, Eurocentric, white majority as a whole has not viewed individuals as having a valuable unique cultural heritage. In the United States, health care assumptions include self-determination, autonomy, independence, right to know, "I" make the decisions about my health care, moral obligations and medical ethics, obligation to tell the truth, duty to give information to the client, and providing the bill of rights of the institution. An important part of cultural context is the method in which individuals communicate verbally and nonverbally. Cultural context can be low, in which the explicit verbal or written message carries the meaning, or high, in which what is written or stated rarely carries the meaning. Cultural differences are highlighted in the following table.

Low-and High-Context Cultural Characteristics

	Low Context	High Context
Countries/regions	United States, Canada, England, Russia, Northwestern Europe	China, Japan, Arabia, Mexico, South America, Pacific Islands
Characteristics	Very verbal	Less verbal or nonverbal
	Individual	Group
	Equality	Individual dignity
	Democracy	Consensus
	Personal freedom	Obligation to others
	Fairness	Fate (karma, joss)
	Achievement	Process/role
	Innovation	Continuous improvement
	Entrepreneurship	Communal
	Competition	Cooperation

Cultural sensitivity and competence can be learned. *Strategies to increase cultural sensitivity and competence* include knowing your own culture, values, and biases; listening and observing; emphasizing the corporate values; developing the ability to be a teacher and learner; holding up the end of the bargain; giving clear directions; delegating the outcomes; giving the big picture; considering the rules and procedures you implement in the workplace; managing your expectations; providing straight forward steps for decision making; being courageous; managing according to values and attitudes of the individual's generation; and providing an opportunity to grow.

Many improvements have been made in health care; however, health care outcomes are not equal for all citizens. *Health disparities* are population-specific differences in the presence of diseases and access to health care (Washington, 2003). *Underserved populations* are those that have less access to health care providers and services than the majority of the population. Racial and ethnic disparities are caused by client-related and system-related factors. Client-related factors include socioeconomic differences, health education differences, and health behavior differences. System-related factors include discrimination, language differences, workforce diversity differences, cultural competence differences, payment/reimbursement differences, insurance coverage differences, and data deficiency. An individual's health is related to health status from lifestyle (50%), the environment (30%), and genetics (20%) (Kent, 2000). Eligibility for public assistance is, in some instances, not available for federal benefits for 5 years from an immigrant's date of entry. This ineligibility makes it difficult to prosper and assimilate into the mainstream of American life.

Leadership and management implications include considering knowledge about generational and cultural parameters. Increasing the number of ethnic minority providers will improve the access to care for the underserved (American Hospital Association, 2002). Another strategy to help meet the nursing shortage in the short run is hiring foreign-born registered nurses. Developing a strategic human resource plan for recruitment and retention of a diverse staff will assist in maintaining a competitive advantage. Nurse administrations can model respect for differences: exploring beyond their comfort zone, withholding judgment of others, emphasizing the positive, and practicing good communication techniques are strategies for success (Grossman & Taylor, 1995). Relationships are important. In the work environment, relationships come down to trust, respect, shared goals, affirming identity, and communication. Everyone should know 10 things about race: race is a modern idea; race has no genetic basis; human subspecies do not exist; skin color really is only skin deep; most variation is within, not between, "races"; slavery predates race; race and freedom evolved together; race justified social inequalities as natural; race is not biological, but racism is still real; and color blindness will not end racism.

A trend in cultural awareness is the attracting of a culturally diverse workforce. The synergy of diverse viewpoints can improve health care knowledge and delivery of services. Strategies for success with cultural diversity in the workplace include respecting differences, exploring beyond the comfort zone, withholding judgment of others, and emphasizing the positive and practicing good communication. Diversity is the "consideration of socioeconomic class, gender, age, religious belief, sexual orientation, and physical disabilities, as well as race and ethnicity" (American Association of Colleges of Nursing, 1997, p. 1). An issue that is becoming increasingly prevalent is that health illiteracy increases with age. Therefore, nursing interventions aimed at effective educational and communication strategies and materials to improve health care knowledge of the elderly are essential in the delivery of services.

LEARNING TOOLS

Activity: Generational Workforce Diversity

Purpose

To identify the characteristics of generational groups or cohorts in order to understand the complexity of generational workforce diversity.

Directions

For each of the four descriptions, identify whether the individual most closely fits the mature, baby boomer, generation X, or millennial cohort. Write your response on the blank line.

1. Katherine Freeman is a 64-year-old registered nurse who works in the coronary intensive care unit. She has been employed in this capacity for the past 44 years and is a graduate of Belleview Hospital School of Nursing. Nurse Freeman is proud of her nursing education and profession and provides quality care to her clients. She is prompt, dependable, and works hard to provide the best possible care to her clients. She is respectful of her colleagues, managers, and other healthcare professionals. Nurse Freeman consistently works extra shifts, if requested, and is dedicated to the coronary care unit.

What Generational Cohort is Nurse Freeman part of? _____

2. Jonathon Addison is a 21-year-old registered nurse who works on neurological unit in a large teaching hospital in Austin, Texas. Nurse Addison is very good with computerized charting and any electronic device. He enjoys his work, but, if you need him, you better catch him before 3:00 PM because he is gone at the end of his shift. Nurse Addison requests help often, and the charge nurse reviews his assignment with him in order to review all unit duties he must complete besides his client care. Once he receives his assignment, he is self-sufficient and provides good client care. Nurse Addison has worked one extra shift since he was employed and did so very reluctantly.

What Generational Cohort is Nurse Addison part of? _____

3. Shelly McDonaldson is a 26-year-old registered nurse who works on the medical surgical unit in a large city hospital in Chicago, Illinois. Nurse McDonaldson provides quality care to her clients and is dependable. She often will challenge the Nurse Manager at staff meetings. Nurse McDonaldson also will challenge her assignment if she thinks it is unfair. She rarely will work extra shifts and often talks about a balanced life.

What Generational Cohort is Nurse McDonaldson part of? _____

4. Sally Radoski is a 45-year-old registered nurse who works on the intermediate care unit. Nurse Radoski is an exceptional nurse, who has strong leadership skills, is an excellent clinician, and is extremely helpful and organized. All of the nurses on the unit respect and look up to her. Every time a Nurse Manager position becomes available she is nominated by numerous nurses and staff, but she declines the position. Nurse Radoski is always trying to involve everyone on the unit using a shared governance model. Nurse Radoski always has new clothes, bought a beautiful cottage, and travels often. She often jokes with her colleagues that she will never be able to retire as she enjoys a nice lifestyle.

What Generational Cohort is Nurse Radoski part of?

_____

CASE STUDY

Dolly Mae Doran, a 62-year-old nurse has worked on the maternity unit for 40 years. She is timely, respectful of clients, administrators, and peers and performs excellent care. She works hard and works fast and is extremely dedicated to the unit. In fact, if she is called by the Nurse Manager and requested to do an extra shift, she always willingly complies. Susan Smith, a 26-year-old nurse was recently hired on the maternity unit. She works hard and provides quality care, but Dolly Mae often notices her challenging the Charge Nurse and Nurse Manager on decisions that they have made. And, to top it all off, Susan has refused all three times she was asked to work an extra shift to cover for a sick colleague. To make matters worse, Abby Delrue, a 21-year-old nurse was hired 6 months ago and Dolly Mae and the other "seasoned" nurses must constantly provide direction and deadlines for her to complete her work. Many of the "seasoned" nurses are becoming frustrated as they feel they are required to do the majority of the unit work.

Case Study Questions

1. Is there a difference in generational characteristics of Dolly Mae, Susan Smith, and Abby Delrue?

2. What are the three generational groups or cohorts?

3. What type of leadership strategies can be used to manage generational workforce diversity?

LEARNING RESOURCES

Discussion Questions

1. How can nurses use information about various cultures to influence health care service delivery?

2. What is cultural diversity? What strategies can be used to increase cultural diversity in the workforce?

3. What is the demographic makeup of the U.S. population? How does the demographic makeup in the United States compare with the demographics of the registered nursing population in the United States?

4. What does the "predominant, Eurocentric, white majority" mean? What are some Eurocentric concepts? How do these concepts affect the provision of nursing services?

5. What should a cultural assessment include?

Study Questions

True or False: Circle the correct answer.

T　F　1. Cultural differences in ways of doing things and in beliefs about health and illness are learned and transmitted via cultural environments.

T　F　2. Examples of cultural differences include eye contact norms, gender issues, touching and physical contact, and food practices.

T　F　3. Japanese clients usually are given lower dosages of medications and have less tolerance of side effects.

T　F　4. The term *Eurocentric* refers to valuing cultural diversity and being sensitive to cultural heritage.

T　F　5. Minority groups obtain parity in positive health care outcomes compared with the general overall health of the American people.

T　F　6. Cultural competence is defined as an ongoing evolution of knowing, respecting, and incorporating the values of others.

T　F　7. The demographics of the U.S. population are similar to the demographics of nurses in the United States

T　F　8. Diversity includes only race and ethnicity.

Matching: Write the letter of the correct response in front of each term.

_____ 9. Cultural awareness

_____ 10. Cultural knowledge

_____ 11. Cultural skill

_____ 12. Cultural encounter

A. The process of seeking and obtaining an educational background about the different worldviews of various cultures

B. A process of directly engaging in cross-cultural interactions

C. The process of learning how to do a cultural assessment, allowing the nurse to identify an individual client's perceptions, beliefs, and practices

D. A deliberate and cognitive process of becoming aware of and sensitive to the client's culture by becoming aware of the influence of one's own cultural values and learning to avoid imposing them on others

REFERENCES

American Association of Colleges of Nursing. (1997). *Diversity and equality of opportunity* (Online). Washington, DC: Author. Retrieved July 15, 2005, from *www.aacn.nche.edu/Publications/positions/diverse.htm*

American Hospital Association. (2002). *In our hands: How hospital leaders can build a thriving workforce.* Chicago: American Hospital Association Commission on Workforce for Hospitals and Health Systems.

American Hospital Association. (2003). *Unequal treatment: Confronting racial and ethnic disparities in health care.* Chicago: AHA news.com. Retrieved November 12, 2004, from *www.aha.org*

Freeman, H. P. (1997). *Concerns of special populations in the national cancer program: The real impact of the reduction in cancer mortality research.* In meeting summary: *President's cancer panel* (Online). Retrieved October 10, 2005, from *www.nci.nih.gov/*

Grossman, D., & Taylor, R. (1995). Cultural diversity on the unit. *American Journal of Nursing, 95*(2), 64-67.

Kent, C. (2000). Perspectives. Disparities: A shadow on U.S. health landscape. *Medicine & Health, 54*(Suppl 35), 1-4.

The Murphy Leadership Institute. (2004, February 25-26). *National conference on transforming the work environment of nurses.* Washington, DC: Author.

U.S. Department of Health and Human Services. (1996). *The registered nurse population.* Rockville, MD: Author.

Washington, D. (2003, October 16). Disparities in health care: The challenges for the new millennium. *Caring Headlines* (pp. 1, 11). Boston: Massachusetts General Hospital.

SUPPLEMENTAL READINGS

Camphinha-Bacota, J. (2003). Cultural desire: The key to unlocking cultural competence. *Journal of Nursing Education, 42*(6), 239-240.

Foley, R., & Wurmser, T. A. (2004). Culture diversity: A mobile workforce command creative leadership, new partnerships, and innovative approaches to integration. *Nursing Administration Quarterly, 28*(2), 122-128.

Hassouneh-Phillips, D., & Beckett, A. (2003). An education in racism. *Journal of Nursing Education, 42*(6), 258-265.

Phillips, M. (2003). The challenge of cultural diversity. *Dermatology Nursing, 15*(4), 311-312.

Walsh, S. (2004). Formulation of a plan of care for culturally diverse patients. *International Journal of Nursing Terminologies and Classifications, 15*(1), 17-26.

Chapter 28: Cultural and Generational Workforce Diversity (pp. 605-624)

1. **Why is cultural competence important for nursing?**

   Cultural competence is important for two primary reasons. One, the workforce of registered nurses in the United States is primarily white female. To encourage others to enter into the nursing profession, nurses must focus on cultural competence in the workplace. Second, culturally competent care practices are essential in providing optimal client care. Lack of understanding of cultural practices may result in longer hospital stays, noncompliance issues, loss of meaningful nurse-client or provider-to-provider communication, and more readmission to health care facilities and emergency room visits (American Hospital Association, 2003).

2. **What are the components of cultural awareness?**

   Cultural awareness is the appreciation of another's race, culture, language, customs, styles, and values. The more that we know about our own cultures and each other's cultures, the better we will be able to provide culturally competent care, to facilitate meaningful communication, and to partner with colleagues in day-to-day work.

3. **How does the nurse apply cultural competence in the workplace?**

   Strategies for applying cultural competence in the workplace include know your culture, listen and observe, develop the ability to be a teacher and a learner at the same time, give clear directions, give a deadline, provide straightforward steps for decision making, manage according to values and attitudes of the individual's generation. These are a few of the strategies that may help the nurse to learn continually from and about differences in cultures.

4. **Where do ideas about race come from? What are the sources of your information?**

   The following is titled "Ten Things Everyone Should Know about Race" and is written to accompany a three-part PBS series *RACE: The Power of an Illusion*. How do these 10 points challenge your thoughts about race?

   1. Race is a modern idea.
   2. Race has no genetic basis.
   3. Human subspecies do not exist.
   4. Skin color really is only skin deep.
   5. Most variation is within, not between, "races."
   6. Slavery predates race.
   7. Race and freedom evolved together.
   8. Race justified social inequalities as natural.
   9. Race is not biological, but racism is still real.
   10. Color blindness will not end racism.

   RACE: The Power of an Illusion was produced by California Newsreel in association with the Independent Television Service (ITVS). Major funding was provided by the Ford Foundation and the Corporation for Public Television Broadcasting Diversity Fund. The program is available on videocassette and DVD from California Newsreel (www.newsreel.org).

29

Staff Recruitment and Retention

The United States is facing a major nursing shortage. This shortage is more severe and is driven by supply-side economics, not just misdistribution of nurses or employers' willingness to hire nurses. *Causes* related to the nursing shortage include decrease in the birth rate since the 1950s, increase in the number of nurses approaching retirement, decrease in the number of students entering nursing in the 1980s, inability of nursing schools to accommodate the students who apply to programs, decreased numbers of faculty, increase in available positions in the workforce, and increase in patient volume related to the aging of the population. Recruitment and retention activities are critically important in meeting the nation's projected need for nursing staff. *Recruitment* is a process by which organizations search for and identify applicants for employment. *Retention* is maintaining employment of qualified individuals in an organization. *Selection* is determining who is most qualified for the job. A *staff vacancy* is a part- or full-time position that is unfilled. *Turnover* is loss of an employee through transfer, termination, or resignation. *Termination* is discharge of an employee for poor performance or a mismatch. *Resignation* is the inability to retain an employee who is performing satisfactorily in a position.

In 2000, the national vacancy rate was 21.3%. The highest vacancy and turnover rates were in the western and southern regions. The Midwest had the lowest vacancy rate, and the Northeast had the lowest turnover rate. The impact of the nursing shortage on organizations includes restriction of admissions, increased waiting time for surgeries, and reduced services. The impact of the nursing shortage on nurses includes increased overtime, higher stress, restricted expansions, changes in recruiting and hiring practices, difficulty in scheduling coordination, and decreased quality of care. One strategy used to fill vacant positions is to recruit internationally for nurses. The two major reasons foreign nurses come to the United States to practice is because

of economic security and professional opportunity. The International Council of Nurses (1999) released a position statement, "Nurse Retention, Transfer and Migration," to discuss ethical and other issues of recruiting internationally. Examples of ethical principles in the International Council of Nurses document include effective human resources planning and development, credible nursing regulation, access to full employment, freedom of movement and freedom from discrimination, good faith contracting, and equal pay for work of equal value.

Several professional nursing associations came together to analyze the nursing shortage and develop a strategic plan titled "Nursing's Agenda for the Future: a Call to Action" (American Nurses Association, 2002). This document identifies 10 domains for action: leadership and planning, delivery systems, legislative/regulatory/policy, professional/nursing culture, recruitment/retention, economic value, work environment, public relations/communication, education, and diversity (p. 7). Five strategies related to recruitment and retention are (1) recruitment of students into nursing education programs and of nurses for health care agencies, (2) development and funding of educational initiatives, (3) creating a desirable image of nursing as a career choice, (4) implementation of professional practice models, and (5) development of comprehensive strategies for recruitment and retention (American Nurses Association, 2002). Recruitment strategies for students and faculty include developing a professional mentoring model, creating curriculum to incorporate diversity, obtaining funding to support minority enrollment, developing recruitment materials to attract individuals from diverse backgrounds, co-op programs, negotiating paid development opportunities, and creating a web for leadership.

The following major factors contribute to the nursing shortage: aging of the workforce, declining enrollment, changing work climate, and poor image of nursing. Strategies for promoting nursing as a career include classroom ambassadors program, job-shadowing experiences, bring your child to work day, volunteer health care opportunities, part-time employment opportunities, presentation to clubs/organizations, participation in community health fairs, advertising campaigns directed at job satisfaction and dynamic websites (Erickson et al., 2004, p. 86). Three major variables of administration, professional practice, and professional development are related to a positive influence on the ability of a hospital to recruit and retain staff. Professional practice models that provide for flexibility in work schedules and staff development, professional autonomy and managerial visibility, and support attract registered nurses. Strategies used to recruit new and experienced nurses include flexible hours, competitive salaries, bonus pay, relocation pay, fixed shifts, weekend option program, part-time pay with bonus hours, flexible benefits packages, scholarships for students, tuition benefit plan, registered nurse specialty internships, career opportunities, shared governance models, clinical ladders, and qualified managerial support.

The *nine major phases of recruitment* are (1) position posting, (2) advertising, (3) screening, (4) interviewing, (5) selecting, (6) orienting, (7) counseling/coaching, (8) performance evaluation, and (9) staff development. Position posting is the process of determining and identifying vacancies in full-time equivalent status and then posting them internally for a period of time (based on organizational or collective bargaining policy) and then posting them externally. Institutional advertising is the process of attracting staff. Screening is a process in which predetermined standards are used to assess applicants for a posted position. Interviewing can be conducted in person, by telephone, in a group or committee, or one on one. The job description serves as the template for assessing an applicant's potential and fit in the organization. Selecting is the process of making a formal offer to a job applicant and facilitating transition for the new employee into the organization. The primary costs associated with selecting the wrong individual include recruitment, replacement and hiring costs; and secondary costs include wasted dollars on training and development, decreased productivity and increased errors, lost opportunities for improvement in processes, and decreased or poor staff morale. Orientation is important in integrating a new employee into the organization. Formal mentoring or preceptor programs are useful in orientation. Coaching and counseling assists with developing a social network for new employees. Organizations that create a non-punitive culture in which staff can learn and grow are called "learning organizations." In a learning organization, individuals expand their capacity, expansive

patterns of thinking are nurtured, and individuals learn continually and together (Senge, 1990). Performance evaluation is a method of giving feedback to employees through *formative* (developmental) or summative (review at the end of orientation and annually) evaluation. Staff development provides individuals the opportunity to improve their practice, increase their competency level, and focus on areas of self-interest. The four areas of personal and professional growth include in-service education, continuing education, formal education, and career development.

Retention of new and experienced nurses is improved when there is a culture of respect and safety, autonomy, interdisciplinary collaboration, and professional care delivery models. Organizations with strong communication tend to have increased stability and retention, higher job satisfaction, higher quality outcomes, and fewer nurse injuries (Aiken et al., 1997; Laschinger & Wong, 1999). Visionary leaders are aware of generational workforce diversity and manage the diversity to improve quality patient outcomes and staff satisfaction. Retaining qualified staff minimizes the costs of turnover, and staff morale is better.

Nursing leadership can facilitate the development and creation of professional practice models; leaders can be visible and can provide staff support (Peterson, 2001). Five themes related to the manager's role in establishing a culture of retention are putting the staff first, forging authentic connections, coaching for—and expecting—competence, focusing on the results, and partnering with staff (Manion, 2004). Effective nurse executives and managers devote considerable time, energy, and resources to developing and implementing quality human resource management systems and processes as an essential long-term investment in positive personnel outcomes. Employees are the greatest asset of a health care organization, and the success of the organization depends on employee performance With the cycles in nursing of shortages and surpluses of registered nurses, marginal organizations react to cyclical trends instead of being proactive and maintaining strong staff selection and development programs.

LEARNING TOOLS

Individual Activity

Purpose

To use and evaluate the components of an interview tool used in staff selection.

Directions

1. Review the interview tool to determine the information requested of the applicant.

2. Determine the purpose of the questions posed in the interview tool. What type of information is each question attempting to elicit?

3. Answer each question on the interview tool. This activity may be used for preparing for the interview process.

4. Partner with a colleague and ask the person the questions on the interview tool and then provide feedback.

5. When finished with the process, reverse roles and have a colleague ask the interview questions to you and provide feedback to you.

Preparing for the Interview

1. Wear appropriate clothing: conservative, not too tight or baggy.

2. Review and answer potential interview questions.

3. Schedule an interview time when you will not be rushed. Do not be late.

4. Develop a list of questions to ask the potential employer.

5. Obtain information on the unit in advance.

6. Be organized.

7. Anticipate and be prepared to interview with several individuals and in a group setting.

8. First impressions are important. Have a strong handshake, smile, establish eye contact, and address each individual by name.

Structured Interview Guide*

1. What are your strongest skills? What are growth areas for you?

2. What motivates and/or rewards you?

3. Describe a situation in which you were able positively to influence the actions of others in a desired direction.

4. If a situation developed where you perceived that communication was ineffective, what steps would you implement to improve the level of communication?

5. What kinds of deadlines do you have in your current position? How do you meet them?

6. Give an example of an important goal you have set in the past and your success in reaching the goal.

7. Describe a situation when you have several things going on all at once and all seemed to be high priority. How did you manage and organize your time?

8. Describe a time when many changes were occurring simultaneously. How did you deal with all the changes?

9. Describe to us a situation you have encountered where "old solutions" did not work and you were instrumental in implementing "new solutions."

10. Give us an example of a time in which you had to go outside of your normal process or procedure to solve a problem. What did you do and why?

11. Tell about a time in which you had to be relatively quick in coming to a decision.

12. What is the most difficult and challenging decision you have made recently? Please describe the situation.

13. Describe the most creative or innovative work project you have completed.

14. What stresses you out at work? What do you do to reduce your stress level?

15. Describe what the word *teamwork* means to you.

16. Tell us about teams you have worked on. Was the team successful? What made it that way?

17. Describe a time when you helped a peer to meet a goal or deadline.

18. What would your co-workers say about you? How important is that to you?

19. Tell us about a time in which you positively dealt with a negative situation and influenced the actions of others.

20. Describe a time when you were not in agreement with a team decision. What was the decision and why did not you buy into it?

21. Tell us about a time when you and a peer disagreed on an issue. What happened? What did you do to resolve the situation?

22. Tell us about a change in management that was unsettling to you. Why?

23. What do you bring to this position that makes you the most qualified candidate?

24. What, if anything, concerns you about this position?

25. What questions do you have for us?

CASE STUDY

Pat Savarnage, is a newly hired director of medical-surgical and ambulatory care units in a large teaching hospital in Pittsburgh, Pennsylvania. She is an experienced manager and feels comfortable in her new role. She was a manager of a small medical-surgical division in a community hospital in Tallahassee, Florida, before accepting her new job. This is her third week in her

This interview guide was developed by Jeanne Roode, RN, MSN, CNA, Director of Neuroscience Services for Spectrum Health, Grand Rapids, MI.

role, and she has sent out seven memoranda to the nurse managers instructing them to do the following:

1. Change the way shift reporting occurs.
2. Provide training on quality improvement initiatives.
3. Implement a new career ladder.
4. Inform staff nurses that she has an "open door" policy.
5. Announce her new role and hands-on approach to managing the staff.
6. Announce a new yet to be announced restructuring.
7. Outline future clinical initiatives.

The nurse managers are concerned, upset, and worried about their jobs and the manner in which Nurse Savarnage is implementing her role. Until now, they have been autonomous, have implemented professional practice models on their units, have high nurse satisfaction and low turnover rates, and have high ratings on quality improvement measures. The managers are concerned that all of their hard work will be destroyed and that they seem to have little if any voice in decision making. To make matters worse, when individual managers have tried to schedule an appointment with Nurse Savarnage, she is "not available" because she is doing "important" work or meeting with key stakeholders. When Sue Port, the nurse manager of oncology, stopped by to visit her office, Nurse Savarnage smiled and greeted her but quickly slipped out and not so politely told Nurse Port that she was too busy just to "chat." To make matters worse, a few staff members from various units have made appointments with Nurse Savarnage and are complaining about individual managers. They seem to get appointments with Nurse Savarnage quickly. The few times Nurse Savarnage has been present on the units, she has focused on the staff and has barely acknowledged the managers.

Case Study Questions

1. What should the nurse managers do? How could they approach Nurse Savarnage?
2. Is Nurse Savarnage demonstrating behaviors that support a "learning community?" Provide rationale for your answer.
3. What types of activities should managers engage in to build strong units and minimize turnover and maximize retention?

4. Describe ways in which Nurse Savarnage could interact with staff and nurse managers in a supportive environment?
5. When a new director or manager enters an organization, that person usually assesses the environment before making numerous changes in a short period of time. What message do you think that Nurse Savarnage sent to the managers and staff when she sent out seven memoranda in her first 3 weeks of employment without getting input from employees?

LEARNING RESOURCES

Discussion Questions

1. Why is the current nursing shortage so severe, and why is it not resolving like the registered nurse shortage cycles usually do?
2. What are some of the causes or reasons that there is such a severe nursing shortage?
3. What are the nine phases of recruitment? Provide a brief discussion of each.
4. Professional nursing organizations joined together to develop a strategic plan to help manage the nursing shortage. What are the 10 domains of action that they described to recruit and retain nurses?
5. What is formative and summative evaluation? Give an example of each.
6. What is a learning organization? Describe the characteristics of a learning organization.

Study Questions

Matching: Write the letter of the correct response in front of each term

_____ 1. Recruitment

_____ 2. Retention

_____ 3. Selection

_____ 4. Staff vacancy

_____ 5. Turnover

_____ 6. Transfer

_____ 7. Termination

_____ 8. Resignation

_____ 9. Learning organization

_____ 10. Formative evaluation

_____ 11. Summative evaluation

A. Discharge of an employee who is performing less than satisfactorily

B. Loss of an employee because of transfer, termination, or resignation

C. Seeking out and identifying individuals for potential employment

D. Developmental assessment of an employee's progress

E. Continuing the employment of qualified staff

F. Assessing the fit and work of an employee at the end of orientation and annually

G. Part- or full-time equivalent employee positions

H. Determining the most qualified applicant for a posted job

I. An organization in which individuals continually expand their talents and work collectively

J. Failure to retain an employee who is performing satisfactorily or better

K. Movement of an employee from one area in the organization to another

REFERENCES

Aiken, L. H., Sloan, D. M., Klocinski, J. L. (1997). Hospital nurses' occupational exposure to blood: Prospective, retrospective, and institutional reports. *American Journal of Public Health, 87*(1), 103-107.

American Nurses Association. (2002). *Nursing's agenda for the future: A call to the nation.* Washington, DC: Author. Retrieved June 20, 2004, from *www.nursingworld.org/naf/indexb.htm*

Erickson, J. I., Holm, L. J., & Chelminiak, L. (2004). Keeping the nursing shortage from becoming a nursing crisis. *Journal of Nursing Administration, 34*(2), 83-87.

International Council of Nurses. (1999). *Nurse retention, transfer and migration.* Geneva, Switzerland: Author. Retrieved June 21, 2004, from *www.icn.ch/psretention.htm*

Laschinger, H. K. S., & Wong, C. (1999). Staff nurse empowerment and collective accountability: Effect on perceived productivity and self-rated work effectiveness. *Nursing Economic$, 17*(6) 308-316.

Manion, J. (2004). Nurture a culture of retention. *Nursing Management, 35*(4) 29-39.

Peterson, C. (2001, January 31). Nursing shortage: Not a simple problem—No easy answer. *Journal of Issues in Nursing, 6*(1), Manuscript 1. Retrieved June 28, 2004, from *http://nursing-world.org/ojin/topic14/tpc14_1.htm*

Senge, P. (1990). *The fifth discipline: The art and practice of the learning organization.* New York: Currency and Doubleday.

SUPPLEMENTAL READINGS

DeJohn, P. (2004). Recruiting, e-commerce use on Broadlane agenda. *Hospital Materials Management, 29*(7), 1, 8-10.

Simpson, R. L. (2004). Recruit, retain, assess: Technology's role in diversity. *Nursing Administration Quarterly, 28*(3), 217-220

West, E. (2004). Back to the basics: Recruitment, retention, and reality. *Medsurg Nursing, 13*(5), 346-350.

Chapter 29: Staff Recruitment and Retention (pp. 625-648)

1. What are the common recruitment practices in your community? Which entice you?

Creative recruitment strategies are being used to market the profession of nursing to nurses, nursing students, and potential nursing students. Shadowing experiences with an experienced nurse through a college of nursing, nurse extern programs, and advertising campaigns that are directed at job satisfaction and "making a difference" are a few examples of recruitment strategies being used by health care and educational institutions. As a nursing student, which are most enticing to you?

2. Which retention strategies are most effective? Do these vary by cohorts of nurses?

Nurses desire employment in institutions that promote professional nursing such as those that promote autonomy, participatory involvement, professional development, and flexible work schedules. Other strategies include having a professional practice model in place, preceptor/mentorship opportunities, low patient-to-registered nurse ratios, collaborative practice environment, Magnet Recognition status, an environment of respect and value, and a competitive compensation model.

3. Who are the logical partners for nurses in recruitment and retention initiatives?

Partnerships between health care organizations, colleges of nursing, and industry/private business sector can assist in improving the image of nursing, which in turn may help with recruitment initiatives. Nurse managers and physician relationships play major roles in the retention of nurses.

4. What areas of the country have the greatest vacancy rates and/or turnover of staff, and what impact does this have on the delivery of services within the region, community, and/or institution?

According to Atencio and colleagues (2003) the western and southern regions of the United States had the highest vacancy and turnover rates with vacancy rates at 12.2% for the West and 11.0% for the South. Turnover rates were at 24% for the southern states and 22.2% for the western regions. These high vacancy and turnover rates have a negative impact on patient care outcomes because of staffing shortages and job dissatisfaction of the nurses working short-staffed. Costs of health care also increase because of overtime usage, hiring and orientation of new nurses, and delays in delivery of care.

5. What are the strengths and weaknesses related to hiring of international nurses as a means of addressing the nursing shortage in the United States?

Countries all over the world are experiencing a nursing shortage. Nurses from other countries come to the United States to enhance professional growth and economic stability. Working in the United States provides learning opportunities for nurses to share in their native country. These nurses also help the United States in combating the nursing shortage; however, migration of nurses to the United States on a more permanent basis contributes to an international nursing shortage. Recruitment of international nurses also is costly and time consuming.

6. What is the view of the American Nurses Association and International Council of Nurses relative to the use of international nurses within the United States?

The American Nurses Association and International Council of Nurses have outlined ethical recruitment practices for institutions to use when recruiting international nurses. Unfortunately, unethical recruitment of nurses in the past has resulted in the exploitation of international nurses.

7. What are the major factors/domains that affect quality care as defined by the Institute of Medicine and American Nurses Association?

The following 10 domains are outlined by the Institute of Medicine and the American Nurses Association:

1. Leadership and planning
2. Delivery systems
3. Legislative/regulatory/policy
4. Professional/nursing culture
5. Recruitment/retention
6. Economic value
7. Work environment
8. Public relations/communication
9. Education
10. Diversity

8. **What are some of the recruitment and retention strategies developed/posed by the American Nurses Association to address quality-of-care concerns?**

The American Nurses Association describes the vision for recruitment and retention strategies as follows:

> Nursing is comprised of a diverse body of individuals committed to promoting and sustaining the profession through addressing diversity, image, education, funding, practice models and environments, and professional development (American Nurses Association, 2002, p. 17).

9. **What impact has the delineation of Magnet characteristics and the movement toward Magnet Recognition had on recruitment and retention of nurses within organizations?**

In the past 10 to 15 years, institutions have been striving to promote initiatives that support job satisfaction and the establishment of a safe and mutually respectful culture. In 2001 the Nursing Executive Center published a study that identified reasons why nurses remained at a hospital. Magnet characteristics such as high-quality care, strong nursing leadership, "meeting the baseline" in terms of compensation, scheduling options, benefits package, and lower patient assignment numbers were identified as strong retention factors.

10. **What is the role of human resource departments relative to recruitment and retention of nurses?**

Human resource departments conduct recruitment processes such as position posting, advertising, screening, and interviewing. In many settings the nurse manager selects the candidate after the interviewing phase has taken place. Depending on the institution, orientation, counseling/coaching, performance evaluation, and staff development are conducted in part by the manager and the staff development/nurse educator department. Retention activities may include monitoring of competitive wages and benefits.

11. **What influence (positive or negative) do nurse managers and registered nurse peers/colleagues have relative to recruitment and retention of nurses?**

Nurses who are happy in their jobs market relate positively to others and tend to stay at the institution. Nurse managers and staff nurses can create a nurturing environment in which the new nurse can feel comfortable.

12. **Why is it important to understand generational difference relative to recruitment and retention of registered nurses?**

Each generation of nurses—mature/silent, Baby Boomers, Generation X, and Generation Y—have different motivators and enticers. To recruit and retain these nurses, leaders must be able to consider differences when developing strategies for change or reward.

13. **What are some of the strategies that have been shown to have the greatest positive impact on recruitment and retention of registered nurses?**

Manion (2004), based on research with nurse managers, identified five themes that contribute to the culture of retention. These are putting staff first, forging authentic connections, coaching for—and expecting—competence, focusing on results, and partnering with staff. These ideas were also present in research on retention conducted by Parsons and Stonestreet (2004) with staff nurses. These same themes are consistent with the Magnet Recognition Program by the American Nurses Association (2003).

14. **What impact have the reports on the current and future nursing shortage had on legislative decisions and public awareness?**

Partnerships with the private business sector that have focused on changing the image of nursing as a career are having a positive impact on students and career switchers. Legislative decisions have been made to assist in funding for nursing education at the state and federal level.

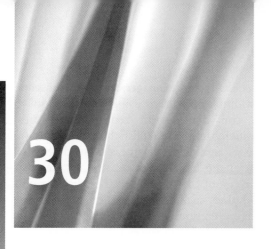

30

Performance Appraisal

STUDY FOCUS

Performance appraisals are an important organizational strategy to manage employee performance and gain a competitive edge in a complex health care environment. An important managerial role is to define roles and expectations for employee performance in return for compensation. *Managerial performance management activities* include providing a sustainable source of motivation, communicating the important issues that affect performance, being available for problem solving, and using critical skills.

Performance is achieving organizational objectives and responsibilities. *Performance management* is an interactive process among performance appraisal, work motivation, and performance rewards. *Performance appraisal* is an integral component of performance management in health care organizations and is the evaluation of an employee's work. A *conventional performance appraisal* is a systematic standardized evaluation of an employee by a superior for the purpose of evaluating quality, effectiveness, and potential for advancement. *Standards* in the form of criteria are applied to the levels of performance as superior, excellent, average, or unacceptable. *Peer review* is the evaluation of practice by an associate. *Self-evaluation* is an employee's assessment of his or her own performance compared with a preset standard.

The *performance appraisal process* includes assessing needs and setting goals, establishing the objectives and the timeframe, and assessing the progress and evaluating performance, and then starting the process over. The *performance appraisal cycle* begins with the hiring of an employee and ends with resignation or termination. Performance appraisal can be *informal* (day-by-day supervision and coaching) and *formal* (written documentation, interview, and follow-up). *Components of a comprehensive appraisal system* are determining the ability required (job description), matching abilities of the employee with job requirements (personnel selection), improving employee's abilities (staff development), and

enhancing employees' motivation (staff development and the reward system).

Typically, individuals' performances combine their ability and their motivation. *Ability* is innate or acquired through learning, and *motivation* is the willingness and desire to perform work. Human resource management is important in performance management processes. Part of human resource management organizationally is establishing work requirements, conducting job analysis, designing compensation administration, engaging in training needs analysis, and determining disciplinary procedures. For employees, human resource management implications include job expectations, compensation policies, mechanisms for performance recognition, and professional development opportunities.

Organizational culture is one method of establishing a context of continual improvement in clinical service performance and client outcomes. Subcultures in organizations often develop to accomplish or streamline work processes. Conflict may arise when biases or work-flow interruption occurs because of subcultural differences. Strong organizational culture and values for quality care are essential to meet consumer and regulatory agency demands of safe client care within a practitioner's scope of practice. The criteria in performance appraisals should reflect the key performance indicators established in an organizational culture to ensure implementation of the key values. One method of evaluating the practice or work of an employee is through annual performance appraisals. Performance appraisals are one important component in managing the quality, efficiency, and effectiveness in the provision of nursing services.

The *goals of a comprehensive appraisal system* include fulfilling the job description requirements, improving on employees' skills, rewarding employee motivation, and matching the right employees with the right job. Evaluations are based on standards. Employer evaluation is often conducted from multiple perspectives by using peer evaluation and self-evaluation to provide an enhanced description of individual quality

215

and competence. *Peer review* consists of written or verbal input by those co-workers who work with the employee being evaluated in the performance appraisal. These are peers who are exceptional clinicians and are knowledgeable about the employee's level of performance. Interdisciplinary team members, even physicians and support staff, also can be asked to provide written data about the employee's performance. By querying multiple stakeholders, a more comprehensive performance assessment is compiled for employee review and discussion. In addition, staff self-appraisal is a good method to promote individual input, personal responsibility, and feedback about job performance. Finally, scheduling an adequate time block for discussion, a quiet environment, and a completed appraisal form is conducive to an effective and productive performance appraisal process.

Commonly, evaluators err in evaluation. The most *common sources of evaluator errors* are the halo, the recent behavior, horn, and similar-to-me effects. The *halo effect* occurs when evaluators rank all categories high when an individual does well in several areas but not all. *Recent behavior* effect occurs when the evaluator rates the employee based on recent events rather than the full year. *Horn effect* is when a manager perceives one negative aspect about an employee performance and generalizes it to an overall poor rating. *Similar-to-me* effect is a higher employee performance evaluation as the manager perceives the employee to have similar characteristics to himself or herself.

Alternative types of performance appraisal to minimize factors of bias in the employee's appraisal process include the 360-degree evaluation, peer review, and management by objectives format. The *360-degree evaluation* includes gathering input from multiple sources (at least four). Examples of evaluation sources include a peer, physician, subordinate, and self-evaluation. *Peer review* is the use of a peer review committee to provide input into the employee's performance. Peers should use objective criteria or standards to provide feedback regarding an employee's performance. *Management by objectives* is a process whereby the manager and employee establish performance goals for the upcoming year. At evaluation time, the feedback is provided around the established goals, and new ones are identified.

As part of any performance appraisal system, reliability and validity in measurement are important. Tools should be developed so that whoever scores or rates the employee performance would obtain the same score and the tool would have a high *interrater reliability*. A test to determine whether the performance criteria are stable over time is to assess *test-retest reliability*. The manager can assess the same person at multiple interviews using the same tool to determine consistency with repeated measures. *Construct validity,* used to establish that the criteria are appropriate, is another useful measure to determine the validity of the tool. Other factors that the rater should be aware of that may affect the reliability and validity of ratings include the manner in which the information is communicated, how the information is organized, the potential influence of the relationship the rate has with the person being rated, and the cognitive ability of the rater.

In organizations, performance appraisals occur in a hierarchical fashion. At the *individual level,* performance is measured by appraisals. At the *unit level,* performance is measured by budget and quality criteria. At the *organizational level,* performance is evaluated by accreditation agencies. Effective performance appraisal systems incorporate and enhance employee knowledge, skills, and abilities. *Counseling* often is used in cases in which performance is substandard and work is poorly completed. *Coaching* often is used with employees to improve performance and teach new tasks or skills. Coaching can be role modeling, providing praise and information, or the employee's attendance at a seminar to learn new skills. *Mentoring* is also useful for employees who shine and demonstrate strong commitment and productivity.

LEARNING TOOLS

Individual Activity

Purpose

To practice writing peer evaluations to include specific measurable data.

Scenario

Hillary Jackson is a hard-working registered nurse who consistently provides excellent quality care to her assigned clients. She always helps others when her work is completed and has good working relationships with physicians, families, and other health care workers. One area Nurse Jackson despises is charting. She charts in a cursory, objective style, but does not always document everything that is needed. Rarely does she contribute to the nursing care plan, which necessitates others completing this work. Nurse Jackson is active in the Oncology Nursing Society and regularly attends continuing educational offerings. She has joined the unit-based quality improvement committee and contributes valuable information.

Directions

The following is a form that you must complete as Nurse Jackson's peer evaluator. Remember to make the notations as objective as possible. Descriptions of each category are listed below the client behavior and Likert scale. A Likert scale is used to rank her performance with a range of 1 for outstanding to 5 for unsatisfactory.

When making comments about Nurse Jackson's performance, use specific measurable objective data. For example, a comment in the professional development section might read as follows:

> Nurse Jackson has been a member of the unit-based quality improvement committee for 4 months and attends regularly. She has brought many ideas for improving processes on the unit, such as walking rounds instead of report, flexible hours for employees, and the need to develop procedures for new oncological treatments.

Clinical Behaviors

Client Care   1   2   3   4   5

Refers to client care activities such as personal care, treatments, medication administration, and coordination of care with physicians and other health care workers.

Comments:

Teamwork   1   2   3   4   5

Works with peers, physicians, clients, and other health care workers to maximize positive client outcomes and improve quality.

Comments:

Client Teaching   1   2   3   4   5

Individualizes a teaching plan for each assigned client, documents the teaching, and reports teaching needs during shift report.

Comments:

Committee Participation   1   2   3   4   5

Actively participates in at least one unit-based committee. Contributes to the committee process by chairing a committee, providing information for committee work, or completing the work of the committee.

Comments:

Charting   1   2   3   4   5

Documents timely, accurately, and comprehensively all client care activities, medications, and treatments.

Comments:

Nursing Care Plans   1 2 3 4 5

Initiates care plans for newly admitted clients during the shift of admission and updates and modifies nursing care plans.

Comments:

Professional Involvement   1 2 3 4 5

Dresses professionally, participates in professional organization activities, attends continuing educational seminars, and provides leadership in unit-based activities.

Comments:

CASE STUDY

Stephanie Kahanals is a nurse manager of a 75-bed oncology unit in large teaching hospital in Atlanta, Georgia. She has been a nurse manager at this hospital for 15 years and has developed a high-performance team on her unit. She personally interviews all applicants for her unit and encourages staff participation in the final selection. Nurse Kahanals frequently volunteers for pilot projects and is able to garner resources for staff projects. She finds performance evaluations difficult and has decided to rank everyone the same this year because they all perform so well as a team. Nurse Kahanals has decided to rank everyone high.

Case Study Questions

1. What type of evaluator error has Nurse Kahanals committed?
2. What are some other methods of evaluation that could assist Nurse Kahanals to make choices about employee ranking?

3. How could Nurse Kahanals use the performance appraisal process to assist the staff to individualize their learning needs and to meet organizational objectives?

LEARNING RESOURCES

Discussion Questions

1. What is the purpose of annual performance appraisals, and how should a nurse manager go about collecting objective data?
2. Is objectivity possible in a performance appraisal system? If so, how can a nurse manager make the appraisal process as objective as possible?
3. What are the current trends in annual performance appraisals regarding who has what kind of input into employee evaluations?
4. In your organization, are employee performance appraisal ratings tied to monetary rewards? Or are the performance appraisal ratings used for self-improvement, and an across-the-board raise is given to employees? Which system of reward would motivate you?
5. Do you feel comfortable in providing and receiving peer evaluation? Do you find peer evaluation useful in upgrading your skills?

Study Questions

Matching: Write the letter of the correct response in front of each term.

_____ 1. Performance appraisal

_____ 2. Peer review

_____ 3. Performance

_____ 4. Performance management

_____ 5. Counseling

_____ 6. Coaching

_____ 7. Standards

_____ 8. Self-evaluation

_____ 9. Formal performance appraisal

_____ 10. Informal performance appraisal

A. A criterion with a designation of superior, excellent, average, or unacceptable performance

B. A part of performance appraisal whereby the employee performs a self-assessment of his or her performance compared with preestablished criteria

C. Day-to-day coaching to improve or refine components of performance

D. A summative performance appraisal with written documentation, interview, and follow-up

E. Evaluating the work of others

F. Assessing the level of work by an associate

G. Addresses problem performance such as substandard work

H. Is used to improve employee performance and ability to do the job

I. Achieving or surpassing organizational and social objectives and responsibilities

J. An interactive process between work motivation, performance appraisal, and performance rewards and developmenter

SUPPLEMENTAL READINGS

Baker, D. L. (2002). Successful performance improvement. *AORN Journal, 75*(4), 825-827.

Carson, E. M. (2004). Do performance appraisals of registered nurses reflect a relationship between hospital size and caring? *Nursing Forum, 39*(1), 5-13.

Nipp, D. A., & Hadfield, P. A. (2002). Worker-designed tools: Developing comprehensive work assessment tools and competencies. *Nursing Economic$, 20*(2), 70-73.

Smith, M. H. (2003). Empower staff with praiseworthy appraisals. *Nursing Management, 34*(1), 16-17, 52.

Wiles, L. L. (2001). Clinical performance appraisal: Renewing graded clinical experiences. *Journal of Nursing Education, 40*(1), 37-39.

Chapter 30: Performance Appraisal (pp. 649-674)

1. **What experiences have you had in the past with performance appraisals? Have those experiences been positive or negative? Why?**

   You may have had experiences with performance appraisals as an employee or as a manager. Recipients of positive performance appraisals cite being given the opportunity to discuss personal, professional, or organizational factors that interfered with or augmented performance. Collaborative goal-setting with the manager results in a motivational process for employee growth and performance enhancement. In addition, positive recipient experiences with performance appraisals may serve as a template for conducting one's own future employee performance appraisals.

2. **Why does the handling of the performance appraisal process leave an aftermath of feelings?**

   A performance appraisal is an evaluative process that is personal. You are being evaluated on your level of performance. The evaluation process used to quantify your performance may be influenced by perceptions, biases, and values of the employee and manager. As a result, the opinions of the evaluator and your opinions may differ. This difference in opinion may be a source of fear and anxiety because the appraisal may not truly reflect your perception of your performance. If the evaluation is positive, you probably will feel rewarded and motivated to continue a high level of excellence.

3. **Think about those times when you were evaluated in a positive and constructive manner. Why was that a good experience?**

   Performance appraisals that have been positive and constructive are those that provide an opportunity for personal evaluation, peer assessment, and collaborative goal setting. The most important component in this type of evaluation process is the ability to conduct a self-assessment. A personal evaluation allows the individual to examine one's accomplishments critically and to identify areas for further growth. The collaborative goal-setting process with the manager can assist the individual to identify and implement strategies for professional development.

4. **How do you feel when you are expected to evaluate others? Why?**

   Evaluating others is a learned skill that requires time and experience to develop. Objectivity is essential, with the focus of the evaluation on counseling, performance improvement, and mutual goal setting. Developing the employee's motivation to excel, stimulating professional growth, and enhancing skill mastery is an ongoing process that requires mentorship and continuous feedback.

5. **How are performance appraisal and quality improvement related?**

   Performance appraisals and quality improvement share many of the same process steps, including data collection, standards comparison, needs assessment, and mutual goal setting. Both processes are concerned with outcomes management and the monitoring of actions that affect the quality of care. Both should reflect the measurement of key performance indicators.

6. **How should pay, promotions, and other rewards be tied to performance and its evaluation?**

   Salaries, promotions, and other rewards should be tied to the individual's performance and should be based on outcomes. Knowledge, skill, professional development, and the individual's accomplishment of goals should serve as the basis for the reward. Data should be collected, quantified, and documented throughout the evaluation period for objective presentation by the evaluator.

7. **How do you evaluate the performance of a team?**

   Although effective team evaluation may be problematic, it is possible. A team evaluation should be based on team strengths, accomplishments, and demonstration of team motivation and cohesion. Instead, the tendency is to evaluate individual performance of the team members; however, this does not appraise how those individuals worked together and solved problems as a team.

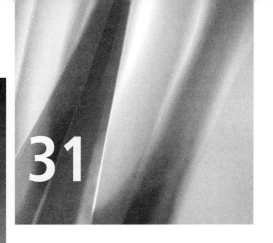

31

Prevention of Workplace Violence

STUDY FOCUS

Violence in the workplace is an important issue for nurses in health care organizations. The rate of workplace violence for nursing and personal care facilities as reported by the Department of Labor is 38 per 10,000 workers. Of the assaults, 27% occurred in nursing homes, 13% in social services, and 11% in hospitals. The two groups of workers with the highest incidence of injuries from workplace assaults are health care and social services (National Institute for Occupational Safety and Health [NIOSH], 1996). Nurses are at risk for violence not only in the United States but also abroad (Henry & Ginn, 2002). A combination of internal and external conditions contribute to workplace violence. Examples of *external conditions* include an increasingly violent society, the availability of handguns, and high-crime neighborhoods. Examples of *internal conditions* include inadequate staffing, large numbers of dangerous patients, poor security for drugs and money, staff members working alone, poorly lit facilities, and unsecured, continuous access to health care agencies.

The nature of nursing jobs place nurses at high risk for workplace violence. Nurses must deal with ill or injured patients; infringe on an individual's personal space; and treat patients' who are in pain or who are emotionally or cognitively impaired, which increases the staffs' risk for an assault or act of violence. Organizations must be convinced of the necessity to institute a workplace violence prevention program as a method of accomplishing a public health objective and organizational work.

Violence can be defined narrowly as acts of violence, such as an assault, battery, manslaughter, or homicide; or broadly as verbal abuse, threats, and harassment (Carroll & Morin, 1998). The cost of violence includes lost productivity from absenteeism, low morale, emotional pain, anxiety, and turnover (Murray & Snyder, 1991; Smith-Pittman & McKoy, 1999). In the short run, bullying can increase productivity by up to 10%

("Violence Threatens the Workplace," 1998), but lawsuits, lost productivity, higher insurance costs, and worker compensation claims cost an estimated $36 billion annually (Jossi, 1999).

The *sources of violence* include criminals, customers, current or former employees, and individuals not employed at the workplace but who have a personal relationship with an employee (Rugala & Isaacs, 2004). *Risk factors for violence* include working with volatile persons, understaffing, long waits, poor environmental design, lack of training, inadequate security, substance abuse, access to firearms, poor lighting, and unrestricted access by the public (NIOSH, 2002). Organizations that are perceived to be unjust, unfair, or unethical are more prone to violence. Centralization is thought to isolate employees from management and dehumanize employees (Ginn & Henry, 2002).

The regulatory background on workplace violence is important from the perspective of NIOSH and the Occupational Safety and Health Administration. The NIOSH recommendations included *three violence prevention strategies:* (1) *environmental designs* (lighting, security escorts, alarm systems); (2) *administrative controls* (reducing waiting times, controlled access); and (3) *behavior modification* (resolving conflicts, hazard awareness) (NIOSH, 2002). The Occupational Safety and Health Administration guidelines suggest that organizations develop a *violence prevention program* that is available to all employees, tracks work-related assaults, and decreases the threat to worker safety (Occupational Safety and Health Administration, 2003). The *major components of a violence prevention programs* are (1) a written plan (which shows commitment that violence will not be tolerated, ensures that no reprisals will occur, and encourages prompt reporting); (2) worksite analysis (search for existing or potential hazards in the workplace); (3) hazard prevention and control (implementation of safe work practices); (4) safety and health training (awareness of hazards and self-protection); and (5) record keeping and evaluation of the program (tracking of work-related assaults).

221

Managerial frameworks for violence prevention include risk management, total quality management, human resource management policies, and employee assistance programs. *Risk management programs* are structured to protect the financial assets of an organization and focus on preventing problems. *Total quality management programs* expect involvement from all levels of the organization in setting standards, collecting information, assessing, and then adjusting policies or procedures. *Human resource management* creates comprehensive violence prevention policies and procedures to guide workplace violence prevention. An example of prevention includes screening of applicants with a propensity for violence. Violent acts often are triggered by being fired, by walking a terminated employee out the front door instead of the back, and by terminating an individual on Monday instead of Friday (Karl & Hancock, 1999). If potential violence is suspected, a *threat assessment* should be conducted to evaluate the threat and the threatener. Then *threat management* should be instituted to determine the course of action to be taken. *Employee assistance programs* are services that assist an employee to cope with home and work stressors.

Not only are nurses subject to violent acts, but also they are subject to acts of intimidation. *Intimidation* is an implied threat; examples include hitting a wall, throwing objects, and glaring at someone. A leadership role is to ensure a nonviolent workplace. The legal implications of workplace violence are multiple. Legal issues include paying higher rates after injuries are sustained, negligence of employers regarding security, failure to warn employees of former employees' criminal propensities, and sexual discrimination (Dolan, 2000). *Legal defense* is taking proactive actions by developing antiviolence policies and procedures to reduce workplace violence. *Damage control* is responding to workplace incidents when prevention fails. *Steps in damage control* include to remain calm, evaluate facts objectively, and call in additional resources (Litke, 1996).

Current issues and trends include predicting violence, highlighting violence prevention in the workplace, and designing environments to minimize or prevent violence. Suggestions for designing safe work environments include installing emergency alarms, designing aesthetic waiting rooms, lighting parking lots, providing escorts, and designing triage systems. Leadership in violence prevention includes worksite analysis, threat assessment, and prevention programs. Not only is there a potential for terrorism and resultant injuries, but also there is a problem of *horizontal violence* (nurse against nurse). The literature shows that nurses are the most common perpetrators of bullying. Bullying most often is directed toward new nurses by experienced ones but can occur between experienced nurses as well. This is a form of psychological harassment and involves a series of incidents that create hostility and discomfort among staff. Consequences of bullying include demoralization, feelings of vulnerability, negative work attitude, loss of confidence, and impaired work performance (McKenna et al., 2003). Nurses should report this form of workplace violence, support colleagues, and encourage managerial support for workplace safety. An important part of violence is *postincident response* in which individuals receive adequate support following the incident. Many types of support can be offered, such as prompt medical treatment, psychological evaluation, support groups, counseling, stress debriefing, trauma crisis counseling, and employee assistance programs.

LEARNING TOOLS

Activity: Environmental Analysis—Hazard Prevention and Control

Purpose

To conduct an environmental analysis of the health care agency in which you are completing your clinical rotation.

Directions

Hazard prevention and control are important aspects of preventing workplace violence. Health care organizations are at high risk for workplace violence. The following is a checklist to use to evaluate your clinical agency on hazard prevention and control. By completing this checklist, you will become more aware of safety and potential dangers in the workplace. Compare your completed checklist with your colleagues, and discuss the prevention systems in place.

Environmental Analysis: Hazard Prevention and Control Checklist

Environmental Assessment Questions

1. Is there good lighting, especially in areas of high risk such as the pharmacy area, or in isolated treatment rooms?

2. Are there safety measures to deter handguns inside the organization; for example, metal detectors?

3. Is there Plexiglas in the payment window in the pharmacy area?

4. Are there security devices such as panic buttons, beepers, surveillance cameras, alarm systems, two-way mirrors, card-key access systems, and security guards?

5. Are there curved mirrors at hallway intersections or concealed areas?

6. Is there controlled access to work areas?

7. Is there training for staff to recognize and manage hostile and assaultive behavior?

8. Is there adequate staffing during the day, evening, and night shifts?

9. Is there adequate staffing in high-risk areas such as the emergency room?

10. Are there close parking areas?

11. Are there security escorts or shuttle services for staff to and from parking lots?

12. Are all assaults documented?

13. Is there evidence of a zero tolerance policy for violence?

14. Are there good relationships with police authorities?

15. Is there a violence prevention plan?

Patient-Related Environmental Assessment Questions

1. Is furniture arranged to prevent staff entrapment in the patient room?

2. Are rooms free of clutter and with nothing available on the countertops for patients to use as weapons?

3. Is there a secondary door for escape in case of entrapment?

4. Is a staff member available to be in the room if a patient threat exists?

Modified from Occupational Safety and Health Administration. (2003). Guidelines for preventing workplace violence for health care and social service workers (Rev. 2003). *Washington, DC: OSHA, U.S. Department of Labor. Retrieved December 9, 2004, from www.osha.gov/SLTC/etools/hospital/hazards/workplaceviolence/checklist.html*

CASE STUDY

Elaine Baringer is a nurse manager of a 45-bed medical-surgical unit in a large teaching hospital in Minneapolis, Minnesota. She was appointed by the director of nursing with no input from the staff nurses. Nurse Baringer had no administrative experience before this position and according to staff, "thinks she knows everything and only her opinion is right or counts, and by all means don't cross her." Nurse Baringer holds monthly staff meetings, and all staff are expected to attend. Nurse Baringer arrives 15 or more minutes late, does not have a prepared agenda, and begins the meeting by introducing a topic, asking for ideas, and then telling everyone how it will be done. Suzy Janis is a seasoned registered nurse who was hired

recently. During the staff meeting, she offered a wonderful solution to the staffing problem, which resulted in Nurse Baringer screaming at her about how horrible her idea was to the entire staff. Nurse Baringer also is making comments about male staff being sexy (with explicit comments). In addition, she frequently talks about staff to other staff members, which is demoralizing. Staff have contacted the director of the medical-surgical unit and shared Nurse Baringer's outbursts and comments with her, but the director laughed and said she likes Nurse Baringer.

Case Study Questions

1. What is horizontal violence?

2. What steps can the staff take to protect themselves from Nurse Baringer's outbursts and demeaning comments?

3. What strategies can the staff take to support one another?

4. What impact does Nurse Baringer's behavior have on morale?

5. Because the staff has approached the director of the medical-surgical unit regarding Nurse Baringer's behavior with no support, with whom should they be sharing this information next?

LEARNING RESOURCES

Discussion Questions

1. What are the sources of violence, and what are the risk factors for violence?

2. Discuss the importance of NIOSH and OSHA, and describe the recommendations and guidelines they suggest.

3. Describe risk management, total quality management, human resource management policies, and employee assistance programs. Then describe which program would be most appropriate for each of the four sources of violence.

4. What are some strategies to use to design a safe work environment?

5. What is horizontal violence? How is this played out in nursing? How can this form of bullying stop? What strategies can a nurse use to decrease this type of violence?

Study Questions

True or False: Circle the correct answer.

T F   1. Health care and social service workers have the highest incidence of injuries from workplace assaults.

T F   2. The cost of violence is relatively low in health care because of the few reported incidence of violence in the workplace.

T F   3. Manager decisions and treatment of employees has little to do with workplace violence.

T F   4. The Occupational Safety and Health Administration is an organization that issues fines for workplace safety violations.

T F   5. The National Institute for Occupational Safety and Health reported that homicide has become the second leading cause of occupational injury death.

T F   6. The main components of a violence prevention program are a (1) written plan, (2) worksite analysis, (3) hazard prevention and control, (4) safety and health training, and (5) record keeping and evaluation of the program.

T F   7. Total quality management is a program to protect the financial assets of an organization from loss by focusing on prevention.

T F   8. Threat assessment is the evaluation of the threat and the threatener.

T F   9. Horizontal violence is common in nursing and is a form of bullying.

T F   10. Intimidation is a form of violence and is an implied threat.

REFERENCES

Carroll, V., & Morin, K. (1998). Workplace violence affects one-third of nurses: Survey of nurses in seven SNAs reveals staff nurses most at risk. *American Nurse, 30*(5), 1. Retrieved July 19, 2004, from *www.nursingworld.org/tan/98sepoct/violence.htm*

Dolan, J. B. (2000). Workplace violence: The universe of legal issues. *Defense Counsel Journal, 67*(3), 332-341.

Ginn, G. O., & Henry, L. J. (2002). Addressing workplace violence from a health management perspective. *S.A.M. Advanced Management Journal, 67*(4), 4-10.

Henry, L. J., & Ginn, G. O. (2002). Violence prevention in health care organization within a TQM Framework. *Journal of Nursing Administration, 32*(9), 479-486.

Jossi, E. (1999). Defusing workplace violence. *Business & Health, 17*(2), 34-49.

Karl, K. A., & Hancock, B. W. (1999). Expert advice on employment termination practices: How expert is it? *Public Personnel Management, 28*(1), 51-62.

Litke, R. (1996). Defusing the workplace time bomb. *Journal of Property Management, 61*(4), 16-21.

McKenna, B. G., Smith, N. A., Poole, S. J., & Coverdale, J. H. (2003). Horizontal violence: Experience of registered nurses in their first year of practice. *Journal of Advanced Nursing, 42*(1), 90-96.

Murray, M. G., & Snyder, J. C. (1991). When staff are assaulted. *Journal of Psychosocial Nursing and Mental Health Nursing, 29*(7), 24-29.

National Institute for Occupational Safety and Health. (1996). *National Institute for Occupational Safety and Health: Current intelligence bulletin 57. Violence in the workplace: Risk factors and strategies.* Washington, DC: NIOSH, Centers for Disease Control and Prevention, U.S. Department of Health and Human Services.

National Institute for Occupational Safety and Health. (2002). *Violence: Occupational hazards in hospitals.* Washington, DC: NIOSH, Centers for Disease Control and Prevention, U.S. Department of Health and Human Services. Retrieved July 19, 2004, from *www.cdc.gov/niosh/2002-101.html*

Occupational Safety and Health Administration. (2003). *Guidelines for preventing workplace violence for health care and social service workers. OSHA publication 3148* (Rev. 2003). Washington, DC: OSHA, U.S. Department of Labor.

Rugala, E. R., & Isaacs, A. R. (Eds.). (2004). *Workplace violence: Issues in response.* Washington, DC: U.S. Department of Justice, Federal Bureau of Investigation. Retrieved July 19, 2004, from *www.fbi.gov/publications/violence.pdf*

Smith-Pittman, M. H., & McKoy, Y. D. (1999). Workplace violence in healthcare environments. *Nursing Forum, 34*(3), 5-13.

Violence threatens the workplace. (1998). *The Internal Auditor, 55*(5), 13.

SUPPLEMENTAL READINGS

McAdams, K., Russell, H., & Walukewicz, C. (2004). Gangstas: Not in my hospital. *Nursing, 34*(9), 32A.

Savage, T. (2004). Decreasing assault occurrence on a psychogeriatric ward. *Journal of Gerontological Nursing, 30*(5), 30-37.

Chapter **31** Prevention of Workplace Violence

Chapter 31: Prevention of Workplace Violence (pp. 675-692)

1. **Why should nurses be vigilant regarding the potential for violence from co-workers?**

   Nurses frequently encounter acts of intimidation: an implied threat when someone hits a wall, throws an object, or glares at someone in the immediate areas as a form of violence (Carroll & Morin, 1998). Hoag-Apel (1999) reported that the toleration of hostile or threatening behavior potentially can escalate to significant physical harm.

2. **When is a threat important enough to report?**

   All incidents of violence, including verbal assaults, should be reported, because it is difficult to predict which events will become more violent, resulting in physical harm. Threat assessment and threat management as part of a violence prevention program. Managers can assess the threat and perform an evaluation of the threatener. Threat management outlines what steps need to be taken once the threat assessment has been completed.

3. **How do you know when an incident has a potential for violence?**

   Persons with a history of violence or situational triggers of potential violence such as employees being fired, acts of bullying, verbal threats, harassment, intimidation, pushing, or slapping may trigger more serious types of violence. The presence of weapons, use of alcohol or drugs also can contribute to violence. Policies and procedures in the violence protection plan should outline potentially violent situations.

4. **What can nurses do about verbal abuse from physicians?**

   Nurses should handle verbal abuse or assaults as any other incident of violence. The incident should be reported and documented according to the policies and procedures outlined in the violence prevention program of the institution.

   Managers should demonstrate commitment by ensuring that no violence will be tolerated and that no reprisals are taken against employees who report or experience workplace violence. Managers should investigate all reports of violence or potential violence immediately.

5. **What laws apply to workplace violence?**

   All federal or state laws and local ordinances apply to workplace violence. This includes assault, battery, attempted murder, rape, and sexual harassment.

6. **What steps should nurse administrators take to secure a safe workplace?**

   Developing written antiviolence policies and procedures is the first step in reducing workplace violence. Policies should address factors such as employees, patients, non–hospital employee providers, and visitors (Smith-Pittman & McKoy, 1999). The National Institute for Occupational Safety and Health (2002), an agency within the Center for Disease Control and Prevention of the United States, recommends three major prevention strategies for employers: environmental designs, administrative controls, and behavior modifications. Environmental designs include signaling systems, alarm systems, monitoring systems, security devices, scrutiny escorts, lighting, and architectural and furniture modifications to improve worker safety. Administrative controls include adequate staffing patterns to prevent personnel from working alone and reducing waiting times, controlled access, and development of systems to alert security personnel when violence is threatened. Behavior modifications provide all workers with training in recognizing and managing assaults, resolving conflicts, and maintaining hazard awareness.

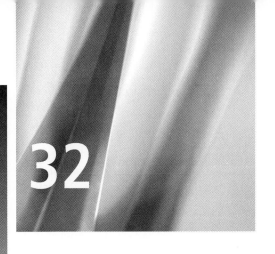

32

Collective Bargaining

STUDY FOCUS

In business and commerce, two groups, management and labor, often interact to resolve conflicts and negotiate over the terms and conditions of employment. Federal and state laws, administrative agency regulation, and judicial decisions regulate collective bargaining. The *National Labor Relations Act* (*NLRA, or Wagner Act*) enacted in 1935 when signed by Franklin Roosevelt is the main body of law for collective bargaining in the United States. The NLRA covers most private nonagricultural employees for the selection of a union for those who wish to engage in collective bargaining. This same legislation prohibits employers from interfering with the employee's selection of a labor union. The *National Labor Relations Board* (NLRB) was created from the NLRA with the two main functions of conducting representative elections and certifying results and preventing employers and unions from engaging in unfair labor practices. The *Federal Service Labor-Management Relations Act* governs federal employees, and the *Railway Labor Act* covers the railway and airline industries for collective bargaining activities.

Areas of concern with the involvement of nursing in collective bargaining include the question of the appropriateness of nurses engaging in collective bargaining, the differences in the public and private sector arenas, and the NLRB and U.S. Supreme Court decisions affecting nurses' inclusion in collective bargaining. Definitions that are important in the collective bargaining process are numerous. *Arbitration (interest)* is the use of an impartial third party to seek a solution to a dispute between parties involving the content of the collective bargaining agreement. The decision by the arbitrator usually is binding on the parties involved. *Arbitration (grievance)* is the use of an impartial third party to settle a dispute between the parties as to the meaning and application of certain language in the collective bargaining agreement. The decision of the arbitrator usually is binding on both parties. *Bargaining agent/representative* is the organization that

the employees in a bargaining unit select to represent the employees in that unit in negotiations with the employer. Frequently there is a local bargaining unit that is affiliated with a national group. *Bargaining unit* is the group of employees who are joined together by the authorized agency to bargain collectively with the employer. *Certification* is the official designation by the labor agency of a bargaining agent as the exclusive representative of employees concerning matters of employment with management. *Collective bargaining* is the process used by representatives of an employer and the certified bargaining agent to write and sign an agreement covering terms of employment. *Contract* is the written agreement between the employees in a bargaining unit and the employer regarding the conditions of employment. *Good faith bargaining* is the performance of the mutual obligation of the employer and representative of the employees to meet at reasonable times and confer in good faith on conditions of employment. *Grievance* is the allegation by an employee or certified bargaining agent that management has violated the collective bargaining agreement. *Grievance procedure* is a written plan outlining the actions to be taken by employees and their certified bargaining agent and the employer to adjust a grievance. *Impasse* is a deadlock in negotiations between management and employee representation over the terms of employment. *Management rights* are policies or practices that the applicable laws indicate are not subject to negotiation. *Mandatory bargaining items* are policies or practices that the applicable laws indicate management must negotiate with employee representatives. *Mediation* is the use of a neutral third party to facilitate negotiations between employees and the employer. *Nonmandatory bargaining items* are policies or practices that applicable law indicates management may negotiate with its employees' agent. *Prohibited bargaining items* are policies or practices that the applicable law indicates management may not negotiate with its employee's agent. *Unfair labor practice* is an allegation made by an individual, an employer, or a labor

227

organization of a violation of the law pertaining to collective bargaining.

The *three categories of work life included in collective bargaining* are mandatory, permissive, and illegal subjects (National Labor Relations Board, 1997). *Mandatory subjects* include wages, overtime, discipline, grievance, seniority, promotion, safety, layoff, recall, discharges, sick leave, and leaves of absence. Other topics covered include pensions for current employees, bonuses, group insurance, grievance procedures, safety practices, seniority, procedures for discharge, layoff, recall, or discipline, and union security. *Permissive subjects* for bargaining include employee rights, management rights, and benefits for retired union members. *Illegal subjects* include closed shop (employers will hire only union members), discriminatory treatment, and the "hot cargo clause" (employees will not be required to handle work during a strike).

In 1947 the *Taft-Hartley Act amendments* maintained the exclusion of not-for-profit hospitals, but in 1974 further amendments to the Taft-Hartley Act removed this exemption. There continues to be the issue of professionalism versus unionization for the profession of nursing. The *American Nurses Association* promotes economic and general welfare for nurses through the state nurses associations' representation of nurses as their labor union. More often than not, nurses unionize because of job satisfaction issues in an oppressive hospital environment. Unionization offers protection of workers, a unified voice, and opportunities to grow professionally.

Nurses must determine who will represent them in collective bargaining and who will be included in the bargaining unit. A *unit* is determined by the community of interest concerning wages, hours, and conditions of employment. The NLRB clearly identifies those activities from which the employer must refrain and the rules that labor unions must keep. The NLRB also describes the scope of bargaining that employees and employers must honor. Collective bargaining units are mechanisms to limit employers' capability of making unilateral actions. In the past, nurses joined unions to enhance job security because major health care reorganizations, layoffs, and downsizing have become the norm. In the 1990s the U.S. Supreme Court ruled that nurses who supervise lower-level personnel were supervisors and therefore were not protected by federal laws on collective bargaining under the NLRA. In 1996 the NLRB ruled that registered nurses, including charge nurses, were not supervisors and therefore were permitted to engage in collective bargaining.

Nursing leadership and management can affect the quality of work life for staff significantly. Work redesign to increase autonomy and clinical decision making helps improve the work climate and nurse satisfaction. Aiken and colleagues (2002) further supported professional nursing practice by demonstrating that there is a relationship between poor registered nurse staffing and poor client outcomes. Nurse leaders are challenged to implement professional practice models that foster a shared governance approach to care delivery. They must provide adequate registered nurse staffing to prevent nurse burnout, foster quality care, and improve client clinical outcomes. Challenges facing staff and management are to perform the following: develop a shared governance model, eliminate mandatory overtime, ensure adequate numbers of well-trained unlicensed assistive personnel, provide professional leadership and management 24/7, reward positive performance and eliminate punitive thinking, develop cooperative labor-management relationships, and use client-focused language. Skilled leadership teams are important in organizations to ensure satisfied employees and positive clinical outcomes.

LEARNING TOOLS

Group Activity

Purpose

To become knowledgeable regarding the collective bargaining activities within health care organizations that affect nursing practice.

Directions

1. Contact your state nurses association and request information about collective bargaining activities within your state.

2. Review the materials that the state nurses association distributes, and have each member of the group interview a nurse that they know using the following professionalism versus unionization worksheet.

3. Be sure to explore the major issues they face in their day-to-day work. Write down the benefits and the limitations that nurses verbalize about unionization. If the nurses do not support unionization, ask them what strategies or mechanisms they will use in the health care setting where they work to resolve conflict and negotiate desirable employment conditions.

Professionalism versus Unionization Worksheet

1. Benefits of Unionization

2. Limitations of Unionization

3. Issues Faced in the Health Care Setting

4. Strategies to Resolve Conflict and Enhance Employment Conditions

4. Review the information that each group member collects and separate into two groups to discuss the pros and cons of professionalism and its relationship to unionization. Use the responses from the nurses who were interviewed to support each position.

CASE STUDY

Suzie Sepland is an exceptional registered nurse on the neurology unit at Billings Hospital in Montana. She is often charge nurse and consistently is able to answer all client-related questions and assist co-workers throughout the day. Whenever Nurse Sepland is in charge, the work flow on the neurology unit is smooth and staff enjoy their work. Nurse Sepland works the 7 AM to 3 PM shift but is well respected on all shifts and on all units in the hospital.

The nurses at Billings Hospital have become dissatisfied with the lack of recognition and control in what they consider to be an oppressive hospital environment.

Wages have been kept low, unlicensed assistive personnel have been replacing registered nurse vacancies, and condition severity levels are high on most units. Administration representatives seem to be ignoring the nurses' concerns. Nurse Sepland has been approached by several of the registered nurses at the hospital about organizing informational meetings with collective bargaining representatives. Nurse Sepland's co-workers would like her to take the leadership initiative for unionization at the hospital.

Case Study Questions

1. What should Nurse Sepland do? Should she take the leadership initiative and assist with informational meetings?

2. What are the issues that the nurses face? Are there alternative solutions to unionization? If so, what are the alternative solutions?

3. What are the advantages and disadvantages of unionization?

LEARNING RESOURCES

Discussion Questions

1. What are the tensions between the views of collective bargaining and its relationship to professionalism?

2. Discuss the history of collective bargaining as it pertains to the profession of nursing.

3. What are the major legislative acts that define collective bargaining?

4. What is the role of the American Nurses Association in collective bargaining?

5. What are factors that may influence nurses to engage in collective bargaining activities?

Study Questions

Matching: Write the letter of the correct response in front of each term.

_____ 1. Collective bargaining	A.	A deadlock in negotiations between management and employee representation over the terms of employment
_____ 2. Grievance		
_____ 3. Mediation	B.	The official designation by the labor agency of a bargaining agent as the exclusive representative of employees concerning matters of employment with management
_____ 4. 1974 amendments to the Taft-Hartley Act		

_____ 5. National Labor Relations Act

_____ 6. Bargaining unit

_____ 7. Contract

_____ 8. Impasse

_____ 9. Arbitration

_____ 10. Certification

C. The use of an impartial third party to settle a dispute between the parties as to the meaning and application of certain language in the collective bargaining agreement

D. The main body of law for collective bargaining

E. The allegation by an employee or certified bargaining agent that management has violated the collective bargaining agreement

F. The use of a neutral third party to facilitate negotiations between employees and the employer

G. The process that is used by representatives of an employer and the certified bargaining agent to write and sign an agreement covering terms of employment

H. The removal of the exclusion of not-for-profit hospitals to engage in collective bargaining

I. Group of employees joined together by the authorized agency to bargain collectively with the employer

J. The written agreement between the employees in a bargaining unit and the employer regarding the condition of employment

True or False: Circle the correct answer.

T   F   11. Under the National Labor Relations Act, procedures are created for the selection of a union or other labor representative for employees who wish to engage in collective bargaining.

T   F   12. The main body of law for collective bargaining in the United States is the federal statute called the National Collective Bargaining Act.

T   F   13. Mediation is the use of a neutral third party to facilitate negotiations between management and the bargaining representative.

T   F   14. The National Labor Relations Act and the Wagner Act are the same acts and were signed into law by President Franklin Roosevelt.

T   F   15. All states have the same requirements for employer bargaining.

REFERENCES

Aiken, L. H., Clarke, S. P., Sloane, D. M., Sochalski, J., & Sieber, J. H. (2002). Hospital nursing staffing and patient mortality, nurse burnout, and job dissatisfaction. _Journal of the American Medical Association, 288_(16), 1987-1993.

National Labor Relations Board. (1997). _A guide to basic law and procedures under the National Labor Relations Act._ Washington, DC: U.S. Government Printing Office.

SUPPLEMENTAL READINGS

Fitzpatrick, M. A. (2001). Collective bargaining: Vulnerability assessment. _Nursing Management, 32_(2), 41-42.

Porter-O'Grady, T. (2001). Collective bargaining: The union as partner. _Nursing Management, 32_(6), 30-32.

Schraeder, M., & Friedman, L. (2002). Collective bargaining in the nursing profession: Salient issues and recent developments in healthcare reform. _Hospital Topics, 80_(3), 21-24.

Steitzer, T. M. (2001). Collective bargaining: A wake-up call. _Nursing Management, 32_(4), 35-37.

Chapter 32: Collective Bargaining (pp. 693-712)

1. What are the attributes of a profession?

The elements of a profession include the following:
- A discrete body of knowledge
- Altruism
- Lifelong learning
- Autonomy
- Peer review

2. Does nursing meet these criteria? If not, why not?

Nursing meets most of these criteria. Nursing has a discrete body of knowledge, requires lifelong learning, and relies on altruism for its practitioners to discharge its responsibilities in a humane manner. Nursing does not meet the criteria in the areas of autonomy and peer review. Until there is one consistent source of educational entry into practice, nursing will continue to be lacking in these areas. Nursing also depends somewhat on following physician orders; therefore, true autonomy is not present. However, nurses do write nursing orders and can develop a plan of care that is consistent with the medical plan, which may suggest nursing autonomy. Nurses who demonstrate autonomous clinical decision making are master's degree-prepared advanced nurse practitioners, or home care registered nurses.

3. Is it unprofessional to join a labor union? Why or why not?

Controversy exists within the nursing profession regarding the congruency between professionalism and unionization. Some argue that unionization diminishes the nursing profession, equating unions to forums for less-educated, blue-collar employees. Management intimidation, management allegiances, and union militancy contributed to the perspective of unionization as nonprofessional. However, others contend that collective bargaining serves to protect nurses and clients while enhancing nurse professionalism, especially when conflict resolution, group solidarity, and collaborative decision making are used as strategies. An important consideration for nurses is the selection of an appropriate bargaining agent to address their professional needs. Nurses may select union representation by a professional organization such as the American Nurses Association or one of its state organizations or by a traditional labor union such as the AFL-CIO. The choice of a bargaining agent that is knowledgeable about professional nursing practice and standards of care provides a better position to address the special interests of nurses than using industrial labor unions.

4. What is the NLRA? The NLRB? Why are they important?

The National Labor Relations Act (NLRA) was originally the Wagner Act, signed into law by President Franklin D. Roosevelt in 1935. The act was designed to protect workers, regulate child labor, and prevent unhealthy and dangerous working conditions. Regarding labor unions, the NLRA also makes it illegal to discriminate against employees to encourage or discourage union membership. The National Labor Relations Board (NLRB) is the governing agency for labor unions. The responsibility of this board is to administer the law as it relates to labor practices and the establishment of a union within an organization.

5. Should nurses be allowed to strike? Why or why not?

A strike is a strategy used when the negotiations between management and the collective bargaining representatives reach an impasse that goes unresolved for an extended period. The decision to implement a strike is often an ethical dilemma for nurses. Typically, when the decision to strike is made, it has to do with more than economic compensation. Most nursing strikes are implemented because nurses believe that client safety and care delivery is being threatened. Although a strike is not the best strategy for conflict resolution, sometimes it may be the only one that will enable nurses to maintain control over nursing practice and ensure the delivery of safe, quality health care.

6. What other options besides unionization are available for labor-management conflict resolution?

Besides unionization, labor-management conflicts can be resolved through effective human resource management and shared governance models. Open communication and employee empowerment in an organizational culture that values its staff will promote a positive work climate, quality client outcomes, and job satisfaction. The frequency of labor-management conflicts will be reduced in an organization that has satisfied employees who participate in the decision-making process.

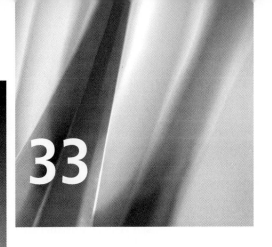

33 Staffing and Scheduling

STUDY FOCUS

Staffing and scheduling are key nursing leadership and management functions. These activities are complex and require considerable time. Staffing and scheduling are important components in the effective provision of cost-effective, client-centered care and in the satisfaction, retention, and recruitment of nurses. Staffing and scheduling also affect issues of safety and quality of client care. The major goal of staffing and scheduling systems is to identify the need and determine the proper type of personnel required to provide client services (Smith, 1994). *Staffing* is the development of a plan to hire qualified workers to fill designated positions in an organization. *Scheduling* is implementing the staffing pattern to assign workers to cover specific shifts and days on specific units. Nurse staffing has three major components: *planning* (number of nurses needed over the long term), *scheduling* (assigning nurses by shift), and *allocation* (adjusting staff shift by shift). The *staffing plan* is a written plan identifying the number and classification of nurses needed to implement the care model by shift. The *care delivery model* is the structure and mechanism for organizing the processes of care, workload, and caregiver assignments. The *staffing strategy* is a comprehensive action plan to determine the future human resource needs of the organization so as to recruit and select the best applicants. *Scheduling* is the ongoing implementation of the staffing pattern by assigning individual nurses to specific shifts and units. *Self-scheduling* is a process by which nurses work together on a unit to construct a schedule (Unruh, 2003). *Staff mix* is the skill level of workers required to provide care. *Nursing resources* include the number and types of workers designated to provide nursing services. The *nursing workload* is a compilation of nursing care needs of clients. In a hospital, workload is a function of the number of client days and hours and the hours of nursing care required per client per day (Kirby & Wiczai, 1985). *Acuity* is the intensity or severity of client illness. *Nursing intensity* is the amount and complexity of care required by clients. Prescott (1991) identified severity of illness, client dependency on nursing, complexity, and time as major dimensions of nursing intensity. *Unlicensed assistive personnel* are workers who complete designated tasks to assist the nurses to care for a larger number of clients or to offer clients a broader selection of services.

Staffing and scheduling are core functions of a nurse manager. They are two major aspects of the allocation of scarce and expensive personnel resources. The following three variables are central to staffing methodology (Abdoo, 2000):

1. Assessing client needs (client classification)

2. Assessing nursing time to meet client needs (workload determination)

3. Developing an algorithm that combines the first two variables

Two documents that address the impact of nursing care on client outcomes and the well-being of nurses are the report of the American Nurses Association and the report by the Institute of Medicine *Nursing Staff in Hospitals and Nursing Homes: Is It Adequate* (Wunderlich et al., 1996). The American Nurses Association (1999) identified nine principles to guide nursing *staff* grouped into *three categories:* (1) client care unit–related (appropriate staffing levels; retire or question the concept of hours per patient day; unit functions support care delivery); (2) staff related (needs of client populations, management support, clinical support); and (3) institutional/organizational related (positive organizational climate, documented competencies of nursing staff, organizational policies that recognize the needs of clients and nursing staff). The American Nurses Association also developed a *matrix for staffing decision making composed of four critical factors:* (1) number of clients with characteristics for whom care is provided; (2) level of intensity of the unit and care; (3) contextual issues to include environmental geography, technology, and architect; and (4) levels of expertise and preparation of care providers.

233

Staffing decisions are complex and require planning and careful consideration for maximum effectiveness. Staffing and scheduling activities are unique to each care delivery setting. There are similarities in scheduling such as ensuring safe, cost-effective care; maximizing resources; managing workload variation; and using a variety of providers (Barratt & Schultz, 1997). *Four essential elements of staffing decisions* include a statement of philosophy, general objectives for the department and specific objectives for the unit, job descriptions for all skill levels, and a statement of the frequency of nursing care along with a designation of who will provide the services. Four key concepts describe variations in intensity of nursing work: (1) client nursing condition, (2) medical condition, (3) caregiver characteristics, and (4) the environment (O'Brien-Pallas et al., 1997). Typically, staffing decisions are based on a measure of volume and/or time. Volume measures include census, visits, births, operations, and client contacts. One method of volume calculation is hours per patient day (or *HPPD*). Hours per patient day is a calculation of nursing hours needed per unit of service.

To measure nursing activities, one must determine the *unit of service,* a volume measure. Time is measured in hours per day or unit. *Standards* often are set for staffing calculations, and *activities* based on time calculations are determined. Two methods used to guide nurse staffing are fixed and variable staffing. *Fixed staffing* is a fixed maximum workload requirement. This type of staffing method is based on the assumption that one will have maximum workload conditions. *Variable staffing* is based on a supplementary approach and involves staffing below maximum workload conditions. A proposed third type of staffing method is a *semiflexible system* whereby 15% of the staff is fixed. In semiflexible staffing, the fixed staff are supplemented based on volume and condition severity.

There are *eleven steps in designing a staffing pattern.* First, select criteria to determine the intensity levels of clients or units of service. Second, determine the time required to complete the work. Third, collect data to determine the validity of a set classification system. Fourth, collect sufficient data (type and quantity) to evaluate your proposed staffing method. Fifth, determine the average number of minutes per activity or task. Sixth, establish a performance time for new functions. Seventh, decide on the staff mix necessary to complete the work. Eighth, determine the amount of time per client type necessary (severity of illness) for each skill level. Ninth, establish a unit of service projection for the year. Tenth, calculate the total number of nursing hours and the number of individuals by skill mix who will be needed per year. Finally, designate the number

of individuals per shift each day and their skill mix. Include a calculation for time off and administrative activities. The components of a clinical labor resource management system are budgeting, scheduling, daily staffing, and management information. The daily work schedule is part of the short-term human resource management. After the minimum number of staff needed is determined, then scheduling of personnel follows. The many types of time scheduling systems include block (fixed, but revised yearly); unstructured (created weekly and changes based on staff need); skeleton (basic staffing with only a portion, such as the weekends fixed); cyclical (pattern is established for each person); and master (cyclical, repetitive schedule) (McKinley & Cavouras, 2000). Oftentimes, daily staffing and management information systems are in place to analyze the most current client and staff mix needs for each unit. This may be done by computerized nurse scheduling programs. Self-scheduling is one strategy that managers are using to improve morale and satisfaction. *Self-scheduling* is a process whereby nurses sign up, using guidelines, for preferred shifts. *Preference scheduling* is a system in which nurses submit preferred shifts before the manager compiles and generates the final schedule.

Many types of client classification systems are in use today. The *three broad types of client classification systems* include (1) prototype, (2) factor, and (3) computerized real-time factor. A *prototype client classification* system is designed to categorize clients by broad categories and characteristics. The *factor client classification* system uses critical indicators to determine individual care needs. In the factor systems, allowances are made for the indirect care activities required. The *computerized real-time factor systems* are based on actual care requirements for individual clients.

Managing human resources is an important leadership and management function because personnel costs are the single largest health care expense item in the operating budget of an organization. During the mid-1980s, diagnosis-related groups and prospective reimbursement were introduced, and during the mid-1990s, health care reform and restructuring occurred in the midst of economic pressures. Layoffs, downsizing, and restructuring created short-term economic gains. Staffing experimentation and redesign were introduced to reduce health care costs. Job uncertainty, low morale, mandatory overtime, and increased workload requirements triggered unionization efforts and concern regarding client safety. A backlash over client safety, emerged from the cost containment and minimal registered nurse shortage. Two reports from the Institute of Medicine, *Nursing Staff in Hospitals and Nursing Homes: Is it Adequate?* (Wunderlich et al., 1996) and *To*

234

Chapter **33 Staffing and Scheduling**

Err Is Human: Building a Safer Health System (Kohn et al., 2000), addressed this issue. Nurse leaders must ensure that adequate, qualified staff is available to care for clients.

LEARNING TOOLS

Activity: Staffing and Scheduling

Purpose

To become familiar with the staffing and scheduling process.

Introduction

Staffing a unit in a hospital or ambulatory care clinic is a challenging process. Different health care organizations handle staffing and scheduling in a variety of ways. One method is self-scheduling in which parameters or principles are given for signing up for specific shifts. When conflicts or shortages occur, managers negotiate with staff members or have staff members negotiate with one another. In other health care organizations, the managers, with input from the staff, create a schedule. The staffing and scheduling exercise that you are about to complete gives you an understanding of the complexity of scheduling staff and covering all shifts and times.

A manager must assess employees' requests for time off, which includes vacation, scheduled days off, and personal time. A manager also must handle the call-ins for sick time. To staff a unit effectively, the manager must establish a skill-mix level and project a unit service figure. The following activity provides you an opportunity to staff a unit and see the complexities of scheduling and staffing.

Staffing and Scheduling Scenario

B6-Oncology unit (25 beds)

Average daily census: 17

Skill mix: 75% Registered nurses (RNs)

25% Unlicensed assistive personnel (UAPs)

The nurse manager has determined that 10 staff members are required for a 24-hour period. The nurse manager must cover 24 hours per week for 7 days a week. The breakdown for percent of nurses needed is as follows: days—45%, evenings—36%, and nights—19%.

RNs: Susie is full-time (7-3); Jen is full-time (7-3); Jon is full-time (7-3); Sylvia is full-time (7-3); Ben is full-time (7-3 and 3-11); Jake is full-time (3-11); Kim is full-time (3-11); Cindy is 24 hours per week (3-11); Jack works on an as-needed basis (3-11 and 11-7); Tom is full-time (11-7); and Jan is full-time (11-7).

UAPs: Jill is full-time (7-3); Joan is 24 hours per week (7-3); Jeremy is as needed (3-11); Jerry is part-time 24 hours per week (3-11); Janet is as needed (3-11); and Jessie is 32 hours per week (11-7). Hiring of some as-needed or pool nurses who are flexible to assist in meeting vacation coverage is important.

RN requests: Susie cannot work Mondays because of school. Jen is getting married and needs September 1 to 17 off for her honeymoon. Jon is going away for a fishing trip and needs the first weekend of September off. Jack does not want to work Tuesdays and Thursdays because of babysitting difficulties and does not want every weekend.

UAP requests: Jessie will be on vacation September 1 to 10. Janet will not be able to work Fridays because of a continuing education course.

Directions

1. Create a schedule with the following requests using the census of 17, and calculate the number of staff needed per shift.

2. First determine how many employees are on each shift: day, evening, and night shifts.

3. Then calculate the number of RNs and UAPs needed per day, evening, and night shift.

4. Next, put all the requests on your calendar.

5. Finally, create a schedule, using the empty schedule grid on the following page (remember, employees do not like to work every weekend).

Questions to Consider

1. How many employees will be scheduled for each shift?

2. What type of employees will be scheduled for each shift? How many of each skill level?

3. Are there any vacation or personal requests?

4. Who works full time and who works part time? What are the part-time employees' hours?

Summary

Working with staffing and scheduling is complex. When individuals call in because of illness or personal crisis, finding an individual to fill the opening may be harrowing. Meeting individual requests in a tight schedule can be problematic. Many units have resorted to self-scheduling to give staff more flexibility to plan their work and personal lives and to encourage them to cover each other's shifts.

One Possible Solution

There should be five staff members on 7-3, three on 3-11, and two on 11-7. Next, calculate how many RNs and

September 7–3 Shift

	F 1	S 2	S 3	M 4	T 5	W 6	TH 7	F 8	S 9	S 10	M 11	T 12	W 13	TH 14	F 15	S 16	S 17	M 18	T 19	W 20	TH 21	F 22	S 23	S 24	M 25	T 26	W 27	TH 28	F 29	S 30
RNs																														
Susie (FT)																														
Jen (FT)																														
Jon (FT)																														
Sylvia (FT)																														
Ben (FT)																														
UAPs																														
Jill (FT)																														
Joan (PT)																														
Jeremy (PRN)																														

September 3–11 Shift

	F 1	S 2	S 3	M 4	T 5	W 6	TH 7	F 8	S 9	S 10	M 11	T 12	W 13	TH 14	F 15	S 16	S 17	M 18	T 19	W 20	TH 21	F 22	S 23	S 24	M 25	T 26	W 27	TH 28	F 29	S 30
RNs																														
Jake (FT)																														
Kim (FT)																														
Cindy (FT)																														
UAPs																														
Jerry (PT)																														
Janet (PRN)																														

September 11–7 Shift

	F 1	S 2	S 3	M 4	T 5	W 6	TH 7	F 8	S 9	S 10	M 11	T 12	W 13	TH 14	F 15	S 16	S 17	M 18	T 19	W 20	TH 21	F 22	S 23	S 24	M 25	T 26	W 27	TH 28	F 29	S 30
RNs																														
Tom (FT)																														
Jan (FT)																														
Jack (PRN)																														
UAPs																														
Jessie (PT)																														

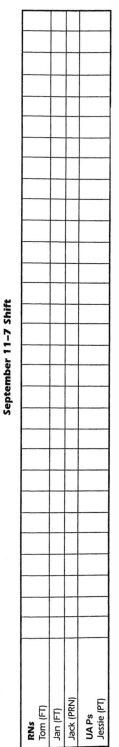

UAPs should be scheduled per shift. On 7-3 there should be four RNs and one UAP; on 3-11 there should be two RNs and one UAP; and on 11-7 there should be one RN and one UAP. Nurse managers have the flexibility to shift the total number of RNs and UAPs within the 24-hour shift, and at times they may alter the skill mix throughout the year to cover vacations and requests.

The key is to keep salaries averaging out over the year (remember, a nurse manager budgets salaries based on the number of RNs and UAPs working per shift). Many times, weekends typically are staffed with fewer nurses to allow staff members every other weekend off. Following is a sample of a completed schedule based on the situation described.

SCHEDULE FOR SEPTEMBER 2005

September 7-3 Shift

	F 1	S 2	S 3	M 4	T 5	W 6	TH 7	F 8	S 9	S 10	M 11	T 12	W 13	TH 14	F 15	S 16	S 17	M 18	T 19	W 20	TH 21	F 22	S 23	S 24	M 25	T 26	W 27	TH 28	F 29	S 30
RNs																														
Susie (FT)	7-3	X	7-3	X	X	7-3	7-3	X	7-3	7-3	X	7-3	7-3	7-3	7-3	X	X	X	7-3	7-3	7-3	X	7-3	X	X	7-3	7-3	7-3	7-3	7-3
Jen (FT)	VAC	X	X	VAC	VAC	VAC	VAC	VAC	X	X	VAC	VAC	VAC	VAC	7-3	X	X	7-3	7-3	7-3	X	7-3	7-3	7-3	7-3	7-3	X	7-3	7-3	7-3
Jon (FT)	X	X	X	7-3	7-3	7-3	X	7-3	7-3	X	7-3	X	7-3	7-3	7-3	X	7-3	7-3	7-3	7-3	X	7-3	7-3	X	7-3	X	X	7-3	7-3	X
Sylvia (FT)	7-3	7-3	7-3	7-3	7-3	7-3	7-3	7-3	X	7-3	7-3	7-3	7-3	7-3	7-3	7-3	7-3	7-3	7-3	X	7-3	7-3	7-3	7-3	7-3	7-3	7-3	X	7-3	X
Ben (FT)	X	3-11	3-11	X	7-3	X	7-3	X	X	7-3	3-11	X	7-3	7-3	7-3	7-3	7-3	X	7-3	7-3	7-3	X	7-3	7-3	7-3	7-3	X	7-3	7-3	3-11
UAPs																														
Jill (FT)	7-3	7-3	7-3	7-3	X	X	7-3	7-3	7-3	7-3	7-3	7-3	X	7-3	7-3	7-3	7-3	X	7-3	7-3	7-3	7-3	7-3	X	7-3	7-3	7-3	7-3	X	7-3
Joan (PT)	7-3	7-3	7-3	7-3	X	X	7-3	7-3	X	7-3	7-3	7-3	7-3	X	X	X	7-3	7-3	X	X	7-3	X	X	X	7-3	X	X	X	X	7-3
Jeremy (PRN)	X	X	X	7-3	7-3	7-3	X	7-3	7-3	7-3	7-3	X	X	7-3	X	X	7-3	7-3	X	X	X	7-3	X	X	X	X	7-3	X	X	X

September 3-11 Shift

	F 1	S 2	S 3	M 4	T 5	W 6	TH 7	F 8	S 9	S 10	M 11	T 12	W 13	TH 14	F 15	S 16	S 17	M 18	T 19	W 20	TH 21	F 22	S 23	S 24	M 25	T 26	W 27	TH 28	F 29	S 30
RNs																														
Jake (FT)	3-11	X	X	3-11	3-11	3-11	X	3-11	3-11	3-11	X	3-11	3-11	3-11	3-11	X	X	3-11	3-11	3-11	3-11	3-11	3-11	3-11	X	3-11	3-11	3-11	3-11	X
Kim (FT)	3-11	3-11	3-11	X	X	X	3-11	3-11	X	X	3-11	3-11	X	3-11	3-11	3-11	3-11	X	3-11	3-11	3-11	3-11	3-11	3-11	3-11	3-11	X	3-11	3-11	3-11
Cindy (FT)	X	X	3-11	3-11	3-11	X	3-11	3-11	3-11	3-11	3-11	3-11	3-11	3-11	3-11	X	3-11	3-11	3-11	3-11	3-11	3-11	3-11	X	X	X	X	X	X	X
UAPs																														
Jerry (PT)	3-11	X	X	3-11	X	3-11	X	X	3-11	3-11	X	X	X	X	X	X	X	3-11	X	X	3-11	X	3-11	3-11	X	3-11	X	X	X	X
Janet (PRN)	X	3-11	3-11	X	7-3	7-3	3-11	X	X	X	3-11	3-11	X	X	X	3-11	3-11	X	X	X	X	X	X	3-11	3-11	X	X	X	X	3-11

September 11-7 Shift

	F 1	S 2	S 3	M 4	T 5	W 6	TH 7	F 8	S 9	S 10	M 11	T 12	W 13	TH 14	F 15	S 16	S 17	M 18	T 19	W 20	TH 21	F 22	S 23	S 24	M 25	T 26	W 27	TH 28	F 29	S 30
RNs																														
Tom (FT)	11-7	X	11-7	11-7	11-7	11-7	11-7	11-7	11-7	11-7	11-7	X	11-7	11-7	11-7	11-7	X	11-7	11-7	11-7	11-7	11-7	11-7	11-7	11-7	X	11-7	11-7	11-7	X
Jan (FT)	11-7	11-7	11-7	11-7	11-7	X	11-7	11-7	X	X	11-7	11-7	11-7	11-7	11-7	11-7	11-7	X	11-7	X	11-7	11-7	X	11-7	11-7	11-7	X	11-7	11-7	11-7
Jack (PRN)	X	11-7	11-7	11-7	X	X	X	11-7	11-7	11-7	X	X	X	X	X	X	11-7	X	X	X	X	3-11	X	X	X	11-7	X	X	X	11-7
UAPs																														
Jessie (PT)	VAC	X	X	VAC	VAC	VAC	VAC	VAC	X	X	11-7	11-7	X	X	X	11-7	11-7	X	11-7	X	X	11-7	11-7	11-7	X	11-7	X	X	X	X

CASE STUDY

Dorothy Viens, a graduate-prepared nurse manager of a 79-bed medical unit, decides to operationalize a professional practice model to maximize the use of each nurse's skills and knowledge base, increase communication, and support autonomous clinical practice. The medical unit is staffed by unlicensed assistive personnel; licensed practical nurses; and diploma-, associate degree-, baccalaureate-, and graduate-prepared nurses. Nurse Viens holds a staff meeting to gather input and discuss possible models of professional practice. She brings articles she had obtained through a literature review to highlight pertinent information and to review successful professional practice models from hospitals with Magnet status. At the meeting there were many different ideas expressed by the staff and no clear consensus on the best model of practice for the medical surgical unit. To continue progress on identifying and implementing a professional practice model, Nurse Viens seeks volunteers to form a task force to identify critical elements, from the staff's perspective, that are needed in a professional practice model.

Case Study Questions

1. Is it possible to establish a professional practice model by involving the entire staff? Is this a good strategy to garner support from the staff and improve client care?

2. What is Magnet status? Describe how Magnet status is important in health care delivery.

3. What are the benefits of implementing professional practice models? What are the barriers of implementing a professional practice model?

LEARNING RESOURCES

Discussion Questions

1. What factors make staffing and scheduling complex?

2. Should clinical nurses be given the opportunity to assist in scheduling? If so, why? If not, why not? Should there be scheduling parameters established by the administration? Or should clinical nurses establish their own scheduling guidelines?

3. How do you calculate hours per patient day? Is this a useful calculation?

4. What must be considered when developing a client classification system?

5. What are the three broad types of client classification, and what are the differences and similarities among them?

Study Questions

True or False: Circle the correct answer.

T   F   1. Staffing is the implementation of a staffing pattern indicating the number and type of workers to be scheduled per shift.

T   F   2. Variable staffing is based on a set maximum workload requirement.

T   F   3. Client classification is the grouping of clients according to nursing care requirements.

T   F   4. Those health care agencies that obtain Magnet status often have improved nurse satisfaction, decreased nurse burnout, and better client outcomes.

T   F   5. There is no correlation between the number of registered nurses per client and positive client outcomes.

T   F   6. Unlicensed assistive personnel assist nurses to perform client care tasks including vital signs and assessments.

T   F   7. Acuity is the severity of a client illness.

T   F   8. Components in determining the severity of illness include client's perceived dependency, complexity, task determination, and the number of workers available.

T   F   9. Staffing decisions are based solely on an individual's philosophy.

T   F   10. Nursing workload is the number of client days and the hours of nursing care required per client day.

REFERENCES

Abdoo, Y. M. (2000). Nurse staffing and scheduling. In L. M. Simms, S. A. Price, & N. E. Ervin (Eds.), *Professional practice of nursing administration* (3rd ed., pp 459-480). Albany, NY: Delmar.

American Nurses Association. (1999). *Principles for nurse staffing.* Silver Spring, MD: Author. Retrieved January 4, 2005, from *www.nursingworld.org/readroom/stffprnc.htm*

Barratt, C. C., & Schultz, M. K. (1997). Staffing the operating room: Time and space factors. *Journal of Nursing Administration, 27*(12), 27-31.

Kirby, K., & Wiczai, L. (1985). Budgeting for variable staffing. *Nursing Economic$, 3*(3), 160-166.

Kohn, L. T., Corrigan, J. M., & Donaldson, M. S. (Eds.). (2000). *To err is human: Building a safer health system.* Washington, DC: National Academies Press.

McKinley, J. W., & Cavouras, C. A. (2000). Evolving staffing measures. In M. Fralic (Ed.), *Staffing management and methods: Tools and techniques for nurse leaders* (pp. 1-33). San Francisco: Jossey-Bass.

O'Brien-Pallas, L., Irvine, D., Peereboom, E., & Murray, M. (1997). Measuring nursing workload: Understanding the variability. *Nursing Economic$, 15*(4), 171-182.

Prescott, P. (1991). Nursing intensity: Needed today for more than staffing. *Nursing Economic$, 9*(6), 409-414.

Smith, M. (1994). Staffing and scheduling: A systems approach. In R. Spitzer-Lehmann (Ed.), *Nursing management desk reference: Concepts, skills & strategies* (pp. 178-197). Philadelphia: W. B. Saunders.

Unruh, L. (2003). The effect of LPN reductions on RN patient load. *Journal of Nursing Administration, 33*(4), 201-208.

Wunderlich, G. S., Sloan, F. A., & Davis, C. K. (1996). *Nursing staff in hospitals and nursing homes: Is it adequate?* Washington, DC: National Academies Press.

SUPPLEMENTAL READINGS

Blegen, M. A., Goode, C. J., & Reed, L. (1998). Nurse staffing and patient outcomes. *Nursing Research, 47*(1), 43-50.

Kirby, M. P., Dkost, P., Holdwick, C. C., Poskie, M., Glaser, D., & Sage, M. (1998). Improving staffing with a resource management plan. *Journal of Nursing Administration, 28*(11), 25-29.

Mooney, M. C. (2004). Stay current with staffing effectiveness standards. *Nursing Management, 35*(2), 14.

Rosen, S. (2004). Web-based staff scheduling. *Nursing Homes, 53*(6), 42-43.

Schuerenberg, B. K. (2004). Making time for scheduling. *Health Data Management, 12*(2), 128-130.

Chapter 33: Staffing and Scheduling (pp. 713-732)

1. Should nursing services be staffed to the minimum, maximum, or mean? Why?

Staffing and scheduling decisions are a challenging yet critical component of the nurse management role. Two general frameworks used to determine staffing include traditional fixed staffing and controlled variable staffing. The traditional fixed staffing model is based on fixed projected maximum workload requirements and workload conditions, using historical census trend data and projections. The controlled variable staffing method is built below maximum workload conditions, with staffing supplementation as needed. Although unique factors may influence staffing and scheduling decisions based on the care delivery context, there are similar factors considered across settings: ensuring safe, cost-effective care; dealing with workload fluctuations; using a variety of caregivers; and implementing effective, responsible resource management.

2. What is the influence of the budget on staffing and scheduling?

The budget is a major influential factor in the development of staffing and scheduling plans. Current economic constraints and limited financial resources have resulted in intense scrutiny of personnel costs and use. The nursing personnel salaries account for a significant proportion of the operating budget of a health care organization. In response to current economic pressures, cost-reduction strategies include strict staffing plans, nursing personnel layoffs, and the introduction of unlicensed assistive personnel.

3. To what extent should staff preferences determine staffing and scheduling? Explain.

Staffing and scheduling is a critical core function for nurse managers that requires a balance between competing interests and needs. Predetermined standards, budget constraints, personal preferences, and legal aspects must be taken into consideration. Staff satisfaction with scheduling is important, especially with varied shift lengths and unorthodox work hours as nurses attempt to meet the demands of their personal lives. A negotiation process may occur to ensure that organizational and personal needs are met.

4. What is the role of the client classification system for staffing and scheduling? Does this vary by setting of care?

The client classification system provides a quantified measure of nursing time and effort required to care for clients. It attempts to identify client condition severity to use as a proxy for workload, which becomes the basis for staffing and scheduling decisions. The three broad types of client classification systems are prototype, factor, and computerized real-time factor systems, all of which have been criticized concerning their reliability, validity, and comparability across settings. Other issues with client classification systems are related to impracticality of some systems, the time involvement necessary for development and maintenance, and the inability to evaluate generated data for usefulness to nursing and the organization.

5. Should a manager do the schedule, or should staff schedule themselves?

Scheduling methods vary and are setting-specific. Scheduling decisions may be limited to nursing personnel and staff, as well as managers and unit secretaries. Scheduling methods may involve computerized scheduling, managerial scheduling, self-scheduling, or a combination of some or all methods. No matter what scheduling method is selected, use of a consensus-building process facilitates meeting hours of care delivery and organizational financial goals. In a shared governance environment, a self-scheduling method may reflect autonomous practice, participation in decision making, and administrative support.

6. What is the "right" mix of registered nurses, licensed practical nurses, and assistive personnel?

What the effective and efficient mix of registered nurses and unlicensed assistive personnel is or should be is not clear. Experimentation is occurring with reconfigurations of personnel, differentiated practice, and the introduction of assistive personnel. Empirical and evaluative efforts have been minimal and without sufficient rigor to document the effect of nurse extenders in health care. It is important that nurses examine the use of nurse extenders and their impact using cost, satisfaction, and quality indicators.

7. **Should nurse-to-client ratios be mandated? Why or why not?**

The mandating of minimum nurse-to-client ratios has been controversial. Many questions arise, such as "What should minimum ratio be?" "How can a rural hospital come into compliance at a given cost and nurse shortage pressure?" "How will costs be covered?" "How will hospitals adjust actual registered nurse staffing?" "How will lunch and breaks be covered?" "Will nurses experience mandated overtime beyond the average 8-hour and 12-hour shift per 24-hour period in order to maintain the minimum nurse-to-client ratios?"

Nurses and lawmakers have been concerned about the quality of care to clients; however, some suggest a better solution would be staffing formulas rather than staffing ratios (Seago, 2002). The best solution to the current staffing problems is unclear.

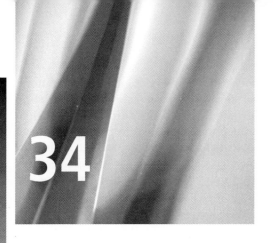

34

Legal and Ethical Issues

STUDY FOCUS

Nurses are becoming increasingly aware of the extensive legal and ethical aspects of nursing practice and nursing management. *Professional autonomy* indicates that the occupational group has control over its own practice. Individuals also have *autonomy* or the authority and accountability for their decisions and actions (Ballou, 1998). The American Nurses Association (1980), in *Nursing: A Social Policy Statement,* identifies the legal regulation of nursing practice by state licensure laws and professional regulation of nursing practice through standards and ethical codes as framing autonomy. As the level of professional autonomy and responsibility increases, so does the level of accountability and liability (Aiken, 1994). Nurses often supervise others in daily activities. *Supervision* entails accountability for assigning tasks based on skill level, monitoring the tasks, and evaluating that the assigned tasks were performed adequately.

The practice of nursing and management of nursing have many legal aspects. In addition to law in federal and state constitutions, U.S. law is composed of statutory, administrative, and common law. *Statutory law* is enacted by the U.S. Congress, state legislatures, and local government bodies. *Administrative law* is promulgated and adopted by federal or state agencies to implement statutory law adopted by Congress or state legislatures. *Common law* is the decisions of courts that set precedent in the jurisdiction of the court. The *two classes of wrongful acts* that can cause harm are (1) criminal and (2) civil acts. *Criminal acts* are activities that are offensive or harmful to society as a whole. *Civil acts* are wrongs that violate the rights of individuals by tort or by breach of contract. Those who are found guilty of crimes are fined or jailed, whereas those who commit civil wrongs often pay monetary damages. Nurse managers may be found legally liable and responsible for harm caused to others by civil wrongs. For nurses and nurse managers, the most common form of legal liability is a tort. A *tort* is a wrongful act,

other than a breach of contract, committed against another person or agency or their property causing harm and remedied by a civil lawsuit. Torts usually give rise to personal or direct liability for the person committing the wrongful act, but nurse managers or organizations can be held vicariously liable for an act they did not commit. The injured party is called the *plaintiff,* and the defense is put forth by the *defendant. Judicial risk* is the aspect of the litigation process that introduces uncertainty and additional cost into the determination of legal liability. The *three categories of torts* are negligence, intentional torts, and strict liability torts. *Negligence* is failing to exercise the proper care required by the situation. Proper care is what a reasonably prudent person would do in the situation to avoid harming others. A special type of negligence is malpractice. *Malpractice* is failing to act as other prudent professionals with a similar background, knowledge, and education would act under similar circumstances. *Ordinary negligence* is the degree of care an ordinary person would apply to a given situation. For example, if a nurse walked by a banana peel and did not pick it up and a client fell, the event would fall under ordinary negligence because no special professional knowledge was required in making the decision of whether to pick up the banana peel. *Intentional torts* are voluntary and willful activities engaged in to cause harm by interfering with another person's rights. Examples include assault and battery, medical battery (performing procedures without client consent), and false imprisonment. *Strict liability* is where the responsibility for certain accidents automatically rests with the defendant.

Contracts also may be a source of liability. Nurses most often work under an *employment-at-will doctrine* for which there are no written contracts specifying the terms of employment. Employers are free to terminate individuals with little notice but must follow guidelines, if published, in employee handbooks or manuals. *Contract-based legal liability* can occur from a (1) breach of contract or (2) an agreement to assume another party's liability. Breach of contract is the most common.

In this situation, one party in the contract fails to perform as promised. An agreement to assume another party's liability is less likely to be encountered by nurses, but an example is in leasing property: part of the agreement may be that if an injury occurs on the property, the individual leasing would assume legal responsibility for the injury.

Nurse managers have an obligation to comply with local, state, and national laws. Nurse managers must be aware of the law in three general areas: personal negligence in clinical practice, liability for delegation and supervision, and liability of health care organizations. Nurses have a duty of *nonmalfeasance* (to do no harm) to their clients. Harm may arise out of unintentional acts such as omission or intentional acts such as defamation or invasion of privacy. *For malpractice to occur, four elements of negligence must be present.* There must be a duty owed to the client, a breach of duty, proximate cause, and damages. A critical component in malpractice is the duty (standard) of care owed by the nursing profession to the client. The standard of care is the average skill and care level given by nurses under the same or similar circumstances (Aiken, 2004). Standards are published by the American Nurses Association, specialty nursing organizations, federal agencies (as guidelines), and agencies (as policies). Common clinical practice areas for which allegations of malpractice arise include treatment, communication, medication, and monitoring/observing/supervising/surveillance. Intentional torts require that the injured client (plantiff) prove that a voluntary and willful act by the nurse (defendant) was intended to interfere with the plaintiff's rights.

Nurses and nurse managers are also responsible for reporting incompetent practices in the delivery of client care. Employers have the job of providing a safe and secure health care environment. The *doctrine of respondent superior,* which means let the master answer, is important for employers because they can be held vicariously liable for negligent acts or omissions of employees. Employers often are named along with the nurse because of their ability to pay larger settlements or judgments. In addition, under the *doctrine of ostensible authority,* organizations may be held liable for negligence of an independent contractor. Nurse managers must know the skills of temporary workers and verify their competence. Managers must consider skills, knowledge, and competencies; awareness of facility policies and procedures; assignment of a preceptor or resource person. The *doctrine of corporate liability* makes the organization legally responsible to ensure a competent practitioner delivers quality of care to clients (Guido, 2001). The spectrum of legal and ethical consideration of nursing management includes the client, provider, and employer rights and obligations. Nurses and health care agencies have legal and ethical obligations to clients through the Patient Self-Determination Act of 1990 to provide informed consent. Nurse managers must take steps to avoid legal liability. One step is to become knowledgeable about the most common errors related to malpractice and legal liability and to provide this information to staff. Reading books, attending conferences, and reading journal articles are good ways to get helpful information on legal liability. Even with knowledge and good clinical practice, it may not be possible to avoid litigation. *Judicial risk* is an aspect of legal liability that is not based solely on the merits of the case or the rules of law applicable to the case. For example, even if a case is not strong, there may be costs for legal fees and procedures or a potential settlement. Cooper (2006) recommends that nurses and nurse managers protect themselves by carrying adequate professional liability insurance. Rationales for purchasing malpractice insurance would be to provide coverage for volunteer or advice when "off duty," coverage if the employer sues the nurse if the nurse is found guilty of malpractice (employer may try to recoup costs), and coverage for personal injuries from libel, slander, or assault.

Ethical issues often arise from the distribution of scarce resources. Ethical dilemmas are decisions that are made about right and wrong when an individual has to make a choice between equally unfavorable alternatives. There may be a clash between ethical duties to clients, between the client's rights and benefits, between duties to self and duties to clients, and between professional ethical provisions and religious ones. There are several important terms in ethical decision making. The four cornerstone principles of biomedical ethical decision making are (1) autonomy, (2) beneficence, (3) nonmaleficence, and (4) justice. *Autonomy* is the client's right of self-determination and freedom of decision making. *Beneficence* is doing good for clients and providing benefit balanced against risk. *Nonmaleficence* is doing no harm to clients. *Justice* is being fair to all and giving equal treatment, including equally distributing benefits, risks, and costs (Aiken, 2004; Beauchamp & Childress, 1994; Guido, 2001). Rules for biomedical ethics that are related to the four fundamental principles include fidelity, veracity, confidentiality, and privacy. *Fidelity* is being loyal and faithful to commitments and accountable for responsibility. *Veracity* is telling the truth and not intentionally deceiving clients. *Confidentiality* prohibits disclosure of information to third parties without the consent of the original source. *Privacy* is the right to limited physical or informational inaccessibility (Aiken, 2004; Beauchamp & Childress, 1994; Guido, 2001).

The *Code of Ethics for Nurses: With Interpretive Statements* from the American Nurses Association (2001) provides standards and ethical obligations and duties of nurses.

Several ethical decision-making models are used to solve problems. Common elements of most ethical decision-making models include a six-step problem-solving model. The six steps in ethical decision making are (1) define the problem, (2) develop alternative courses of action, (3) evaluate each alternative course of action, (4) select the best course of action, (5) implement the selected course of action, and (6) monitor the results.

At times a clash between the professional caregiver and organizational financial goals occurs. Other conflicts include disappointment with the quality of care, staffing issues, and concerns about closings or layoffs. Nurses are urged to become active in ethical discussions and venues (ethical activism). They are encouraged to become ethically assertive by participating in ethical decisions and discussions even when not invited. Berger and colleagues (1991) reported that the most frequent ethical issues encountered by registered nurses were inadequate staffing, inadequate life support measures, inappropriate resource allocation, inappropriate discussion of clients, and irresponsible actions by co-workers. Inadequate staffing was the most frequently reported ethical problem. Nurses constantly juggle ethical conflicts because of competing pressures from co-workers, clients, and the organization.

LEARNING TOOLS

Group Activity: Discussing Moral Issues in Nursing

Purpose

To gain a clear understanding of the ethical aspects of problem solving and to use an ethical decision-making model in problem resolution.

Directions

1. Discuss the ethical issues that affect nurses who work on the units to which you are assigned.

2. Identify one ethical dilemma that the group would like to solve.

3. Use the MORAL model described by Crisham (1985) or the general six-step problem-solving model for ethical decision making (Aiken, 2004; Guido, 2001) to guide your discussions.

MORAL Model

1. Massage the dilemma and define the conflicts and interests.

2. Outline the potential options.

3. Review criteria for problem resolution, and resolve the dilemma.

4. Affirm a position and act on the judgment.

5. Look back to evaluate the effectiveness of the decision.

General Six-Step Problem-Solving Model for Ethical Decision Making

1. Define the problem.

2. Develop alternative courses of action.

3. Evaluate each alternative course of action.

4. Select the best course of action.

5. Implement the selected course of action.

6. Monitor the results.

Group Activity: Identifying Current Ethical Issues

Purpose

To identify current ethical issues in nursing management and nursing practice settings.

Directions

1. Each individual selects one nurse manager and one registered nurse to interview.

2. Ask each of the selected individuals the following question:

   What are the most pressing and difficult ethical issues you face in your work?

3. The group should meet at a set time and place and review the answers from the participants using the following questions as guidelines:

   • What were the common ethical issues encountered by the managers and by the registered nurses?

   • Were there any differences in the ethical issues between the two groups?

   • How might you respond when faced with similar ethical issues?

CASE STUDY

Jo Ellen McGee is a registered nurse on a 45-bed orthopedic unit in a community hospital. She works the 3-to-11 PM shift as a full-time employee. Nurse McGee is 32 years old and has three small children ages 2, 4, and 7.

She elects the 3-11 shift so that the children do not have to be in day care. Her husband is an electrical engineer and is able to get home at 4 PM, and Nurse McGee's mother watches the children for $1\frac{1}{2}$ hours during the week. For the past 6 months the community hospital administration has enacted mandatory overtime for nurses because of a nurse shortage. Nurse McGee has been working approximately two to three mandatory shifts per week. She is upset with working so much overtime, and it is beginning to affect her family. She is so tired all the time and tries to nap while the children play during the day.

Case Study Questions

1. What options does Nurse McGee have in relation to working the mandatory overtime?

2. What ethical decision-making concepts are important in Nurse McGee's predicament of mandatory overtime?

3. Use the MORAL model to solve Nurse McGee's ethical dilemma.

LEARNING RESOURCES

Discussion Questions

1. What are ethical problems that have emerged around managed care organizations?

2. What are examples of reportable occurrences that registered nurses must manage?

3. What are the four types of laws that must be dealt with to handle human resource decisions properly?

4. What is the registered nurse's role in supervision and delegation of activities?

5. What is the doctrine of respondent superior?

6. What are the six steps in the general ethical decision-making model? Identify an ethical dilemma in health care delivery, and use this model to reach a decision strategy.

Study Questions

True or False: Circle the correct answer.

T   F   1. As professional autonomy and responsibility increases, the level of accountability and liability decreases.

T   F   2. Administrative law includes those regulations promulgated and adopted by federal or state agencies to implement statutory law adopted by Congress or state legislatures.

T   F   3. *Nursing: A Social Policy Statement* is a mandate for standards of conduct of nurses.

T   F   4. Physicians govern the legal practice of nurses.

T   F   5. When there is conflict between federal and state statutes, the federal statute will usually, but not always, take precedence.

T   F   6. Beneficence means doing no harm to clients.

Matching: Write the letter of the correct response in front of each term.

_____ 7. Autonomy

_____ 8. Fidelity

_____ 9. Values

_____ 10. Veracity

_____ 11. Nonmal-feasance

_____ 12. Justice

A. Norm of telling the truth; not intentionally deceiving

B. Clients' right to self-determination and freedom of decision making

C. Strongly held beliefs that are thought to be freely chosen

D. Doing no harm to clients

E. Being loyal and faithful to commitments and accountable for responsibilities

F. Norm of being fair to all and giving equal treatment

References

Aiken, T. (1994). *Legal, ethical and political issues in nursing.* Philadelphia: F.A. Davis.

Aiken, T. D. (2004). *Legal, ethical and political issues in nursing* (2nd ed.). Philadelphia: F.A. Davis.

American Nurses Association. (1980). *Nursing: A social policy statement.* Kansas City, MO: Author.

American Nurses Association. (2001). *Code of ethics for nurses: With interpretive statements.* Washington, DC: Author. Retrieved November 28, 2004. from *www.nursingworld.org/ethics/code/ethicscode150htm*

Ballou, K. A. (1998). A concept analysis of autonomy. *Journal of Professional Nursing, 14*(2), 102-110.

Beauchamp, T., & Childress, J. (1994). *Principles of biomedical ethics* (4th ed.). New York: Oxford University Press.

Berger, M., Seversen, A., & Chvatal, R. (1991). Ethical issues in nursing. *Western Journal of Nursing Research, 13*(4), 514-521.

Cooper, R. (2006). Legal and ethical issues. In Huber, D. (Ed.), *Leadership and nursing care management* (3rd ed). Philadelphia: Saunders.

Crisham, P. (1985). Resolving ethical and moral dilemmas of nursing interventions. In M. Snyder (Ed.), *Independent nursing interventions* (pp. 25-43). New York: John Wiley & Sons.

Guido, G. W. (2001). *Legal and ethical issues in nursing* (3rd ed.). Upper Saddle River, NJ: Prentice-Hall.

Supplemental Readings

Crigger, N. J. (2004). Always having to say you're sorry: An ethical response to making mistakes in professional practice. *Nursing Ethics, 11*(6), 568-576.

Evans, M., Bergum, V., Bamforth, S., & MacPhail, S. (2004). Relational ethics and genetic counseling. *Nursing Ethics, 11*(5), 459-471.

Haegert, S. (2004). The ethics of self. *Nursing Ethics, 11*(5), 434-443.

Liang, B. A., & Coulson, K. M. (2002). Legal issues in performing patient safety work. *Nursing Economic$, 20*(3), 118-125.

Slettebo, A., & Bunch, E. H. (2004). Solving ethically difficult care situations in nursing homes. *Nursing Ethics, 11*(6), 543-552.

Summers, J., & Nowicki, M. (2004). System failures and ethical issues for rehabilitation nurses. *Rehabilitation Nursing, 29*(2), 42-44, 61.

Chapter 34: Legal and Ethical Issues (pp. 733-754)

1. **What governs the practice of nursing?**

Nurse practice acts and professional regulation govern the practice of nursing. Nurse practice acts from each state govern the legal practice of nursing, including delegation and supervision, whereas professional standards and ethical codes regulate nursing practice. Licensure assures the public that individuals are properly prepared and competent to deliver nursing services.

2. **Why do nurses and nurse managers need to understand how legal liability relates to their clinical practice activities and their responsibilities in delegating and supervising?**

Nurses and nurse managers are responsible for the supervision of others, who are often unlicensed assistive personnel. Supervision includes monitoring the tasks performed, ensuring that functions are performed in an appropriate fashion, and ensuring that assigned tasks and functions do not exceed competency or require a license to perform. Nurses and nurse managers are accountable for their own acts and decisions, as well as delegated acts. Nurse and nurse managers are subject to malpractice lawsuits.

3. **What are the various grounds on which nurses, nurse managers, and health care organizations can be found legally liable for injuries to others?**

Nurses and nurse managers are legally liable for injuries to others resulting in malpractice in clinical practice and negligence in delegation and supervision of care. Health care organizations are legally liable for the actions of their employees, negligence of independent contractors, corporate negligence arising out of the facility's responsibilities to hire qualified employees and monitor and supervise their activities, and failure to comply with numerous laws and regulations.

4. **What actions can nurse managers take in an effort to protect against legal liability?**

Many prevention activities are available to help protect against legal liability such as facility guidelines, adequate orientation of staff members, and generally, anticipating the most common problems related to malpractice and developing a plan to prevent them.

5. **What resources are available to nurses and nurse managers for dealing with ethical dilemmas encountered in clinical practice?**

Nurses and nurse managers apply the concepts of autonomy, beneficence, nonmaleficence, and justice when making biomedical ethical decisions. Other resources for nurses and nurse managers include the American Nurses Association Code of Ethics for Nurses (2001) in addition to the nurse's personal moral values and standards, professional publications on ethics, and discussion of ethical issues with other professionals. Some institutions have ethics committees, which help guide ethical decisions.

6. **How do the ethical dilemmas encountered as a result of the clash between clinical and organizational ethics differ from those encountered in clinical practice?**

Ethical dilemmas as a result of differences between clinical and organizational ethics may be due to organizational budget cuts. Examples such as refusing to purchase equipment or provide support services on off-shifts are related to financial constraints. Others include the lack of time for teaching, which may not be available to staff nurses because of staffing practices. Other instances may be politically driven. Nurses may be told that there is no additional money for nursing care needs while the hospital takes over a space occupied by nursing services offices to renovate for a new physicians' lounge and private dining room. Ethical dilemmas related to clinical practice are more client-driven such as the client's right to die.

7. **What responsibilities do nurse managers have to prepare themselves and those reporting to them for dealing effectively with ethical dilemmas?**

Nurse managers have a responsibility to prepare themselves and those reporting to them to deal effectively with not only the yet unresolved issues of clinical ethics, such as full disclosure and end-of-life care, but also the many unresolved dilemmas arising from the ongoing conflict between clinical and organizational ethics. Nurse managers can help develop an organizational culture of respecting each other's ethical standards and not asking nurses to compromise their ethics. Nurse managers also can provide clear communication of appropriate ethical behavior.

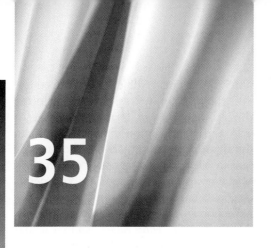

35

Financial Management

Health care services are costly, and pressures to control spiraling costs are growing. Nurses must increase their knowledge and become sophisticated in financial management. Nurses need to be able to develop and justify budgets, use computerized information systems and technology, and use staff and supplies judiciously. The target of financial management is to allocate scarce resources efficiently and effectively. *Financial management* is a set of activities involving the allocation of resources to complete organizational objectives and ensure viability. *Four phases of financial management* are budgeting, recording, reporting, and evaluating. The goal of financial management is to meet the financial needs of the organization. To maximize the use of limited resources, organizations engage in planning. *Operational plans* are those activities determined necessary for meeting day-to-day organizational goals. Strategy formulation or *strategic planning* is important in organizations. *Strategic management* is more long term and entails analyzing and projecting future organizational goals. A budget puts planning into financial terms and provides direction for managers. A *budget* is a written plan of revenues and expenditures. *Expenses* are those costs incurred to meet organizational goals. *Revenues* are payments made by clients and insurance companies for services rendered or an amount still owed for a service that was provided. *Profits* occur when revenues exceed costs of labor, materials, and overhead expenses.

Financial management of any organization occurs in the context of the broader community. The *key factors to assess in communities* are the major employers, provider groups, and health care facilities in the area. A population-based approach to planning health care services is essential. *Other factors important in financial management* include the structure of the health care organization, economic principles, and accounting and finance. *Economics* is based on principles related to the finite and limited nature of resources coupled with

competing needs. The *two major financial statements* are (1) the balance sheet and (2) the statement of revenues and expenses for a nonprofit organization or an income statement of profits and loss for a for-profit organization. *Balance sheets* are a single page following a standard form that has line items with dollar amounts and gives a snapshot of the financial health of the organization on a given date. The *revenue and expense report* is a summary financial report showing activity over a specified period. *The two types of accounting* are managerial and financial. *Managerial accounting* is the generation and evaluation of financial information needed to manage the organization. *Financial accounting* is providing information to external sources for investments, money lending, or control. *Cost accounting* or *cost analysis* is measuring and reporting costs. A *unit of service* is the basic measure of the product or service being produced. *Costs* may be *fixed* where they do not change as the volume changes, *variable* where they vary directly with volume changes, or *marginal* where there is extra cost of one more unit of service.

There are many health care financial strategies to use scarce resources judiciously. Key concepts include utility, marginal cost, supply and demand, market efficiency, and redistribution of resources (Finkler & Kovner, 2000). Finance, focusing on a several-year period, and accounting, focusing on a one-year period, are important financial components. The fundamentals of financial management include understanding the balance sheet and operating statement, assets, equities, revenues, and expenses and recording and reporting processes and fund accounting. The core of organizational financial efforts are in planning and controlling resources through strategic planning, budgeting, and control of operating results. The elements of health care finance include taxes, philanthropy, operating finances, and capital financing. Strategies to avoid further escalation of overall health care costs include cost containment, avoidance, and reduction strategies. Problems faced in health care organizations include cash shortages, overstaffing, poor use of present staff, low productivity, and equipment breakdown. Research has shown that the reliability of service is the most important factor in judging service quality. Organizations depend on trust and credibility of the services to maintain customer loyalty and survive.

Cost-effectiveness analysis can be used as a tool to evaluate the cost impact of new models of care. Nurse managers are assuming more accountability for financial management on the work units. As consolidation and elimination of managers occur, individual nurses assume more responsibility and accountability. Decentralization is one strategy to empower and to motivate employees to increase accountability and productivity. A *cost center* is the smallest functional unit that generates revenues and expenses. Administration is one cost center that does not generate revenues. A *charge* is the price asked for services provided. *Cost* is the actual amount of money to cover direct production of expenses associated with the provision of the service. A *profit* is the money earned in excess of the charges over costs for providing a service.

Nursing service costs in the 1980s were 25% to 35% of the total budget. Because of the large size of nursing services in health care organizations and the view that nursing services are costs rather than revenue streams, nursing services often are targeted when cuts are made. Nurses must design new approaches to capturing revenues and demonstrating nursing contributions. Although administration costs have been estimated at 22.9% to 34% of the total budget, they have not faced the same scrutiny as nursing when cost cuts are made. Nurses need to identify services for which physicians are reimbursed and for which nurses actually complete the work (Ott et al., 1989) and methods of capturing revenue and communicating this information.

The nurse manager's role in financial management includes determining resource requirements, justifying resources, evaluating technology, and holding down expenses. The staff nurse's role in financial management includes contributing data and rationale for resource needs, practicing cost awareness in nursing care delivery, and understanding the basic techniques of financial management. In all organizations, there will be competing demands for scarce resources.

Conflicts and ethical dilemmas over competing demands for finite resources will abound. Examples of scarce resources in organizations include money, personnel, space, and time. Ethical obligations of *fidelity,* an obligation to act in good faith, and to uphold trust and confidence can create conflicts for the nurse with the client, physician, and organizational needs competing for the nurse's loyalty. *Professional fidelity or loyalty* is upholding the clients' interests as a priority. This also is called *advocacy* for clients. Nurses have the ethical obligation of stewardship to oversee and allocate scarce resources. *Stewardship* is the balancing of clients' needs and organization financial survival. Potential ethical problems that nurses may face include rationing care to clients, avoiding costly outliers and unprofitable clients to maximize revenue, and determining what clients receive scarce resources. *Aspects of an ethical practice environment* include autonomy, trust, and communication. *Three values that were drivers of sustainable success* are (1) control of destiny, (2) trust-based relationships, and (3) investment in employee success (Berry, 1999). Great service companies build a humane, ethical, and value-driven community.

LEARNING TOOLS

Group Activity

Purpose

To examine and use financial management principles in the initial stages of developing a nurse-based business.

Directions

1. Work as a group to determine the key components of financial management when initiating a business.

2. After group members determine the *business* and *services* that will be the *core* of the organization, use financial management principles to determine whether the services will be used in the community. Use a population-based assessment to determine community needs.

3. Use the four phases of financial management to assist in organizing and planning for the furture of your company:

    - Determine for each service provided the actual cost of producing the service, the charge you will collect, and the profit that will be generated.

    - Determine the likely volume, and then multiply it by the charge to determine revenues.

    - Deduct all expenses: personnel, materials, overhead, and uncollectible amounts for services to determine potential viability.

    - Do not forget to include the amount of start-up costs that will be needed to cover the period of time before revenues are generated.

4. Once the group has worked through financial management of a new business venture, discuss the following questions:

    - What are the similarities and differences in costs for a new business versus an existing business?

    - How can strong financial management assist in maintaining the viability of an organization?

- What factors are important in financial management?
- What are businesses that nurses could initiate and own that would be profitable and serve community needs?
- Which websites provide data that can assist with financial management?

CASE STUDY

Holly Meriweather, a nurse director of inpatient and outpatient medical-surgical services and the emergency room in a large teaching hospital in Santa Fe, New Mexico, has reviewed financial documents and is aware of a potential deficit in revenues in the emergency room cost center. Factors contributing to the projected deficit are an increase in uncompensated visits in the emergency room, increased turnover of registered nurses, and a relatively flat payment schedule from third-party payers on nonurgent client visits. The volume in the emergency room has increased for nonurgent visits by 12%. Uncompensated visits account for the majority of this increase. Nurse Meriweather must make recommendations to the vice president of nursing to prevent the emergency room costs from getting out of control. She identifies the following three potential options:

1. Hire nurse practitioners to staff a "fast track" for nonurgent clients.
2. Partner with a free-standing urgent care center to refer nonurgent clients to their facility.
3. Institute a cost-cutting program in the emergency room.

Case Study Questions

1. What is the problem in this case study?
2. What financial management strategies could Nurse Meriweather implement?
3. What are other options that Nurse Meriweather might consider implementing in the emergency room?
4. What strategies would be useful to motivate staff to assist in implementing a potential solution?
5. Should financial data be shared with emergency room staff to assist in understanding the situation?

LEARNING RESOURCES

Discussion Questions

1. What is the role of the nurse manager and staff nurse in financial management?
2. Are the terms *budgeting* and *financial management* interchangeable? Why or why not?

3. What are the phases of financial management? What is included in each phase of financial management?
4. What are the types of accounting? Provide a definition and example for each.
5. What are scarce resources in organizations?

Study Questions

Matching: Write the letter of the correct response in front of each term.

_____ 1. Profit

_____ 2. Cost

_____ 3. Charge

_____ 4. Financial accounting

_____ 5. Managerial accounting

_____ 6. Unit of service

_____ 7. Cost center

_____ 8. Cost-effectiveness analysis

_____ 9. Strategic planning

_____ 10. Financial management

A. The smallest functional unit that generates revenues and expenses

B. The price asked for services or goods

C. The actual amount of money required as payment to cover direct production inputs used in producing the services

D. Money gained as excess of charges over outlay costs in producing a service

E. Focused on the generation and evaluation of financial information needed by managers to manage the organization

F. Targeted to provide information to external sources of investments, money lending, or control

G. Focused on cost measurement and reporting

H. The basic measure of the product or service being produced

I. A series of activities designed to allocate resources and plan for the efficient operation of an organization

J. Process of assessing the organization and its departments

251

True or False: Circle the correct answer.

T   F   11. The managerial process of planning is linked closely with financial management.

T   F   12. Costs may be fixed, variable, or marginal.

T   F   13. Administration in nonprofit hospitals is the largest cost item in the organization.

T   F   14. Professional fidelity or loyalty is upholding the clients' interests as a priority in care provision.

REFERENCES

Berry, L. L. (1999). *Discovering the soul of services: The nine drivers of sustainable business success.* New York: The Free Press.

Finkler, S. A., & Kovner, C. T. (2000). *Financial management for nurse managers and executives* (2nd ed.). Philadelphia: Saunders.

Ott, B., Griffith, H., & Towers, J. (1989). Who gets the money? *American Journal of Nursing, 89*(2), 186-188.

SUPPLEMENTAL READINGS

Geer, R., & Smith, J. (2004). Strategies to take hospitals off (revenue) diversion. *Healthcare Financial Management, 58*(3), 70-74.

Krugman, M., MacLauchlan, M. Riippi, L., & Grubbs, J. (2002). A multidisciplinary financial education research project. *Nursing Economic$, 20*(6), 273-278.

Leeth, L. (2004). Are you fiscally fit? *Nursing Management, 35*(4), 42-48.

McIntosh, E., Nagelkerk, J., Vonderheid, S. C., Poole, M., Dontje, K., & Pohl, J. (2003). Financially viable nurse-managed centers, *The Nurse Practitioner, 28*(3), 40, 46-48, 51.

Vonderheid, S. C., Pohl, J., Barkauskas, V., Gift, D., & Huges-Cromwick, P. (2003). Financial performance of academic nurse managed primary care centers. *Nursing Economic$, 21,* 167-175.

Chapter 35: Financial Management (pp. 755-777)

1. **How does financial management relate to leadership? To management and control?**

   Financial management is a series of activities designed to meet the economic needs of the organization. Visionary leadership is needed to incorporate financial data into a budget, to develop a strategic plan to manage scarce resources, and to control organizational costs.

2. **How much effort should nurses place on financial management activities?**

   The role of nurses in financial management has expanded over the years. As such, nurses play an integral role in the determination and justification of resources, the evaluation of technology, and the implementation of cost-containment strategies. Staff nurse awareness of the "financial health" of the institution and effort into practicing judicious financial management will reduce monetary losses so that cost savings may be allocated to care delivery and service quality.

3. **What strategies can nurses use to influence financial decision making?**

   Nurses can use their clinical knowledge and expertise to influence financial decision-making. As coordinators of care, nurses can minimize the duplication of services and reduce wasted health care resources. Nurses who are knowledgeable about the financial management process can use innovative strategies to design care delivery systems that enhance productivity, cost-effectiveness, and customer satisfaction.

4. **How can nurses gauge the financial effectiveness of their practice?**

   Nurses can gauge the financial effectiveness of their practice by using measurable outcomes. As nurses begin to identify the cost of their services, the positive outcomes of their care, and the resultant cost savings, they will be able to demonstrate financial effectiveness.

5. **In what ways can nurses address legal or ethical issues arising in financial management?**

   Nurses can address legal or ethical issues associated with financial management by advocating for quality health care and client safety, by upholding professional practice standards, and by following organizational policies and procedures. This process will be facilitated in organizations that foster autonomy, trust, and communication among their employees.

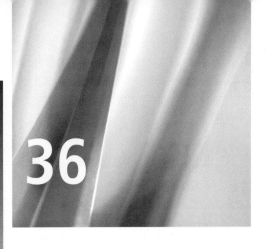

36 Budgeting

STUDY FOCUS

Budgeting and financial management are crucial skills for nurses. In health care, resources are scarce, reimbursement structures have changed, and organizations are seeking methods to cut costs. How then can a nurse manager justify expenses, garner new resources, and compete with other health care managers for limited dollars? A strong foundation in financial management is essential.

The first phase of the financial management process is budgeting. *Budgeting* is a major aspect of the planning process of an organization. A budget is a detailed plan in dollar amounts. A *budget* is the projected plan for revenues and expenses for a specified period. *Expenses* are the cost of activities undertaken in the operations of an organization. *Revenue* is the income generated for services provided, and expenses are the cost of producing the services. *Total operating expenses* is the total cost of all resources to produce services. *Income* is revenue over expenses. A *variance* is a difference between budgeted and actual amounts. A budget is a written financial plan aimed at controlling the allocation of resources in organizations. The budget is a key aspect of the planning process that identifies funds necessary for implementing programs and services. Budgeting is a component of cost accounting, is essential for providing a road map, and is a guide to assist individuals in successfully meeting goals.

There are seven general types of budgets (Finkler & Kovner, 2000). The *operating budget* is the plan for the daily operating revenue and expenses for a specified unit or organization for a designated period. *Elements included in the operational budget* are a workload budget with activity reports, units of service, and workload calculations; expense budgets for personnel, staffing requirements, and labor costs; expense budgets for supplies, equipment, and overhead; and a revenue budget. A *long-range budget* is a strategic plan that establishes goals over long periods, often 3, 5, and 10 years. A *program budget* evaluates a specific program that

often involves more than one department over a period of several years. A *capital budget* tracks the purchase of large assets such as buildings, land, or large costly pieces of equipment. In many organizations, a capital purchase is any item greater than $500. A *product-line budget* is the revenues and expenses associated with a defined group of clients. A *cash budget* logs the cash receipts and disbursements on a monthly basis. A *special purpose budget* is developed for programs or services that were not included in the annual budget.

Familiarity with the two basic types of budgets will assist nurse managers when interacting with financial personnel. *Traditional budgets* are based on expenses for the previous year with an inflation factor added. *Zero-based budgets* require the manager to rebuild the budget each year and to justify all line items. For nurses, capital and operating budgets are related directly to service delivery. The *operating budget* covers the fiscal year and is the plan for day-to-day service operations. Nurse managers are responsible for preparing three aspects of the operating budget: (1) expense budget for personnel, (2) expense budget for costs other than personnel, and (3) revenue budget. The first step in developing the expense budget is forecasting the volume of work for the coming year. The work often is measured in units of service. Calculation of staffing, which is a complex process, must be done to determine expenses. To determine staffing, calculate the average daily census and occupancy (or utilization); determine the number of full-time employees by type and shift; adjust for benefits and downtime (productive versus nonproductive hours); calculate the staff mix, add administrative and other fixed staff; and add in straight versus overtime, differentials, premiums, and fringe benefits (Finkler & Kovner, 2000).

The basics of budgeting include understanding the two major types of budgets: (1) capital and (2) operating. A *capital budget* is planning and identifying major investments for the organizations, which includes large equipment, long-term investments, and physical plant or program expenditures. The operating budget is the

255

more detailed budget a nurse manager will be managing. The *operating budget* is the day-to-day budget that the nurse manager will monitor and make appropriate supply purchasing and staffing adjustments. Managers also track direct and indirect expenses. *Direct costs* are those items that result in providing physical care to the client. *Indirect costs* include overhead and supportive and administrative expenses. Nurse managers also measure the intensity of care by examining the amount, type, and cost of nursing care for client groups.

The budgetary process involves four phases: disseminating instructions, preparing the first budget draft, reviewing and adjusting, and appealing. The two key components of budgeting are (1) volume and (2) cost measures. Volume measures are activity standards based on a workload measure for the organization. The cost measure is commonly a salary standard. *Two major issues of indirect and overhead costs* are accuracy and control. *Accuracy* is assigning specific costs to the correct departments, whereas *control* refers to the nurse managers autonomy to make appropriate supply purchases and staffing levels while being held responsible for cost control goals.

Three phases of the budgeting process are (1) establishing the basis for budget preparation, (2) preparing the first draft, and (3) reviewing and rebudgeting (Finkler & Kovner, 2000). Multiple financial forms can be used for displaying and tracking financial data such as cash budget, general expenses (operating) budget, labor or personnel budget, and capital equipment budget. Two key components for budgeting are (1) a volume measure and (2) a cost measure. Some of the largest expenses in health care organization budgets are nursing personnel and supply usage. The large size of nursing departments puts nurses at risk for layoffs and downsizing. Nurses will be called on to contain costs and provide high-quality health care. In the twenty-first century, the two major themes for nursing practice are (1) cost and (2) quality. *Suggestions for nurses that promote cost control* include doing a job efficiently, motivating clients to recover, using supplies carefully, and maximizing the use of time. Nurse managers may use internal and external benchmarking as a mechanism to evaluate their budgeting and staffing. Nurse managers also may cost out nursing services to determine the actual "cost" of care provided by client type. Nurses must be able to identify and charge for services provided instead of being invisible in hospital charges. Other issues and trends include developing business plans and costing out nursing services.

LEARNING TOOLS

Reporting Exercise

Purpose

To identify the important categories of a monthly manager's report and to identify important data for each category.

Introduction

Nurse managers have 24-hour accountability for the staffing, management, and leadership of their assigned unit(s). They are fiscally responsible and must manage their resources to stay within budget or within the adjusted budget based on client days, adjustments in condition severity, and length of stay. Most managers are held accountable in four major categories: financial, material, human, and unit goals. The financial data category reflects the actual versus budgeted expenses for each line item (such as equipment, supplies, and salaries). Positive and negative variances are reported and justified. The material data category reports changes in products or supplies, any equipment trials or examinations, and any changes in procedures for the unit(s). The human resource category reflects any concerns, issues, accomplishments, and critical incidents as well as any unit news or individual education, or professional achievement. The last column is for unit goals established by the nurse manager and reported monthly and annually. These goals may include budget variance predictions, staffing issues, or procedural changes.

The following is a form that could be used to report monthly data:

Monthly Report

I. *Financial indicators:* List any variances for line items and provide rationale for the positive or negative variance.

II. *Material issues:* Describe any changes in materials or supplies, any equipment trials, or any changes in procedures requiring changes in materials.

III. *Human relations:* Describe any concerns, critical incidents, issues, accomplishments, or personal and professional achievements.

IV. *Unit goals:* Describe accomplishments toward your established unit goals and provide data on your progress.

Directions

Use the data in the following case study to complete the monthly report.

CASE STUDY

Susan Brinion is the nurse manager for a 46-bed general surgical unit in Palm Harbor, Florida. She has just received her revenue and expense report for the month. Nurse Brinion has been speaking with the chief financial officer about the possibility of receiving biweekly revenue and expense reports because she feels that problems cannot be corrected quickly with such a delay in reporting. In response, the chief financial officer is working out the mechanics to issue reports every 2 weeks to help managers react more quickly to fiscal issues. (See the following revenue and expense report.)

Nurse Brinion also is testing new syringes on her unit, and Cam Smith, a registered nurse on 7-3, has streamlined the procedure for collecting and sending specimens to the laboratory. She has been tracking the critical incidents of the unit and discovers three medication errors for the same nurse within a 2-week period. Sally Simons, a registered nurse on 3-11 has just completed an RN-BSN program, and Ron Gerber, a registered nurse, has just passed a certification examination. Nurse Brinion's unit goals were to stay within 2% of budget; to assist nurses to continue their education through certification, continuing education, or formal education; and to analyze the activities that could be completed by nursing assistants to decrease their down time.

Cost Center: 611 General Surgery **Report For June 2000**

This Month			Account	Year to Date		
Actual	Budget	Variance	Number/Description	Actual	Budget	Variance
			311. Revenue			
(371,026)	(365,800)	5,226	0110 Routine	(3,244,410)	(3,221,400)	23,010
(2,987)	(3,153)	(166)	020 Other	(27,590)	(27,768)	(178)
(374,013)	(368,953)	5,060	Total Operating Rev	(3,272,000)	(3,249,168)	22,832
			411. Salary Expense			
85,115	85,127	12	010 Salaries-Regular	730,881	749,665	18,784
2,758	0	(2,758)	020 Salaries-Per Diem	2,758	0	(2,758)
3,209	4,101	892	030 Salaries-Overtime	40,128	36,115	(4,013)
10,885	11,220	335	040 Salaries Differential	97,995	98,810	815
7,168	7,066	(102)	050 FICA	61,285	62,222	937
7,235	7,363	128	060 Health Insurance	62,125	64,846	2,721
2,212	2,358	146	070 Pension	19,855	20,766	911
1,896	1,915	19	080 Other	17,228	16,868	(360)
120,478	119,150	(1,328)	Total Salary Expense	1,032,255	1,049,292	17,037
			611. Supply Expense			
4,976	4,084	(892)	010 Patient Care Supplies	41,692	35,961	(5,731)
118	202	84	020 Office Supplies	1,097	1,780	683
371	366	(5)	030 Forms	3,111	3,224	113
0	127	127	040 Supplies Purchased	1,210	1,122	(88)
250	191	(59)	050 Equipment	1,553	1,683	130
125	149	24	060 Seminars/Meetings	1,163	1,309	146
25	17	(8)	070 Books	145	150	5
0	112	112	080 Equipment Rental	385	987	602
31	64	33	090 Miscellaneous	388	561	173
5,896	5,312	(584)	Total Supply Expense	50,744	46,777	(3,967)
			911. Interdepartmental Expense			
934	921	(13)	010 Central Supply	7,828	8,114	286
1,137	1,121	(16)	020 Pharmacy	9,527	9,868	341
1,915	1,888	(27)	030 Linen/Laundry	16,046	16,628	582
105	297	192	040 Maintenance	977	2,618	1,641
211	212	1	060 Telephone	1,962	1,870	(92)
0	21	21	070 Photocopy	124	187	63
0	13	13	090 Miscellaneous	165	112	(53)
4,302	4,473	171	Total Interdepartmental Expense	36,629	39,397	2,768
130,676	128,935	(1,741)	Total Operating Expense	1,119,628	1,135,466	15,838
(243,337)	(240,018)	3,319	Contributions from Operations	(2,152,372)	(2,113,702)	38,670
65.1%	65.1%		Contributions % of Revenue	65.8%	65.1%	

Budgeting Exercise*

Introduction

A basic understanding of budgeting and financial management is important for a clinical nurse. This section will provide definitions of terms, simple calculations, and answers to the calculations.

I. A unit of service is a measurement that describes an activity in an organization. The units of service are what determine the revenue or income of the organization and describe the needed resources to offer the service.

The following definitions are basic to budgeting and financial calculations:

Beds = number of beds available for occupancy

Census = number of clients occupying beds at a specific time of day (usually midnight)

Percent occupancy = census divided by beds available × 100

Client day = one client occupying one bed for 1 day

Average daily census = client days in a given period divided by the number of days in the period

Average length of stay = client days in a given period divided by number of discharges in the period

II. How do client classification systems work? Classification systems are based on instruments that reflect critical indicators of care requirements. Based on the absence or presence of indicators, clients are assigned a score. The following is a printout of a classification.

Required Care Hours in 24 Hours

Client Type	Range	Average	Relative Value
1	0.5-2.9	2.0	0.4
2	3.0-6.9	5.0	1.0
3	7.0-15.4	10.0	2.0
4	15.5-24.0	22.0	4.4

In this example, the client type is simply a descriptor of the classification categories. A type 1 client has the least workload requirements and a type 4 the most. The range indicates the amount of care required, and the average is the assigned value of care for all type 1 clients. The relative value scale puts the hours of care required for each type of client in a workload measure. type 2 clients are arbitrarily assigned a workload value of 1.0 taking 5 hours of care on average; and type 3 therefore are assigned a double workload factor because of the 10 average hours of care required.

III. How are condition severity levels calculated? The following list is a census of 18 clients with client types identified. The calculation for condition severity level is workload divided by census equals condition severity ($24.0 \div 18 = 1.33$).

Client Type	Number of Clients	Relative Value	Workload
1	4	0.4	1.6
2	8	1.0	8.0
3	5	2.0	10.0
4	1	4.4	4.4
TOTAL	18	-	24.0

What would the average condition severity level be for this population? The calculation for average condition severity is workload divided by census equals condition severity ($120.0 \div 18 = 6.67$).

Client Type	Required Average in 24 Hours	Number of Clients	Workload
1	2.0	4	8.0
2	5.0	8	40.0
3	10.0	5	50.0
4	22.0	1	22.0
TOTAL	-	18	120.0

Employers frequently discuss the terms FTEs (full-time equivalent employees) and positions or position control. These are common terms used to discuss the personnel needs of a unit or an organization. Most organizations hire at least 60% to 80% of their workforce with full-time equivalent employees. A full-time equivalent in hours per year is 2080. A full-time equivalent per week is 40 hours. Job positions that the unit/organization has or will hire are part time, full time, or per diem. Each unit is allocated a number of full-time and part-time positions, which then is referred to in some institutions as a *position control*. The position control, or number of full-time, part-time, and per diem employees, is allocated, as well as the type (registered nurse, licensed practical nurse, unlicensed assistive personnel) that they are permitted to hire to cover the workload of the unit.

---

* *Definitions and budgeting calculations from Finkler, S. A. (1992). Budgeting concepts for nurse managers. Philadelphia: W.B. Saunders.*

LEARNING RESOURCES

Discussion Questions

1. Describe the two different types of budgets: zero-based and traditional.
2. Describe the seven general types of budgets.
3. Discuss the types of budgets: capital and operating budgets.
4. Define *direct* and *indirect costs.*
5. What are the three phases of the budget process.

Study Questions

Matching: Write the letter of the correct response in front of each term.

_____ 1. Budget

_____ 2. Expenses

_____ 3. Strategic planning

_____ 4. Revenues

_____ 5. Cash budget

_____ 6. Capital budget

_____ 7. Expense budget

_____ 8. Indirect costs

_____ 9. Traditional budget

_____ 10. Zero-based budget

A. A form of budgeting in which the whole budget is built from scratch

B. A form of budgeting in which baseline data for the budget are determined from previous costs plus an inflation factor

C. Expenses related to overhead, administration, or building

D. Income for the provision of services

E. A financial plan that guides resource use

F. Costs incurred for services provided

G. Formulation of strategy for the organization

H. Indicates receipts and disbursements

I. Indicates major purchases of $500 or more

J. Indicates payment of wages, benefits, and maintenance

True or False: Circle the correct answer.

T   F   11. Zero-based budgeting is a method of identifying expenses and including indirect costs.

T   F   12. A cost center is the smallest functional unit that generates expenses and revenues.

REFERENCE

Finkler, S., & Kovner, C. T. (2000). *Financial management for nurse managers and executives* (2nd ed.). Philadelphia: W.B. Saunders.

SUPPLEMENTAL READINGS

Henderson, E. (2003). Budgeting: Part one. *Nursing Management, 10*(1), 33-37.

Henderson, E. (2003). Budgeting: Part two. *Nursing Management, 10*(2), 32-36.

Kirby, M. P. (2003). Number crunching with variable budgets, *Nursing Management, 34*(3), 28-33.

Pinkerton, S. E. (2004). Budget!! Budget$!! Budget!! *The Journal of Continuing Education in Nursing, 35*(2), 52-53.

Rose, V. L. (2004). Budgeting: It's everyone's responsibility, *Nursing Homes, 53*(8), 28-30.

Chapter 36: Budgeting (pp. 771-788)

1. **How does budgeting relate to leadership, control, and management in health care?**

A budget is a written document used to forecast revenues and expenditures in order to control costs and to allocate resources. Although the development of the budget and the evaluation of its effectiveness is a managerial responsibility, staff nurse leadership also is needed to motivate other individuals to implement the financial plan and accomplish the objectives of the budget.

2. **Do nurses raise health care costs or lower them?**

Health care agencies are the largest employers of nurses, with a large proportion of the personnel budget being allocated to their salaries. Although nurses' salaries may result in substantial expenditures, nurses can reduce health care costs through responsible and well-informed clinical decision making, efficient care provision, and astute resource management. Without constant attention to these details by nurses, health care costs will escalate.

3. **How would a nurse manager manage a revenue budget?**

Operating revenues are calculated by multiplying the services provided by the charges for the services. Nurse managers can manage the revenue budget by making sure that all services are charged for, that all charges are appropriate, that reimbursement is maximized, and that new methods to increase revenue are investigated.

4. **What leadership roles and activities are important in budgeting?**

Creative leadership is needed to justify, secure, and allocate scarce resources; influence employees to find innovative ways to work efficiently and effectively; and to explore creative resource venues. Leaders model cost-conscious behaviors, analyze expenditures, and mentor employees to facilitate financial goal attainment.

5. **What activities of budgeting are appropriate at the staff nurse level?**

Appropriate budgeting activities for nurses include providing information concerning equipment requests, supply usage, and product evaluation. By knowing the costs of supplies, nurses carefully can select cost-effective materials, substituting less expensive items as appropriate. Budget conscious nurses can decrease the length of hospitalization by motivating clients toward recovery, minimizing scheduling errors, and encouraging interdisciplinary collaboration to optimize positive client outcomes.

6. **How can staff nurses best acquire knowledge and skills in budgeting?**

Nurses acquire valuable knowledge and skills from leaders that take the time to educate their staff about the budgeting process. Further knowledge is gained as nurse leaders model fiscally responsible behaviors and provide opportunities to learn budgeting skills. Participation in committees, quality improvement programs, continuing education, and college courses are other sources for gaining valuable knowledge about budgeting.

7. **How is budgeting like balancing a personal checkbook?**

Consider your personal checkbook as your budget, reflecting your personal financial plan. You have predetermined deposits (revenues) and you write checks to cover your expenses (expenditures). How you manage your account will determine whether you will maintain a positive balance. Planning, organizing, acquiring, and controlling money and resources are essential elements that are inherent in personal and organizational budgeting.

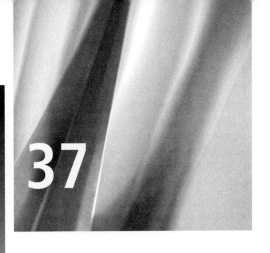

37

Productivity and Costing Out Nursing

STUDY FOCUS

Productivity is key to organizational financial viability. Nurses often are expected to minimize costs and increase productivity while maintaining safe, quality care. This is in part due to the fact that nursing is the largest health profession and the single most costly line item in hospital budgets. *Productivity* is measuring outputs produced using a quantity of inputs. *The production process* is the relationship between outputs and the inputs used to produce them. *The production process has five related concepts:* (1) *marginal productivity* (additional output gained by adding additional input); (2) *economies of scale* (increasing inputs resulting in increase volume and decrease cost per unit); (3) *short-run distinctions* (time period during which there can be limited change to the inputs); (4) *long-run distinctions* (time period during which all inputs can be varied); and (5) *substitution* (replacing a higher-cost input with a lower one). The term *costing of nursing services* refers to the cost of services or interventions carried out by nurses. *Economic evaluation* is the cost and consequences of activities (inputs and outputs) (Drummond, et al., 1997). Economic evaluations often are done to assess the choices individuals make about scarce health care resources. *Four basic techniques of economic evaluation* are (1) *cost analysis* (determining the cost of producing a good or service), (2) *cost-benefit analysis* (measuring the worth of a program in dollars), (3) *cost-effectiveness analysis* (comparing the cost of two or more methods of achieving the same outcome), and (4) *cost utility analysis* (considering the preferences of an individual for alternative types of treatment). *Effectiveness* is doing the right things correctly to achieve established outcomes. *Efficiency* is providing the necessary services quickly and inexpensively. A *charge* is the dollar amount billed to a customer for a service before discounts are taken. The *price* is the dollar value of each of the inputs. *Total cost* is the resultant dollar value of the production process.

The *National Health Expenditures* is an important measure of spending for health care in the United States by type of service (Heffler et al., 2003). In 1998, the National Health Expenditures exceeded $1 trillion, and by 2012, it is projected to be $3.1 trillion. Rising labor costs are the major contributing factor to this increase. Nurses must ensure that supplies and equipment are used wisely.

Nurse managers must be cognizant of productivity levels and the cost of nursing services in order to manage a health care organization effectively. An important concept in productivity is the production process that was used first in industrial applications. The *production process* is composed of a relationship between outputs and inputs to produce a given quantity of output. Transferring this concept to health care can assist with understanding of the inputs required to produce the services associated with patient care. Inputs in health care can be registered nurse (RN) time, laboratory tests, and medical equipment. The generic equation for representing the production process is as follows:

$$Qq = f(I_1, I_2, I_3, Z \ldots)$$

where Qq is the amount of the service being produced; f is the output; and I_1, I_2, I_3, and Z represent all inputs used.

An example of a health care equation for surgical nursing patient care is:

$Qsnpc = f(time\ of\ RNs,\ time\ of\ licensed\ practical$
$nurses,\ time\ of\ nursing\ assistants,\ computer\ hardware,$
$equipment,\ Z \ldots)$

Once inputs are identified, a cost analysis can be conducted. *Cost analysis consists of three* steps: (1) identifying inputs, (2) determining the total cost of the production process, and (3) determining the average cost of each unit of output. *The total cost* (total value of the production process for the service) is equal to the *price* (dollar value of an input) multiplied by the quantity of the inputs used. When performing calculations for the cost of the production process, inclusion of fringe benefit costs is important.

261

Five characteristics of the production process are (1) *economic efficiency* (minimizing the cost of production); (2) *substitutability of inputs* (using a comparable input to replace the original one); (3) *marginal productivity* (additional output by increasing an input); (4) *long-run* (all inputs may be varied) and *short-run* (only some inputs may be varied) distinctions; and (5) *economies of scale* (increase in inputs, but the output volume increases by a larger percent).

Nursing productivity is a combination of nursing care hours and the provision of nursing care services. To increase productivity, nurses can provide services with fewer nursing care hours or complete more interventions in a shorter time. The challenge is to increase productivity, ensure quality, and empower employees to improve processes. Substituting equipment for labor, improving work methods, removing unproductive practices, and improving human resource management can increase employee productivity.

Multiple measures of productivity involve a relationship between volume of inputs and costs. The most critical input in the production of nursing care is nurses' time. Calculating *hours per patient day* is the oldest nursing productivity index and is imprecise because of the wide variation in patient condition severity. In this formula the input is nursing hours worked and the output is the number of hospitalized patient days. The reasons why productivity measurements are complex include (1) measuring nursing care outcomes is difficult and controversial, (2) relationships among care processes and nursing outcomes are not fully understood, and (3) the most efficient combinations of resources for performing care are not known (Edwardson, 1989).

Activity-based costing is an approach to service costing that is different from traditional methods and may be useful in settings such as home health. This costing approach reflects what it costs to provide services and why costs were incurred. The *two steps to activity-based cost assignment* are (1) identifying activities that consume resources and (2) assigning activities to cost categories. Assignment of costs for activities is based on actual time spent by activity. Costs follow a four-level cost hierarchy of unit, batch, business, and enterprise levels. The purpose of costing out nursing care is to facilitate health policy and reimbursement decisions.

The *Medicare Cost Report* also may be used as a resource for costing out nursing services in hospitals. Hospitals being reimbursed with Medicare funds are required to submit annual data on cost-to-charge ratios. Hospital bills can be unbundled, and a cost and price for nursing services may be established.

Current health care issues and trends influencing productivity in health care services are (1) the national nursing shortage, (2) integration of economics into the practice of clinical nursing, and (3) a multigenerational nursing workforce. A shortage of 800,000 nurses is projected to occur by the year 2002. An increased demand for RNs is occurring at the same time that the RN workforce is aging and interest by young persons to choose nursing as a career is decreasing. A strategy to increase nursing productivity is the use of technology to assist with documentation (computerized) and medication administration (systems) and use of monitoring devices that can detect deviations from normal and communicate this information to nurses. Heavy recruitment of young persons and career switchers is needed to help increase the number of nurses in the workforce.

Economic analysis is important as one factor in making decisions about health care programs and policies. Resources for citizens are limited, and choices will need to be made about where scarce health care resources are spent. The *cost-effectiveness model* can be useful in examining different methods of obtaining desired outcomes. The model examines different programs with objectives that vary in order to determine the most productive method of providing services. An understanding of the use and definition of terms is important so that researchers conducting studies and professionals reading the results can compare findings and build upon existing work. The following table provides a description of types of economic evaluations used in research:

Types of Economic Evaluation

Type of Study	Answers the Question
Cost analysis	What does it cost?
Cost-benefit analysis	Is the program worthwhile, as measured in dollars?
Cost-effectiveness analysis	What is the cost of Method A versus Method B for achieving the same outcome?
Cost minimization	What is the least costly alternative of two programs?
Cost utility analysis	What are the preferences the individual has for the outcomes of a treatment?

Another issue and challenge for nurse leaders is to manage a multigenerational nurse workforce. Four generations of nurses are employed in health care settings, which makes management complex because each generation holds different values about work, recreation, professional activities, and financial rewards and resources. Clearly a menu of economic and work life reward options must be available to attract and retain a diverse workforce. In addition, managers must build teams, coordinate work activities, and foster strong communication networks to design a supportive work climate for workers with diverse values.

LEARNING TOOLS

Cost Analysis Assignment

Purpose

To explore cost analysis by performing a three-step calculation.

Introduction

Cost analyses involves three steps: (1) identifying the inputs, (2) determining the total cost of the production process, and (3) determining the average cost of each unit of output. This assignment begins by explaining each of the three steps in cost analysis and then provides the student an opportunity to use the three steps by reading a brief case study and answering the questions posed. Answers to the questions are found at the end of this assignment.

Directions

1. Step A: General Production Process Formula

$Qonpc = f(time\ of\ RNs,\ time\ of\ licensed\ practical\ nurses,\ time\ of\ nursing\ assistants,\ computer\ hardware,\ equipment,\ Z...)$

Explanation: In this example, Q is a quantity of obstetrical nursing patient care (output), and f is a function of the inputs that include labor (i.e., RNs, licensed practical nurses, unlicensed assistive personnel, and secretaries), supplies, equipment, and overhead expenses for the building. All inputs must be calculated and accounted for in order to establish an accurate and reflective price for the service. For example, careful review of the line items in a budget can assist with ensuring that all inputs are calculated. Examples include wage and salary costs, fringe benefits, postage, mileage costs, telephone charges, and supplies. This simple calculation provides insight into the total cost for the inputs and clearly identifies the quantity of care provided.

2. Step B: Total Cost of Production Process Formula

$$TCoq = (PI_1 \times QI_1) + (PI_2 \times QI_2) + (PI_3 \times QI_3) + (PZ... + QZ...)$$

where P is price of the input and Q is quantity of the input.

Example: Input I_1 is the RN's time to care for a person having a total hysterectomy, and 8 hours of time are used. The price of the input is 8 multiplied by the hourly salary of the nurse, which is $26.00, for a total cost of $208.

Chapter **37** Productivity and Costing Out Nursing

3. *Step C: Average Cost Per Case Formula*

$$ACC = TC/OQ$$

where *ACC* is average cost per case, *TC* is total cost (derived in Step B), and *OQ* is output quantity.

Example: If a health care organization wishes to implement a day care geriatric program and a cost analysis reveals the operational costs to be $125 per day per patient, and reimbursement is only $75 per patient, it is unlikely that the program will be initiated.

Practice Problem

Jane Arsalo, a nurse manager in an inpatient mental health facility, is proposing implementing a treatment program for adolescents with mental illness. She has developed a rough estimate for the costs of the program and number of patients she feels would be enrolled daily. The costs associated for the program per day are $25.00 per hour for RN wage and fringe benefits; $10.00 per hour for a secretary's wage and fringe benefits; $30 per hour for a psychologist's wage and fringe benefit; $10 per day per patient for food; $10 per day per patient for supplies; and $10 per day per patient for overhead expenses. Nurse Arsalo proposes charging $250 per day and plans on a daily census of 10.

Questions

1. What are the inputs in the general production process?
2. What is "the total cost of production" (Step B)?
3. What is "the average cost per case" (Step C)?
4. Will the health care agency make, lose, or break even if the cost estimates and revenue estimates are accurate?

Answers

1. What are the inputs required for the general production process? The following formula provides a structure in which to identify each of the inputs:

   Qonpc = f(time of RNs, time of licensed practical nurses, time of nursing assistants, computer hardware, equipment, Z ...)

   The inputs are the following: RN hourly wage and fringe benefits + Secretary wage and fringe benefits + Psychologist wage and fringe benefits + food + supplies + overhead

2. The total cost of production, as calculated using the formula in Step B—TCoq = $(PI_1 \times QI_1) + (PI_2 \times QI_2) + (PI_3 \times QI_3) + (PZ ...+ QZ ...)$—where *P* is price of the input and *Q* is quantity of the input:

   ($25 × 8 hours) + ($10 × 8 hours) + ($30 × 8 hours) + ($10 × 10 patients) + ($10 × 10 patients) + ($10 × 10 patients) = $820

3. The average cost per case, as calculated using the formula in Step C is ACC = TC/OQ—where *ACC* is average cost per case, *TC* is total cost (derived in Step B), and *OQ* is output quantity—is $820 ÷ 10 patients = $82.00.

   The program would cost $82.00 per day per patient to implement.

4. If Jane is able to enroll 10 patients each day of the week and charge $250.00 per day, she would make (250 - 82) or $168.00 profit per patient per day.

   This program would be profitable.

CASE STUDY

Karen Smoneski, a nurse manager of a 23-bed step-down unit in a medium-size hospital in El Paso, Texas, prides herself on the fact that her unit has the highest quality scores in the hospital. The clinical staff who work on the step-down unit consistently document all nursing interventions and pertinent patient data, carry out procedures according to protocol, and go out of their way to facilitate the patient's journey to health and wellness. Many physicians use the step-down unit as an example of excellence in patient care. The only problem that Nurse Smoneski has is keeping the unit on budget and maintaining a high level of productivity. Compared with the other units, the step-down unit has a low productivity level and a high budget.

Case Study Questions

1. Is the unit Nurse Smoneski manages efficient?
2. Is the unit Nurse Smoneski manages effective?
3. What would you do if you were the manager? Would you maintain status quo or try to improve productivity? Provide a rationale for your decision.

LEARNING RESOURCES

Discussion Questions

1. What type of activities could help leaders increase employee productivity? What type of activities could help managers increase employee productivity?

2. What is productivity? How do you measure productivity?

3. What are some changes that could be made on your unit to improve productivity?

4. What is the cost-effectiveness model? What is the cost-benefit model? Give an example of a situation in which you would use each of these models.

5. What is activity-based costing and in what clinical setting would it be used? Provide a rationale for your answer.

Study Questions

True or False: Circle the correct answer.

T   F   1. Productivity is measured by calculating the cost of nursing care multiplied by the unit of output.

T   F   2. Effectiveness is how fast or inexpensive a service is provided.

T   F   3. Efficiency is doing the right things to improve quality.

T   F   4. Costing out nursing services is the actual cost of providing services by nurses.

T   F   5. Time and motion studies are no longer valuable in determining workload requirements.

T   F   6. The cost-benefit model is goal-focused and examines different methods to achieve outcomes.

T   F   7. The cost-effectiveness model is a budgetary model that determines costs and assists managers with determining the proper skill mix for a unit.

T   F   8. Economies of scale refer to the productivity of units.

T   F   9. Nurse managers may need to be more creative in constructing a menu of economic and work life reward options for a multigenerational nursing workforce.

T   F   10. Nurses are in a prime position in the changing health care environment and need only to sit and wait for expanded roles in managed care environments.

T   F   11. The use of technology and computerization improves productivity and increases accuracy.

T   F   12. Activity-based costing is a useful approach to use in the hospital setting.

T   F   13. Techniques for measuring productivity include time and motion studies, patient care requirements, and standards of care.

T   F   14. Larger hospitals have an advantage in purchasing supplies and equipment over rural hospitals because they can buy in large quantities.

T   F   15. Nurses have clearly defined their contributions to health care services and readily can identify the costs and outcomes associated with their care.

REFERENCES

Drummond, M. F., O'Brien, B., Stoddart, G. L., & Torrance, G. W. (1997). *Methods of economic evaluation of health care programmes* (2nd ed.). New York: Oxford University Press.

Edwardson, S. (1989). Productivity measurement. In B. Henry, C. Arndt, M. Di Vincenti, & A. Mariner-Tomey (Eds.), *Dimensions of nursing administration: Theory, research, education, and practice* (pp. 371-385). Boston: Blackwell.

Heffler, S., Smith, S., Keehan, S., Clemens, M. K., Won, G., & Zezza, M. (2003, February 7). *Health spending projections for 2002-2012 [Online exclusive]. Health Affairs: The Policy Journal of Health Sphere.* Retrieved January 3, 2005, from *http://content.healthaffairs.org/cgi/content/full/hlthaff.w3.54v1/DC1?maxtoshow=&HITS=10&hits=10&RESULTFORMAT=&author1=heffler&fulltext=spending+projections&andorexactfulltext=and&searchid=1122307546478_1546&stored_search=&FIRSTINDEX=0&resourcetype=1&journalcode=healthaff*

SUPPLEMENTAL READINGS

Brown, C., Bagby, R., Neiswinder, J., & Helmuth, A. (2004). Computer-based data collection boosts productivity, regulatory compliance, *Nursing Management, 35*(2), 40B-40D.

Fitzpatrick, M. A., (2002). Let's bring balance to health care, *Nursing Management, 33*(3), 35-37.

Hall, L. M. (2003). Nursing intellectual capital: A theoretical approach for analyzing nursing productivity, *Nursing Economic$, 21*(1), 14-19.

McNeese-Smith, D. K. (2001). Staff nurse views of their productivity and nonproductivity, *Health Care Management Review, 26*(2), 7-19.

Quittenton, A. (2002). Improving productivity through the use of portable radios, *Orthopedic Nursing, 21*(2), 67-72.

Chapter 37: Productivity and Costing Out Nursing (pp. 789-802)

1. Why does quality of care suffer when nursing care hours are reduced?

The quality of care services is influenced by a number of factors including the staff mix, the care delivery system, condition severity levels, and the number of caregivers assigned to provide direct and indirect care. When nursing care hours are reduced, there is less time to perform all of the required patient care activities. As a result, nurses are required to work faster, streamline documentation, or decrease patient-centered activities. When nursing care hours are reduced drastically, the nurse may have to prioritize patient care, completing the most urgent care first and leaving many patient care needs unmet.

2. Do more experienced nurses work more productively? Why or why not?

Productivity is based on many factors including knowledge, experience, motivation, administrative support, and commitment to quality care. Experienced nurses are generally more productive than novice nurses because they have more experience and a stronger knowledge base to make astute clinical judgments. If experienced nurses are not motivated, lack administrative support, or have serious personal problems, their productivity level may decline. As novice nurses gain experience, efficiency, and confidence in their clinical decisions, their productivity level increases.

3. Why should nurses worry about productivity?

Nurses compose the largest expenditure for health care organizations. When cost-cutting strategies are implemented, areas with large expenditures are targeted for reductions. If nurses are unable to demonstrate that they are productive members of the health care team and that they positively influence patient outcomes, they will be targeted for workforce reductions.

4. What issues in productivity are most urgent? Why?

It is important for nurses to standardize the measurement of productivity. Productivity measures are complex because quantifying nursing care outcomes is difficult, there are no clear relationships between care process and nursing outcomes, and the most efficient resources for performing care are unknown. Without standardization of productivity indices, meaningful comparisons among nursing units and facilities are not possible.

5. How do nurses determine whether their care is effective and efficient?

Effectiveness is doing the right things and achieving quality outcomes, whereas efficiency is how fast a service or product is completed in the most cost-effective manner. Nurses have established quality improvement programs that monitor indicators of care for compliance. Quality programs determine how effective the care has been. Efficiency usually is monitored by productivity measures. Costs are tracked by examining actual expenditures compared with budgeted projections, with adjustments for units of service or patient days.

6. Why should nurses cost out their services?

Costing out nursing services is important so that nurses know the actual costs of services to patients. This knowledge is used for reimbursement decisions and to facilitate health policy formation. To obtain third-party reimbursement, nurses must be able to cost out nursing care, clearly articulate the outcomes of care delivery, and negotiate services for a set fee. Through these processes, nurses will be able to demonstrate their effectiveness and worth to the organization.

7. **How can nurses control health care costs? Nursing costs?**

Several strategies can be used to contain costs. Effective leaders can motivate and collaborate with employees to find innovative methods to be productive, effective, and efficient in accomplishing the goals of the organization. Case management of high-risk populations can control health care expenditures. Other health care costs can be controlled by providing community-based care and by using advanced practice nurses in primary care settings. Evaluating skill mix and care delivery systems, facilitating interdisciplinary collaboration, maximizing reimbursement, and using critical pathways to reduce redundancy can control nursing costs.

8. **What is the ideal ratio of nurses to patients?**

Unfortunately there is no ideal ratio of nurses to patients. Nurse-to-patient ratios depend on the condition severity of the patients, the education and experience of the nurses, the technology required for care provision, the work methods, the care delivery system, and information technology. Evaluating standards of care, conducting time and motion studies, and assessing patient care requirements provide a foundation to determining the ratio of nurses to patients.

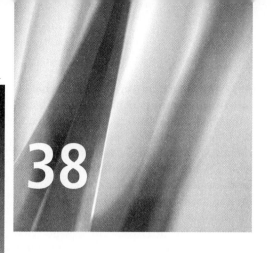

38 Change and Innovation

STUDY FOCUS

Change is a pervasive element in health care today. The perspectives on change—making something different—are positive and negative. Even when change is positive, it can create tensions and anxiety. Change is a process that is inevitable in our personal and professional lives. Change ranges on a continuum from haphazard to planned. *Change* is an alteration to make something different. *Planned change* is intentional intervention. A *change agent* is an outside helper who facilitates planning and implementing change. *Four types of systems* that become the focus for change are (1) individuals, (2) face-to-face groups, (3) organizations, and (4) communities (Lippittt et al., 1958). *Change can be viewed from four levels:* (1) knowledge, (2) attitudes, (3) individual behavior, and (4) group or organizational behavior or performance (Hersey et al., 2001). The *three strategies for organizational change* are the *rational-empirical* (reward and referent power are used to motivate change; individuals will support change if it benefits them and resist it if they lose something), the *normative-reeducative* (expert power is used to motivate change; support or opposition occurs based on the impact on society), and the *power-coercive* (legitimate and coercive power is used to motivate change; individuals will support change if powerful figures initiate it) (Bennis et al., & Corey, 1976).

Tiffany and Lutjens (1998) have proposed *seven categories of change strategies:* (1) educational, (2) facilitative, (3) technostructural, (4) data-based, (5) communication-related, (6) persuasive, and (7) coercive. Strategies must be chosen carefully to match the change process and to enhance effectiveness. *Change occurs within two frameworks:* (1) first-order change (occurs in stable systems with adaptation and incremental change made with purposeful adjustments) and (2) second-order change (change that is discontinuous and radical that occurs when fundamental properties are changed) (Hersey et al., 2001). *Factors to*

consider in assessing the probability of successful change implementation include the following: (1) characteristics of organizational management, (2) system users, (3) collaboration between users, (4) the project itself, (5) the project team, (6) the team's approach, (7) the project solution, (8) the readiness of the organization to change, (9) level of dissatisfaction with the status quo, (10) a desired future state, (11) first step needed, and (12) perceived costs of changing (Gustafson et al., 2003). No matter what change is implemented, the amount and rapidity of change has the propensity to disrupt and disorganize people. Therefore, planned change in nursing management can be viewed as an intervention strategy. Part of planning change is examining the situational elements of organizational structure, people, and resources before implementing a change strategy. *Two basic types of change theory are* (1) those that help people watch change and (2) those that help people cause change. When the process of change in groups is engineered deliberately, it is called *planned change. Planned change theory* is a logical set of interrelated concepts that help explain how change occurs, predict effects, and help planners control variables in the change process. The three change theories popular in nursing and one nonnursing model are the following (Tiffany & Lutjens, 1998): (1) Lewin's (1947, 1951) planned change theory, writings by Bennis and colleagues (1961, 1976), and Rogers' (2003) theory of diffusion of innovations.

Many theories can be used to facilitate the change process. The most widely used theory is *Lewin's change theory.* Lewin provides a framework from which a force field analysis is conducted. The *three elements* of his theory are unfreezing, moving, and refreezing. Unfreezing, a process in which individuals become ready to change, occurs first. During the *unfreezing* process, individuals become aware of unmet expectations and feel discomfort over action or inaction, causing them to remove obstacles to change. The second stage is *moving,* which is when cognitive redefinition occurs. During the moving phase, a pretrial or testing occurs. The final

269

stage, *refreezing,* is when the change occurs and is integrated and stabilized. During refreezing, leaders provide positive feedback, encouragement, and motivation to reinforce the new change. Education, motivation, and enthusiasm are leadership strategies in the change process. Unmet expectations, discomfort about action or inaction, and removal of an obstacle to change creates awareness of the need for change.

Lewin's theory has formed the foundation for change theory. Another theory is Lippittt's (1973) who expanded Lewin's work by describing seven phases of change: diagnosing the problem, assessing motivation and the capacity to change, assessing motivation and resources, selecting change objectives, choosing roles for change agents, maintaining change, and terminating the helping relationship with the change agent. Havelock (1973) described six elements of the process of planned change: (1) building relationship, (2) diagnosing the problem, (3) acquiring relevant resources, (4) choosing the solution, and (5) gaining acceptance. Many similarities exist in the change process, nursing process, and problem-solving process, as indicated in the table below:

Similarities of Change Process, Nursing Process, and Problem-Solving Process

Change Process	Nursing Process	Problem Solving
Unfreezing	Assessing	Problem identification
Moving	Planning and implementing	Problem analysis and seeking alternatives
Refreezing	Evaluation	Implementation and evaluation

Data from Workman, R., & Kenney, M. (1988). The change experience. In S. Pinkerton & P. Schroeder (Eds.), *Commitment to excellence: Developing a professional nursing staff* (pp. 17-25). Rockville, MD: Aspen.

The *steps change agents follow in the process of change* are articulating a clear need for the change, getting the group to participate by leaving details to the individuals who implement the change, getting reliable information to those who implement the change, motivating through rewards and benefits, and not promising things that cannot be delivered. Individuals respond differently to change. Some individuals are exhilarated, whereas others are depressed, confused, and angry. Being aware of the emotional responses to a change can assist leaders to manage and facilitate change in a positive manner. Perlman and Takacs (1990) identified the *10 stages of the emotional voyage* during change. The 10 stages are equilibrium, denial, anger, bargaining, chaos, depression, resignation, openness, readiness, and reemergence. Manion (1995) identified *seven stages individuals go through during personal transition:* (1) lose focus, (2) minimize the impact, (3) the pit (feelings of anger, discouragement), (4) let go of the past, (5) test the limits, (6) search for meaning, and (7) integration. Individuals may view change in a positive framework or negative. Those who view change as positive are more optimistic. *Four positive responses to change* are (1) uninformed optimism, (2) informed pessimism, (3) hopeful realism, and (4) informed optimism. The ability to manage one's attitude and perceptions are key skills for success.

Resistance is another important characteristic of individuals experiencing the change process. Resistance occurs for many different reasons. Some individuals are afraid of disorder and the interruption of their daily routine, whereas others are fearful of losing their job, power, or resources. *Four ways resistance to change can be manifested* are (1) active resistance through frustration and aggression, (2) organized passive resistance or resisting change collectively, (3) indifference by ignoring or attempting to divert attention elsewhere, and (4) acceptance on the surface (Asprec, 1975). Resistance can be useful if structured positively. Encouraging individuals to discuss change openly and to identify opportunities and barriers can create a smooth transition. Driving resistance underground by censuring, controlling, or punishing is counterproductive. *Techniques to increase the probability of effectiveness in the change process* are explaining the rational for the change, allowing emotions to work out, giving participants information, and helping individuals cope with change. *Actions to avoid in implementing change in organizations* include simply announcing the change, ignoring or offending powerful individuals, violating authority and communication lines, relying only on formal authority, overestimating your formal authority, making poor decisions about what change is needed, communicating ineffectively, putting others on the defensive, underestimating the perceived magnitude of change, and not dealing with others' fears.

Implementing change strategies effectively leads to positive outcomes. Effective leaders have good diagnostic skills and the ability to adapt the leadership style to the situation and to change some or all of the situational variables during the change process. *Action steps to maintain momentum* include emphasizing managerial support, answering questions and personal concerns, and exercising tolerance. Leaders should focus on their employees and consider the following factors when implementing changes: the time and effort it takes to

Chapter **38 Change and Innovation**

adjust, the possibility of less desirable outcomes, fear of the unknown, tolerance for change capacity, trust levels, needs for security, leadership skills, vested interests, opposing group values, how coalitions form, strongly held views, and existing relationship dynamics disruptions. Leaders also need to be aware of the *nine common mistakes that individuals make in coping with organizational change:* (1) assuming management should keep them comfortable, (2) expecting someone else to reduce the stress, (3) shooting for a low-stress work setting, (4) trying to control the uncontrollable, (5) failing to abandon the expendable, (6) fearing the future, (7) picking the wrong battles, (8) psychologically unplugging from the job, and (9) avoiding new assignments (Davidhizar, 1996). Savvy leaders will learn how to manage people through periods of change and make transitions and implementations of new changes as seamless as possible. To assist managers in implementing change, Smith's (1996) identified *10 change management principles:* The management principles to manage people through a period of change are (1) keeping performance results the prime objective, (2) increasing the numbers of individuals involved, (3) ensuring individuals know why their performance matters, (4) learning by doing, (5) embracing improvisation, (6) using team performance, (7) concentrating designs on the work people do, (8) focusing energy and meaningful language, (9) sustaining behavior-driven change, and (10) practicing leadership based on the new changes.

Innovations are the creation of something new. Innovation often entails a systematic, purposeful, and organized search for solutions to existing problems. Careful analysis and research occur before innovation. *Organized abandonment* is the process of eliminating the obsolete and unproductive efforts of the past. *Seven sources of innovation* include the following: (1) examining the unexpected, (2) incongruity, (3) process needs, (4) changes in industry or market structure, (5) demographics, (6) new knowledge, and (7) change in perceptions or moods (Drucker, 1992). Helpful leader *skills in innovations* include (1) getting outside the organization for facts and perspectives, (2) taking responsibility for one's own information needs, (3) focusing for effectiveness, and (4) building learning into the system. The *five stages of innovation-decision are as follows:* (1) first knowledge of the existence and functions of an innovation, (2) persuasion to form an attitude toward the innovation, (3) decision to adopt or reject, (4) implementation of the new ideas, and (5) confirmation to reinforce or reverse the innovation decision. Adoption of innovation typically follows a normal, bell-shaped curve when plotted over time on a frequency basis. The individuals fall into five categories (innovators, early adopters, early majority, late majority, and laggards) (Rogers, 2003). Leaders can use this information to identify individuals in relation to accepting the innovation and using strategies to decrease resistance.

Strong leadership in nursing is needed to be proactive to the continuous learning and adapting required in an era of unprecedented change. *Five factors that determine successful planned change include* (1) relative advantage, (2) compatibility, (3) complexity, (4) trialability, and (5) observability (Rogers, 2003). Transformational change ignites passion in people, stirs creativity, and encourages innovations. *Elements to consider in an innovation diffusion are* (1) the innovation itself, (2) communication channels, (3) time, and (4) members of the social system (Romano, 1990). McCloskey and colleagues (1994) identified *five categories of nursing innovations:* (1) introducing new technology, (2) creating personnel development strategies, (3) changing the organization of work, (4) changing rewards/incentives, and (5) implementing quality improvement mechanisms.

Leaders create supportive learning organizations to nurture staff and care for clients. They create innovations and design structures to support change. *Five principles and processes that build a systematic approach to change are* (1) no extraneous jobs, (2) as few managers as possible, (3) managerial focus on the context of work and the worker's relationship to it, (4) commitment to change and learning, and (5) better and more meaningful use of data (Porter-O'Grady, 1994). Health care is in a paradigm shift. *Six interconnected transformations compose the major areas of change and include* (1) from person as customer to the population as customer, (2) from illness care to wellness care, (3) from revenue management to cost management, (4) from autonomy of professionals to their interdependence, (5) from client as nonconsumer of cost and quality information to consumer, and (6) from continuity of provider to continuity of information (Issel & Anderson, 1996). Nurse leaders are positioned strategically to create new environments and systems to shape health care. *Change drivers in health care and nursing* are cultural diversity, aging U.S. population, new services and technologies, and the public policy of posting information about quality care (Wakefield, 2003). Leaders are challenged to implement strategies that develop a proactive culture. *Strategies to foster creativity and change* include promoting conversations and dialogue, providing access to information, building relationships, teaching rethinking, questioning, and innovation, creating a culture of innovation, and orchestrating and executing (Kerfoot, 1998).

LEARNING TOOLS

Individual Activity

Purpose

To examine and use a change theory evaluation instrument to assess the utility of a specific change theory for your proposed change.

Introduction

Change is inevitable, occurring continuously in our daily lives. By taking charge of change and planning change activities, you can maintain control over a turbulent environment. Many change theories are in the literature. By evaluating the theory you wish to use with a specific planned change, you will have a clear sense of the utility of the change theory for your proposed change. The following tool will assist you with evaluating change theories.

Identify a pet project that you would like to institute at work. Select a planned change theory that you would like to use to assess the readiness for the change, guide the process of change, and assist you at the evaluation of the change. Several change theories are described in Chapter 38 of the textbook. Use the Tiffany/Lutjens Planned Change Theory Evaluation Instrument to assess the utility of the change theory for your pet project.

The Tiffany/Lutjens Planned Change Theory Evaluation Instrument*

The scoring for this tool is 0 for "I fully disagree" to 4 for "I fully agree."

Directions: Choose a change theory. Write a number from 0 to 4 on the line in front of the statement that reflects your beliefs about the utility of this theory to your specific change.

I. Significance

_____ 1. The planned change theory addresses targets for change.

_____ 2. This theory has an assessment process that could help a change agent identify a problem in a social system.

_____ 3. The theory has a clear process for evaluating the total change event.

_____ 4. The theory accounts for emerging problems and/or goals throughout the change process.

_____ 5. The theory prompts nursing change agents to ask if the proposed change is important for nursing.

_____ 6. The theory encourages the ethical use of power.

_____ 7. The theory encourages close cooperation between change agents and target populations.

_____ 8. The theory encourages change agents to help people in the target population make informed decisions.

_____ 9. The theory stresses social justice.

_____ 10. The theory looks at the world as a whole.

_____ 11. The theory views the world as changing rather than nonchanging.

_____ 12. The theory prompts change agents to consider whether the strategies they plan will agree with expectations of the social unit targeted for change.

II. Clarity and Consistency

_____ 13. This theory has a clear process for planning change.

_____ 14. This theory has a clear process for implementing change (causing change to occur).

_____ 15. This theory clearly defines planned change.

_____ 16. The definition of planned change fits with the remainder of the content of the theory.

_____ 17. Key ideas are clearly defined.

_____ 18. Relational statements are clearly stated.

_____ 19. Key ideas and relational statements avoid unnecessary repetition.

_____ 20. Key ideas are used consistently as defined throughout the theory.

_____ 21. The theory clearly states what it accepts as truth (assumptions).

_____ 22. Key ideas are related to one another.

_____ 23. Any diagrams offered increase the reader's understanding of planned change and its processes.

_____ 24. The planned change theory contributes to an understanding of planned change beyond what could be obtained from everyday experience or formal study of other planned change theories.

III. Generality

_____ 25. The planned change theory could help agents plan change.

_____ 26. The theory focuses only on the processes of planned change, not on unplanned change.

* From Tiffany, C. R., & Lutjens, L. R. J. (1998). Planned change theories for nursing: Review, analysis, and implications. *Thousand Oaks, CA: Sage.*

_____ 27. The purpose of the theory allows a change agent to carry out plans for change in any one of a number of clinical settings rather than in one specific setting or area.

_____ 28. This theory could apply to individuals.

_____ 29. This theory could apply to groups.

_____ 30. This theory could apply to communities.

_____ 31. This theory could apply to society.

_____ 32. This theory could apply to different cultures within and outside the United States.

_____ 33. Nurses could use this theory as a foundation for research.

_____ 34. The theory could be tested through research.

_____ 35. Hypotheses that can be tested could be developed from the theory.

_____ 36. Key ideas and processes of the theory can be observed in the real world.

IV. Practicality

_____ 37. The theory prompts change agents to consider timeframes.

_____ 38. The theory prompts change agents to consider the people (including experts) available to make the change.

_____ 39. The theory prompts change agents to consider space, equipment, and supplies.

_____ 40. The theory prompts change agents to consider financial resources.

_____ 41. The theory prompts change agents to consider organizational support.

_____ 42. The theory promotes change agents to consider whether they can obtain needed political resources for implementing change.

_____ 43. The theory prompts change agents to consider whether they can obtain needed legal resources for implementing change.

V. Applicability

_____ 44. Nurse change agents could use this theory to create change in clinical settings.

_____ 45. Nurse change agents could use this theory to create change in nursing education.

_____ 46. Nurse change agents could use this theory to create change in nursing administration.

VI. Foresight

_____ 47. The theory helps change agents to foresee possible procedural pitfalls in planning change.

_____ 48. The theory helps change agents to foresee possible cultural pitfalls in planning change.

_____ 49. The theory suggests ways to deal with possible procedural pitfalls in planning change.

_____ 50. The theory suggests ways to deal with possible cultural pitfalls in planning change.

_____ 51. The theory helps change agents to foresee immediate resistance to change.

_____ 52. The theory helps change agents to foresee long-term resistance to change.

_____ 53. The theory helps change agents to foresee the immediate results of adopting the proposed solutions.

_____ 54. The theory helps change agents to foresee the long-term results of adopting the proposed solutions.

Scoring: This tool helps you to see how well the change theory fits your specific change situation. As you score the statements, you are able to tell how well the theory meets your change process needs. Overall, the higher the total score (adding up each number for all 54 items = highest total score, 216), the better the fit between the change theory and your change situation.

CASE STUDY

Evelyn Viens, a nurse manager of a 47-bed oncology unit in a large teaching hospital in Cincinnati, Ohio, decides to implement a new system of shift reporting because the current system is too lengthy. She first introduces the idea at a staff meeting and discusses several different options and the problems with the current system. She discusses the difficulties of providing high-quality client care for the first 45 minutes of each shift. Nurse Viens then opens the meeting for discussion. She encourages objections and support for each idea. She elicits volunteers to work on the planned change. After 2 months, Nurse Viens asks the task force to report back their findings and propose a new method for the reporting structure for the unit. Individuals are again encouraged to critique and support the proposal. After this meeting, modifications in the new reporting format are made, and the plan is implemented. Nurse Viens and the task force make a point to reinforce the change with the staff and to provide them with encouragement and support when any difficulties arise.

Case Study Questions

1. Did Nurse Viens use a change theory? If so, which one?

2. What steps of the change theory do you see in this case study?

3. Why did Nurse Viens and the task force encourage the staff to raise concerns and verbalize resistance?

LEARNING RESOURCES

Discussion Questions

1. Discuss the similarities and differences of Lippitt's and Rogers' change theories.

2. What is an innovation? Discuss nursing innovations with which you are familiar.

3. Discuss potential emotional responses to change, and describe how you would facilitate the change process when encountering these responses.

4. What are four major changes occurring in the health care industry today? What are some strategies to manage these changes effectively?

5. How can resistance positively affect change? What should a leader do when encountering resistance?

Study Questions

True or False: Circle the correct answer.

T   F   1. Change is inevitable and is necessary for organizational viability.

T   F   2. Resistance can be useful and should be listened to and analyzed.

T   F   3. Lippitt's change theory involves the phases of unfreezing, moving, and refreezing.

T   F   4. Change is a linear process requiring a series of discrete steps.

T   F   5. Resistance most commonly arises because individuals are trying to gain more power.

T   F   6. Changing individual behavior requires considerable time and energy.

T   F   7. Individuals become aware of the need for change when needs are unmet.

T   F   8. Position power can be used effectively to initiate change.

T   F   9. Change occurs in a logical, planned manner.

T   F   10. Too much change is disruptive and can create disorganization.

REFERENCES

Asprec, E. (1975). The process of change. *Supervisor Nurse, 6*, 15-24.

Bennis, W. G., Benne, K. D., & Chin, R. (Eds.). (1961). *The planning of change: Readings in the applied behavioral sciences.* New York: Holt, Rinehart & Winston.

Bennis, W., Benne, K., Chin, R., & Corey, K. (1976). *The planning of change.* New York: Holt, Rinehart & Winston.

Davidhizar, R. (1996). Surviving organizational change. *Health Care Supervisor, 14*(4), 19-24.

Drucker, P. (1992). *Managing the future: The 1990s and beyond.* New York: Truman Talley Books/Plume.

Gustafson, D. H., Sainfort, F., Eichler, M., Adams, L., Bisognano, M., & Steudel, H. (2003). Developing and testing a model to predict outcomes of organizational change. *Health Services Research, 38*(2), 751-776.

Havelock, R. (1973). *The change agent's guide to innovation in education.* Englewood Cliffs, NJ: Educational Technology Publications.

Hersey, P., Blanchard, K. H., & Johnson, D. E. (2001). *Management of organizational behavior: Leading human resources* (8th ed.). Upper Saddle River, NJ: Prentice-Hall.

Issel, L. M., & Anderson, R. A. (1996). Take charge: Managing six transformations in healthcare delivery. *Nursing Economic$, 14*(2), 78-85.

Kerfoot, K. (1998). Leading change is leading creativity. *Nursing Economic$, 16*(2), 98-99.

Lewin, K. (1947). Frontiers in group dynamics: Concept, method, and reality in social science; social equilibria an social change. *Human Relations, 1*(1), 5-41.

Lewin, K. (1951). *Field theory in social sciences: Selected theoretical papers.* New York: Harper & Row.

Lippitt, G. (1973). *Visualizing change: Model building and the change process.* La Jolla, CA: University Associates.

Lippitt, R., Watson, J., & Westley, B. (1958). *The dynamics of planned change: A comparative study of principles and techniques.* New York: Harcourt, Brace & World.

Manion, J. (1995). Understanding the seven stages of change. *American Journal of Nursing, 95*(4), 41-43.

McCloskey, J., Maas, M., Huber, D., Kasparek, A., Specht, J., Ramler, C., et al. (1994). Nursing management innovations: A need for systematic evaluation. *Nursing Econimic$, 12*(1) 35-44.

Perlman, D., & Takacs, G. (1990). The 10 stages of change. *Nursing Management, 21*(4), 33-38.

Porter-O'Grady, T. (1994). A systems approach to managing transformation. *Seminars for Nurse Managers, 2*(4), 191-195.

Rogers, E. M. (2003). *Diffusion of innovations* (5th ed.). New York: Free Press.

Romano, C. (1990). *Diffusion of innovations* (5th ed.). New York: Free Press.

Smith, D. K. (1996). *Taking charge of change: 10 principles for managing people and performance.* Reading, MA: Addison-Wesley.

Tiffany, C. R., & Lutjens, L. R. J. (1998). *Planned change theories for nursing: Review, analysis, and implications.* Thousand Oaks, CA: Sage.

Wakefield, M. (2003). Change drivers for nursing and health care. *Nursing Economic$, 21*(3), 150-151.

Supplemental Readings

Dodd-McCue, D., Tartaglia, A., Myer, K., Kuthy, S., & Faulkner, K. (2004). Unintended consequences: The impact of protocol change on critical care nurses' perception of stress. *Progress in Transplantation, 14*(1), 61-67.

Domagala, S. E., & Rowles, C. J. (2002). Capacity for change. *Nursing Management, 33*(7), 34-35.

Lokk, J., & Arnetz, B. (2002). Work site change and psychosocial well-being among health care personnel in geriatric wards: effects of an intervention program. *Journal of Nursing Care Quality, 16*(4), 30-38.

Porter-O'Grady, T. (2003). Of hubris and hope: Transforming nursing for a new age, *Nursing Economic$, 21*(2), 59-64.

ANSWERS TO TEXT STUDY QUESTIONS

Chapter 38: Change and Innovation (pp. 803-826)

1. How do individuals in organizations get the information resources that they need to effect change?

Individuals in organizations get the information needed to effect change through regulatory agencies, legislative mandates, professional organizations, scientific investigations, and collegial networks. With an organization, information may be disseminated through formal channels of communication or through informal networks known as "grapevines."

2. How can informal leaders be used for successful change?

The successful implementation of a change process cannot be achieved solely by management or formal leaders. Informal leaders can be valuable assets to the change process in that they are able to enlist the support of their contemporaries. The active participation of informal leaders can promote acceptance to change while minimizing resistance.

3. What changes need to take place in nursing? Why?

Several changes need to take place in nursing. First, nursing must present itself as a profession based on a solid body of knowledge. Clinical judgments made by nurses are rooted in science and involve the diagnosis and treatment of human responses. The development of and accessibility to large databases will promote collaborative scholarly activity that will influence nursing practice and client care. Second, nurses must be politically and socially active if they are to have control over professional practice and input into the delivery of quality client care. Proactive efforts aimed at advancing the professional and financial status of nursing may serve as a catalyst to recruit more individuals into nursing and to deter others from leaving its ranks.

4. How does resistance manifest itself? What should the manager do?

Resistance may manifest itself in several ways. It may present in the form of frustration, aggression, or even indifference. However, resistance may belie fears such as loss of employment, power, or control. Misunderstanding the purpose and need of the change combined with the dissemination of inaccurate information may serve to escalate resistance and thwart efforts necessary for the successful enactment of change. Managers can assist by reevaluating the change, clarify the purpose, or increase communication. Even though resistance is an expected phenomenon of change, the manager or change agent also should determine why the resistance is occurring and what the resistant person is trying to protect.

5. How can nurses' perceptions be changed to result in empowerment? Why is this important?

Nurses must be active participants in the change process. Allowing feelings and fears to be aired allows for dialogue and the exchange of ideas while fostering autonomy and creativity. Through this process nurses will perceive their input as valuable. Individuals who feel empowered are more apt to enact changes that challenge the status quo.

6. How should nursing education change? Why?

Nursing education must prepare nurses with the leadership skills necessary to initiate and enact change. Nurses must be prepared with the leadership skills necessary to interact with others, resolve conflicts, and to promote collegial relationships to build consensus and enact change. By educating novice nurses in this manner, the profession of nursing will be able proactively and creativity to take advantage of opportunities to effect changes that will improve nursing care, professional practice, and service delivery.

7. Do we have too much change? What can be done about this?

Change is inevitable. Change is a constant process that can be planned or unplanned. Unplanned change may precipitate feelings of fear or loss of control. However, if one can move along the continuum from haphazard to planned change, feelings of control are regained as individuals plan, examine, and adapt to the impending change. Providing information, open communication, and the active involvement of the participants supports a sense of control necessary to adapt to and accept change.

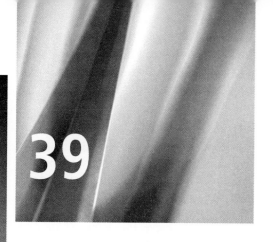

39

Quality Improvement and Health Care Safety

STUDY FOCUS

Health care quality is an important aspect of care provision. The Institute of Medicine reports have highlighted issues in safety and quality of care in health care agencies. Nurses are in good positions to take a leadership role in quality and performance improvements. Quality improvement is an essential component of health care and is linked with evaluation and accountability. Tremendous pressure is put on health care organizations to deliver high-quality care at lower costs in order to compete successfully in a competitive environment. *Benchmarking* is a tool to measure what exists against the best practices in the industry. *Best practice* is a service, function, or process that is implemented to produce superior outcomes. *Continuous quality improvement* (CQI) is a multidisciplinary process to improve systems by analyzing performance, collecting data, and changing archaic or inefficient systems. The *four main principles of CQI* are (1) having a customer focus, (2) identifying key processes to improve quality, (3) using quality tools and statistics, and (4) involving people and departments in problem solving (Bohnet et al., 1993; Miller & Flanagan, 1993). *Evidence-based practice* is judiciously using current best evidence to make decisions about care of individual patients (Sackett et al., 1996). *Indicators* are valid and reliable quantitative measures of structure, process, or outcomes related to one or more dimensions of performance. *Performance indicators* measure competence or productivity. *Clinical indicators* are focused on service, practice, or governance. *Performance measurement systems* are automated databases that facilitate performance improvement in disseminating and collecting process and outcome measures (Joint Commission on Accreditation of Healthcare Organizations, 1998). *Quality* is the provision of excellent care that is effective, efficient, and appropriate in the pursuit of excellence. *Quality of care* refers to the delivery of health care services and the belief that using up-to-date professional knowledge likely will result in positive outcomes. *Quality improvement*

programs are implemented organization-wide to ensure accountability to patients and payers. *Risk adjustment* is the process in which differences among patients or variables are weighted or are adjusted in outcomes analysis or benchmark efforts (Maas & Kerr, 1999). *Risk management* is an interdisciplinary process developed to protect the financial assets of an organization and promote quality health care (Velianoff & Hobbs, 1998). *Risk management programs* are organization-wide processes to identify, evaluate, and control the risks to the institution. *Sentinel events* measure a low-volume but serious, undesirable, and potentially avoidable process or outcome. *Standards* are written value statements. The *three basic types of standards for health care* are structure, process, and outcome. *Total quality management* is a method of including all employees in the improvement of services to ensure patient satisfaction.

Central to nursing practice is the provision of evidence-based, consumer-oriented care. To that end, health care professionals in the past 20 years have embraced quality improvement concepts. Donald M. Berwick, MD, was a pioneer in identifying and transferring the concepts of industrial total quality management programs to health care (Berwick et al., 1990). In 1991, under Berwick's direction, the National Demonstration Project on Quality Improvement in Health Care was conducted, and as a result, the Institute for Health Care was born. During this same period (mid-1990s), the Joint Commission on Accreditation of Healthcare Organizations (JCAHO) started to incorporate CQI into its standards. In 1996 the Institute of Medicine, through its Committee on Health Care Quality in America, convened the nation's health care leaders to improve access and care. These health care leaders embraced the following tenets: processes and systems are the problem, not people; standardization of processes is key to managing work and people; quality can be enhanced in safe, nonpunitive work cultures; quality is everyone's job; quality is part of the organizational culture; consumers and stakeholders must be involved in quality improvement; consensus among stakeholders must be gained; and health policy should include a focus on quality. The specific aims of the Institute of Medicine for health care improvement include safe, effective, patient-centered, efficient, and equitable care.

Collaboration is important in any workplace interaction. Collaboration is about partnerships.

Industrial models have influenced the way quality is measured in health care. Shewhart examined variations in workplace processes and developed a PDCA model that is used widely today: *P,* plan; *D,* do; *C,* check; and *A,* act (Deming, 2000). W. Edward Deming built on Shewhart's work and was influential in alerting Americans to the necessity of commitment to quality and listening to the customer's concerns. He used a unit-based approach focused on using higher quality to entice loyal customers. Key principles necessary for CQI include organizational commitment, an understanding of individual patient needs, continuously improving process, commitment to high-quality services, use of data, commitment by top management, benchmarking, and the formation of long-term relationships with a few suppliers. Deming's 14 points for quality are as follows (Deming, 2000):

1. Create constancy of purpose toward improvement.

2. Adopt the new philosophy.

3. Cease dependence on inspection to improve quality.

4. End the practice of awarding business on cost alone.

5. Improve constantly.

6. Institute training on the job.

7. Adopt and institute leadership aimed at helping individuals do their jobs better.

8. Drive out fear by promoting two-way communication.

9. Break down barriers between departments.

10. Eliminate exhortations in the form of posters and slogans.

11. Eliminate numerical quotas for productivity.

12. Permit pride in workmanship.

13. Encourage education and self-improvement.

14. Define management's commitment to CQI.

Juran (1989) used a three-pronged approach to quality: (1) planning, (2) control, and (3) improvement. Crosby approached quality in terms of zero defects and measured quality in relation to conformance to standards. He emphasized doing the right thing the first time to prevent waste. *Standards* are established by professional organizations and regulatory agencies and can be written in terms of *structure, process,* or *outcomes* (Donabedian, 1980). Professional organizations are the authoritative source for professional standards of practice. Standards define quality from which outcomes and performance can be measured. *Structural standards* focus on the internal organization and personnel. *Process standards* measure activities, and *outcome standards* measure whether the services made a difference. A *standard of care* is outcome-oriented and identifies what the patient can expect. A *standard of practice* is process-oriented and identifies what the provider must do to achieve the standard of care. Common performance selection criteria are being developed as a first step in designing comprehensive performance measurement systems. Common performance measurement selection criteria include relevance, meaningfulness and interpretability, scientific or clinical evidence, reliability or reproducibility, feasibility, validity, and health importance (Pelletier & Hoffman, 2002).

Some of the industry-based models of quality management have been adapted to health care. These models include Six Sigma, Lean Enterprise, the National Malcolm Baldrige Award, ISO 9000, and the concept of high-performance organizations. *Six Sigma* was developed by Motorola and was implemented successfully at General Electric and AlliedSignal Companies to reduce variation and error rates. The goal is to reach an error or defect rate of 3.5 per 1 million. *Lean Enterprise's* premise is that operational waste needs to be eliminated in the following areas: unnecessary processing, errors/defects, waiting, overproduction, inventory, excess motion by people, transportation by product, and underutilized people (Martin, 2003). *The Baldrige National Quality Award* establishes a set of performance standards in seven areas of excellence: (1) leadership, (2) strategic planning, (3) customer and market focus, (4) information and analysis, (5) human resource focus, (6) process management, and (7) business results. *ISO 9000* represents the International Organization for Standardization, a network of 148 countries that agree on quality requirements in business and service industries. Organizations that continue to evolve their quality models and strive for continual improvements are embracing the concept of *high-performance organizations.* Attributes of high-performance organizations are communicating a strong and clear mission and vision to employees, thinking strategically to anticipate customer's needs and market changes, committing to ongoing identification of problems, resiliency, flexibility, and creative and improvisational problem solving to address failures or "near misses."

Costs associated with medical errors are substantial: disability, lost income, and health care costs total about $29 billion annually (Quality Interagency Task

Chapter **39 Quality Improvement and Health Care Safety**

Force, 2000). The Institute of Medicine report *To Err Is Human: Building a Safer Health Care System* describes the number of medical errors in the nation as unacceptable (Kohn et al., 2000). The Quality Interagency Task Force was established in 1989 to ensure that federal agencies involved in health care services worked in a coordinated manner to improve quality. The Quality Interagency Task Force defined a four-tiered approach: establish a national focus to create leadership and tools to improve the knowledge base about safety, identify and learn from voluntary and mandatory reporting systems, raise standards and expectations, and implement safe practice (Quality Interagency Task Force, 2000). Another Institute of Medicine report, *Crossing the Quality Chasm: A New Health System for the 21st Century* was the impetus for Congress to establish the Health Care Quality Innovation Fund. This fund supported projects that (1) achieved six aims of safety, effectiveness, patient-centeredness, timeliness, efficiency, and equity and/or (2) produced improvement in quality in the priority conditions (Institute of Medicine, 2001). The intent of the funding was to produce programs, tools, and technology that could be used nationwide by health care agencies to improve quality care. In 2002 the third Institute of Medicine report, *Leadership by Example: Coordinating Government Roles in Improving Health Care Quality,* was published and addressed the patchwork of federal quality oversight programs in place (Corrigan et al., 2002). The committee was convened to (1) provide protection to beneficiaries, (2) provide strong incentives for quality, and (3) improve oversight by eliminating redundancy (Institute of Medicine, 2002). The major findings of the study were (1) lack of consistency in performance requirements in government programs; (2) lack of use of standardized measures; (3) no well-thought-out conceptual framework to guide selection of performance measures; (4) lack of computerized data at Medicare, Medicaid, and the State Children's Health Insurance Program; and (5) lack of transparency in openly sharing safety and quality information (Omenn, 2002).

Leadership in planning for health care quality is important. Leaders who develop and nurture a culture of CQI will position their organizations strategically for excellence in care and quality. Part of developing a culture of CQI is to articulate this concept clearly in the mission, vision, and value statements of the organization. This is important to send the message that quality and continuous improvement are important, as is involving internal and external stakeholders. The paradigm has shifted from quality assurance to CQI, which includes strong leadership, commitment to customer's needs, understanding processes, and the use of data collection and analysis in problem solving using a multidisciplinary team to drive change and improvements. Tools and techniques that nurses can use in CQI include data collection tools (checksheets and checklists); control chart (data points on a graph to depict variation—illustrates whether variation is expected [common cause] versus unexpected [special cause]); cause-and-effect diagram or fish bone diagram (resembles a diagram of sentences with the effect in a box at the end [fish head] and the causes in four to five categories indicating the possible contributors so that the root cause can be found more easily); flowchart (work flow process is depicted and is the cornerstone of process improvement planning and analysis; Pareto diagram (helps depict the "80/20" rule/the vital few causes of the problem); and scatter diagram (shows the relationship between two variables that are continuous; data are plotted along the vertical and horizontal graph to show correlations).

Health care agencies must meet the requirements of federal and state reimbursement regulations (Medicare and Medicaid and state licensure rules). The standards of the JCAHO, the Commission on Accreditation of Rehabilitation Facilities, and the National Committee for Quality Assurance and other performance standards are universally adopted quality standards. Of these, the JCAHO has the greatest impact on the health care industry. The JCAHO is a private, not-for-profit organization that was founded in 1951. The JCAHO has evolved continually and adjusted its performance standards for quality. The JCAHO has evolved from the "10-Step Process for Quality Assurance" to the "Agenda for Change," which organized the standards into cross-functional processes of care and services. Then "Improving Organizational Performance" was added to incorporate CQI. In 1998 the JCAHO required organizations to participate in the ORYX initiative. This initiative required organizations to select six outcome measures and have an outside vendor aggregate the data. The JCAHO refined the ORYX initiative by specifying specific measures that organizations must assess, including three measures from the Center for Medicare and Medicaid Services "Scope of Work," which includes process and outcome data. Since 1980 the Center for Medicare and Medicaid Services has mandated that its recipients be evaluated by its peer review organization.. The peer review organizations have evolved into state and regional quality improvement organizations and have continued their mandate through the "Statement of Work" projects. In 2001 the JCAHO introduced a new standard for accredited hospitals to implement a formal patient safety program. The components of a health care safety program are leadership in allocation of resources to safety initiatives, assignment of individuals to manage the program, education of patients and families about safety, disclosure of unanticipated outcomes to patients and families, education of staff on safety issues, data collection and analysis in safety-related areas, definition of terms related to safety, management of sentinel events, adherence to national patient safety goals, and establishment of a risk-reduction process. By 2006 the JCAHO will be conducting its surveys on an unannounced basis.

Leadership in providing resources, guidance, and a culture of quality improvement is essential. Nurse leaders can create an environment emphasizing safety by learning the concepts of risk identification, analysis, and error reduction; embracing the concept of nonpunitive error reporting; encouraging staff to identify potential environmental risks; creating a sense of partnership; and becoming a role model in practicing health care safety concepts. Nurse leaders must handle sentinel events, those unexpected occurrences that involve death or serious physical or psychological injury, or risk thereof, in a systematic and formal way. Often a root analysis is conducted by the staff to "drill down" to the common causes and to identify activities that could prevent the occurrence in the future. The JCAHO requires a detailed reporting and submitting of certain types of sentinel events. The events that are reviewable by the JCAHO include unanticipated death, permanent loss of function, suicide of a patient in a setting where the patient received around-the-clock care, unanticipated death of a full-term infant, infant abduction or discharge to the wrong facility, rape, hemolytic transfusion involving major blood group incompatabilites, and surgery on the wrong patient or body part. The JCAHO further requires that annually at least one RCA process will undergo a formal process of failure modes effects and criticality analysis. This process starts with flowcharting of the steps of the process and assists in developing preventive strategies for future error. The JCAHO also publishes a newsletter on sentinel event alerts to disseminate "lessons learned" by others. The JCAHO also has approved six national patient safety goals.

Risk management is an interdisciplinary process designed to protect financial assets of an organization and to maintain quality care (Velianoff & Hobbs, 1998). A *risk management program* is instituted to identify risks, control occurrences, prevent damage, and control legal liability. *Risk managers* are often the first responders in a serious or sentinel event. *Enterprise risk management* is evaluation of all risks faced by an organization to maximize safety and risk reduction. Risk managers perform the following functions: assessing ongoing risk potential; ensuring individuals are removed from immediate threat; securing equipment as appropriate; investigating the facts; determining whether the event is sentinel; making reports to appropriate agencies; communicating with staff, patients, families, and administration; collecting data and ensuring follow-up; and if necessary conducting a root analysis. A tool for risk identification is an incident report, which is a factual account of the adverse event. This document alerts the risk manager of a potential problem and triggers an investigation. Clearly, the public, employers, and reimbursement organizations are aware of the need for improved quality and safety in health care processes. High-performing organizations will adopt cultures of CQI and safety awareness and management.

LEARNING TOOLS

Activity: Organizational Quality Improvement Assessment

Purpose

To assess the level of CQI in the organization in which you work.

Directions

Read each of the following statements, and then circle the number that best describes your assessment.

Key: 1, Not at all; 2, To a small extent; 3, To a moderate extent; 4, To a great extent; 5, To a very great extent.

1. Employees clearly understand who the customer is.	1 2 3 4 5
2. All employees clearly understand the customer's needs.	1 2 3 4 5
3. There is regular contact with the customer.	1 2 3 4 5
4. There is ongoing quality assessment of the customer's needs and what actually is provided.	1 2 3 4 5
5. Employees work in interdisciplinary teams.	1 2 3 4 5
6. Employees independently identify problems and seek to improve them.	1 2 3 4 5
7. Employees handle customer complaints autonomously.	1 2 3 4 5
8. Employees are valued and treated with respect.	1 2 3 4 5
9. Employees are allowed to do what it takes to do a high-quality job.	1 2 3 4 5
10. Employees are encouraged to handle work problems.	1 2 3 4 5

11. Employees do not need managerial approval to handle problems.	1 2 3 4 5	
12. Experimentation and risk taking is valued and encouraged.	1 2 3 4 5	
13. Change is viewed positively by employees.	1 2 3 4 5	
14. Employees are encouraged to meet and discuss work.	1 2 3 4 5	
15. Employees feel free to discuss matters openly and have no fear about disagreeing or offering alternative solutions.	1 2 3 4 5	
16. Failures are viewed as learning opportunities and are not punished.	1 2 3 4 5	
17. Managers facilitate employees' work and encourage input into work activities and consumer needs	1 2 3 4 5	
18. Communication is open, and employees are kept informed of changes.	1 2 3 4 5	
19. Group members work cohesively and share recognition for team accomplishments.	1 2 3 4 5	
20. Individuals in top management positions are visible and encourage employee input into organizational matters.	1 2 3 4 5	
21. Employees enjoy and have fun at work.	1 2 3 4 5	
22. Innovation is encouraged, facilitated, and supported.	1 2 3 4 5	

Scoring

Add up the total score for all 22 items. The higher the score, the more apt your organization is to have a quality improvement program or strong elements of a program in place. Organizations that have CQI programs tend to value employees, satisfy customers, and continually improve the process and services provided. Innovations are prized and risk taking is encouraged.

CASE STUDY

Pat Neimeyer is a master's-prepared nurse who has been asked by the chief executive officer of a medium-sized community hospital in Waterloo, Tennessee, to decrease the amount and number of malpractice claims. Nurse Neimeyer knows that there is an incident report system currently in place at the hospital, but the only persons who see the reports are the managers. She decides to centralize the incident report system, identify and track major occurrences, and develop programs to minimize incidents. Nurse Neimeyer creates a task force composed of employees and managers to relate her concerns and to elicit feedback. The chief executive officer expects a monthly report of Nurse Neimeyer's progress and malpractice claims.

Case Study Questions

1. What type of program is Nurse Neimeyer designing?

2. Is the program Nurse Neimeyer is designing a component of quality improvement?

3. Should incident reports be used in a punitive manner?

4. What type of a culture should Nurse Neimeyer create in dealing with sentinel events?

LEARNING RESOURCES

Discussion Questions

1. Describe what CQI is, and identify key elements of a CQI program.

2. Why do health care organizations seek accreditation from the JCAHO?

3. What is a sentinel event, and why is it important?

4. What type of approach should be taken with employees when a sentinel event occurs?

5. What is the role of the JCAHO in accreditation, and what is its focus?

6. What are the different types of outcomes collected?

7. Identify tools that nurses can use in quality improvement activities.

8. Describe at least one emerging health care quality model.

9. Define risk management and the role of the risk manager.

Study Questions

True or False: Circle the correct answer.

T   F   1. A standard of care is outcome-oriented and focuses on the nurse as a provider.

T   F   2. The three areas in which quality can be measured are structure, process, and cost.

T   F   3. Risk management programs are designed to ensure a high level of quality.

T   F   4. Once an incident report is filled out, it absolves the person from responsibility for the occurrence.

T   F   5. Standards can be set only by professional organizations.

T   F   6. Today, emphasis is on outcomes rather than process.

T   F   7. Continuous quality improvement aims to develop long-term relationships with a few suppliers and is responsive to customer needs.

T   F   8. Medicare and Medicaid reimbursement will not be paid to health care organizations that are not accredited.

T   F   9. The JCAHO, founded in 1951, is a private, not-for-profit organization that is an accrediting body for hospitals and health care organizations.

T   F   10. Structure standards measure whether the services provided by the organization make any difference.

T   F   11. A fish bone diagram is a graphic tool indicating that 80% of the problems result from 20% of individuals.

References

Berwick, D. M., Godfrey, A. B., & Roessner, J. (1990). *Caring health care: New strategies for quality improvement.* San Francisco: Jossey-Bass.

Bohnet, N., Ilcyn, J., Milanovich, P., Ream, M., & Wright, K. (1993). Continuous quality improvement: Improving quality in your home care organization. *Journal of Nursing Administration, 23*(2), 42-48.

Corrigan, J. M., Eden, J., & Smith, B. M. (Eds). (2002). *Leadership by example: Coordinating government roles in improving health care quality.* Washington, DC: National Academies Press.

Deming, W. E. (2000). *Out of the crisis.* Cambridge, MA: MIT Center for Advanced Engineering Studies.

Donabedian, A. (1980). *Explorations in quality assessment and monitoring: The definition of quality and approaches to its assessment* (Vol. 1). Ann Arbor, MI: Health Administration Press.

Institute of Medicine, Committee on Health Care Quality in America. (2001). *Crossing the quality chasm: A new health system for the 21st century.* Washington, DC: National Academies Press.

Institute of Medicine. Committee on Enhancing Federal Health Care Quality Programs (2002). *Project description.* Washington, DC: National Academies Press. Retrieved October 30, 2002, from *www.iom.edu/iomhome.nsf/pages/ Fed+Qual+Home?OpenDocument*

Joint Commission on Accreditation of Health care Organizations. (1998). *Glossary of terms for performance measurement.* Oakbrook Terrace, IL: Author. Retrieved January 11, 2005, from *www.jcaho.og/accredited+organizations/behavioral+ health+care/oryx/glossary+of+terms/glossary.htm*

Juran, J. M. (1989). *Juran on leadership for quality: An executive handbook.* New York: The Free Press.

Kohn, L. T., Corrigan, J. M., & Donaldson, M. S. (Eds.). (2000). *To err is human: Building a safer health care system.* Washington, DC: National Academies Press.

Maas, M. L., & Kerr, P. (1999). Risk adjustment in nursing effectiveness research. *Outcomes Management for Nursing Practice, 3*(2), 50-52.

Martin, K. (2003). On lean enterprise and its potential health care applications [Editorial]. *Journal for Healthcare Quality, 25*(5), 2, 43.

Miller, S., & Flanagan, E. (1993). The transition from quality assurance to continuous quality improvement in ambulatory care. *Quality Review Bulletin, 19*(2), 62-65.

Omenn, G. (2002). *Opening statement: Leadership by example: Coordinating government roles in improving health care quality.* Public briefing presented at the Institute of Medicine, Washington, DC, October 30, 2002.

Pellletier, L. R., & Hoffman, J. A. (2002). A framework for selecting performance measures for opioid treatment programs. *Journal for Healthcare Quality, 24*(3), 24-35.

Quality Interagency Task Force. (2000). *Doing what counts for patient safety: Federal actions to reduce medical errors and their impact. Report of the Quality Interagency Task Force (QuIC) to the President of the United States.* Rockville, MD: Author. Retrieved June 8, 2004, from *www.quic.gov/report/errors6.pdf*

Sackett, D. L., Rosenburg, W. M. C., Gray, J. A. M., Haynes, R. B., & Richardson, W. S. (1996). Evidence-based medicine: What it is and what it isn't. *British Medical Journal, 312*(7023), 71.

Velianoff, G. D., & Hobbs, D. K. (1998). Designing a patient care risk management system. In J. A. Dienemann (Ed.). *Nursing administration: Managing patient care* (2nd ed., pp. 91-99). Stamford, CT: Appleton & Lange.

Supplemental Readings

Johnson, T., & Ventura, R. (2004). Applied informatics for quality assessment and improvement. *Journal of Nursing Care Quality, 19*(2), 100-104.

Kinsman, L. (2004). Clinical pathway compliance and quality improvement. *Nursing Standard, 18*(18), 33-35.

Larrabee, J. H. (2004). Advancing quality improvement through using the best evidence to change practice. *Journal of Nursing Care Quality, 19*(1), 10-13.

Rubeor, K. (2003). The role of risk management in maternal-child health. *Journal of Perinatal & Neonatal Nursing, 17*(2), 94-100.

Scott-Cawiezell, J., Schenkman, M., Moore, L., & Vojir, C. (2004). Exploring nursing home staff's perceptions of communication and leadership to facilitate quality improvement, *Journal of Nursing Care Quality, 19*(3), 242-252.

Smith, T. C. (2004). Performance improvements tips and strategies. *Journal of Nursing Care Quality, 19*(1), 1-4.

Chapter **39** **Quality Improvement and Health Care Safety**

Chapter 39: Quality Improvement and Health Care Safety (pp. 827-868)

1. Who is responsible for quality management?

Quality management is a continuous, ongoing measurement and evaluation process within an institution. All levels of management and care providers are accountable for the knowledge of and adherence to standards of care. The professional nurse is responsible for monitoring her or his own practice relative to improving care delivery and can be involved in some aspect of the process, be it gathering data or acting as a representative on a quality improvement committee in addition to using standards of care.

2. What are the differences between institutional and professional responsibilities for quality? Why does this occur?

Institutional responsibilities for quality are linked directly to organizational efforts to provide a quality health care system. These responsibilities often include meeting external mandates for accreditation and reimbursement requirements. The professional responsibility for quality is related more directly to practice issues, patient outcomes, and standards of care. The organizational focus is to provide care in the most efficient and cost-effective manner possible, whereas health professionals tend to focus more on people or patient outcomes.

3. How is quality defined? How is it measured?

Quality is defined as the characteristics manifested in the pursuit of excellence. Quality has been defined in terms of effectiveness and efficiency, benefits and harms, or appropriateness of care. Quality exists when outcomes compare favorably with standards and is measured by continually by evaluating structure, process, and outcomes; relating outcomes to standards; and measuring performance. Structure focuses on the internal characteristics of an organization and its personnel; process examines the activities and interventions used to attain outcomes; and outcomes are measured by evaluating the services.

4. List and describe four tenets embraced by members of the Institute of Medicine Committee on Quality of Health Care in America. How are these incorporated in nursing practice?

The Institute of Medicine Committee on Quality of Health Care in America lists the following tenets:

1. Processes and systems are the problems, not people.
2. Standardization of processes is key to managing work and people.
3. Quality can be enhanced only in safe, nonpunitive work cultures.
4. Quality measurement and monitoring is everyone's job.
5. The impetus for quality monitoring is not primarily for accreditation or regulatory compliance but is a planned part of the organizational culture to enhance and improve services continuously, based on continuous feedback from employees and customers.
6. Consumers and stakeholder must be included in all phases of quality improvement planning.
7. Consensus among all stakeholders must be gained to have an impact on quality.
8. Health policy should include a focus on continuous enhancement of quality.

Some of the aforementioned tenets are inherent in the nursing process. Assessment is used to collect patient data. In the quality improvement methodology, data are collected to assess the state of optimal health care within, and perhaps outside the walls, of the institution. Steps of quality improvement processes using the methodology of PDCA (plan-do-check-act) are similar to the nursing process. Continuous quality improvement methodologies include the customer and the patient, as does nursing, in mutual goal setting. Standardization of processes is found in nursing diagnoses and interventions. Nurses are members of the multidisciplinary CQI teams. They also identify issues to be considered in process improvement and conduct research to identify best practice standards.

5. **Why is it important to have standardized performance measures?**

Standardized performance measures provide a means of measurement with other health care systems against the "gold standard." These measurements are established guidelines of structural standards, process standards, and outcome standards. Using standardized performance measures assists the organization in setting quality goals.

6. **Describe JCAHO national patient safety goals. Pick one safety goal and describe how it has been implemented in your organization.**

The JCAHO national patient safety goals are listed on the website listed in Box 39-5 of the Huber text. There are several goals listed under each category, one being Ambulatory Care and Office-based Surgery, one being "Improve the safety of using infusion pumps." Many institutions have changed infusion pumps to ones that have a safety device to prevent a sudden continuous infusion if the pump is jarred and the infusion door is opened inadvertently.

7. **List four ways nurse managers personally can create an environment that is devoted to health care safety.**

Nurse managers can establish a culture that is consistent with the standards of the Institute of Medicine Committee on Health Care Quality in America, which promote that care is safe, effective, patient-centered, timely, efficient, and equitable. Nurse managers can develop a nonpunitive work culture, examine processes and systems issues for problems rather than people, mentor others toward the goals of "excellence" in health care and in the evaluation of data, and provide positive feedback and rewards for achievement of these goals.

8. **What is a FMECA, and how does it contribute to improving patient safety?**

Failure modes effects and criticality analysis (FMECA) is a formal process to assess high-risk processes. This process now is required by the JCAHO to be conducted at least annually in order to evaluate the health care risk reduction and management programs of an institution.

9. **Describe strategies that a nurse manager can use to avoid or prevent a sentinel event from occurring in his or her areas of responsibility.**

The implementation of the JCAHO national patient safety goals can assist in decreasing sentinel events. Some of these safety goals include the following:

- Improve the accuracy of patient identification.
- Improve the effectiveness of communication among caregivers.
- Improve the safety of using medications.

Education of staff and others of newly documented sentinel events and proactive planning will assist in the prevention of a sentinel event occurrence.

10. **List at least one public reporting system to which your organization submits data. Describe the outcomes from one of these measures.**

Organization can submit data to several public reporting systems: HEDIS, the Commission on Accreditation of Rehabilitation Facilities, and the JCAHO core measures program. Data can be collected from different institutions on various high-priority health issues and related measures. Data then are collated, and institutions can be compared with other institutions of similar characteristics.

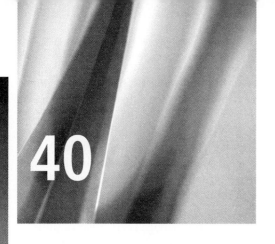

40

Measuring and Managing Outcomes

STUDY FOCUS

Outcomes research is important to help nurses understand the results of clinical practices and health care interventions (Agency for Healthcare Research and Quality, 2004). Beginning with Florence Nightingale, nurses have focused on outcomes. Florence Nightingale was the pioneer of systematic client outcomes evaluation through the collection and analysis of data on mortality for the improvement of health care in a hospital in Crimea. Today, it is imperative for nurses to collect data on outcomes measurement in order to provide evidence of effectiveness, efficiency, and cost benefits of services performed. The benefits of measuring health care outcomes include surviving in an unstable job market, improving the quality of care, informing health care consumers, and ensuring the perspective of nursing is represented. Consumers are demanding to know the extent to which clients are benefiting from and satisfied with health care services provided.

Key terms in outcomes measurement and management include outcomes, indicators, outcomes measurement, and outcomes management. An *outcome* is the result of an effort to accomplish a goal. *Outcomes* are the end results of an effort (Huber & Oermann, 1998). *Indicators* are valid and reliable measures. Accrediting, regulatory, and health care quality assessment organizations have designed standardized health care performance indicator data sets to evaluate quality. Often, these data sets use process (i.e., pressure ulcer) and structure (i.e., staff mix) indicators to evaluate the nature and amount of care provided to clients. Examples of national quality indicator data sets include the Joint Commission on Accreditation of Healthcare Organizations ORYX initiative (JCAHO, 2004a, 2004b), the American Nurses Association (2004) National Database of Nursing Quality Indicators (NDNQI), and the National Committee for Quality Assurance indicator measurement system, the Health Plan Employer Data and Information Set (HEDIS).

Outcomes measurement is data analysis related to indicators. The process of measuring outcomes is multifaceted and is initiated with the identification of the indicators of interest. Data are aggregated, analyzed, and interpreted. Changes then are implemented based on the outcomes, and the process cycles with evaluation activities implemented. *Outcomes monitoring* is ongoing surveillance and repeated quantification of data based on observation as opposed to measurement. *Outcomes management* is a multidisciplinary process to provide quality services, enhance outcomes, and constrain costs by using process activities to improve outcomes. The goals of outcome management are to improve quality, reduce risks, decrease fragmentation, and constrain costs. The process of managing outcomes includes the following five steps: (1) data are collected, (2) trends are identified, (3) variances (deviation from what is expected) are investigated, (4) appropriate service delivery changes are determined, and (5) changes are implemented and reevaluated. This process relies on variance analysis, an outcomes management tool. Variances, positive and negative, are important and useful to track over time and to make comparisons.

Benchmarking is one method that can be used for comparison purposes. *Benchmarking* is a continual measuring of what exists in one system to the best practices of the industry. *Best practices* are processes or services that provide superior outcomes. Best practices activities generate the benchmarks on key indicators for others to use and monitor outcomes. Factors influencing the demand for outcome measurement included the lack of existing outcome studies, the need for quantifiable health care data, and the variation among medical practices in the diagnosis and treatment of clients. In addition, employers are demanding to know not only the costs of health care but also what client outcomes were achieved for the dollars invested. Potential questions that outcomes studies can answer in nursing include the following: What nursing interventions will achieve the best outcome for a specific

285

symptom in a given client population? What educational intervention is most effective in preparing clients for diagnostic interventions? What method for teaching clients and preparing family members about postoperative care is most effective? What clinical pathway is most cost-effective while maintaining high-quality care for the delivery of services for a specific population group?

Mortality data were the main client outcome data from the Nightingale period to the early 1960s. Morbidity data became the next common outcome measure. In the 1980s the classic Medical Outcomes Study framework included end points, functional status, general well-being, and satisfaction with care. In the early 1960s, Aydelotte (1962) included client welfare as an outcome in nursing care. In the 1970s, many important projects were initiated that formed the underpinnings for measuring outcomes in nursing practice. Early projects included the following: the Joint Commission on Accreditation of Healthcare Organizations recommended using outcome criteria in nursing audits; health care agencies began to develop and use criteria for measuring quality of services; Hover and Zimmer (1978) established five outcomes for use in measurement of nursing care quality (client's knowledge, medications, skills, adaptive behaviors, and health status); Horn and Swain (1978) developed outcome measures; and Daubert (1979) developed a client classification system. Also, in the 1970s the Omaha System was developed by the Visiting Nurse Association of Omaha. As part of this improvement system, the Problem Rating Scale for Outcomes was developed to include knowledge, behavior, and status. The Omaha System has developed and now is used as a practice, documentation, and information management system.

A continual emphasis on outcome measurement as a mechanism to assess quality continued to gain momentum in the 1980s. The Health Care Financing Administration, now called the Centers for Medicare & Medicaid Services, instituted an initiative to measure the effectiveness and appropriateness of health care services provided to Medicare and Medicaid clients. In 1989 the Agency for Health Care Policy and Research was created to review the effectiveness of various treatments for medical conditions. The name of the agency is now the Agency for Healthcare Research and Quality. In the 1980s the Joint Commission on Accreditation of Healthcare Organizations developed the *Indicator Measurement System* to evaluate the quality of care provided by health care organizations, which later evolved into the ORYX. The *Outcomes and Assessment Information Set* (OASIS) was developed to collect outcomes data in home care agencies. In the 1980s the OASIS project was significant in bringing about a partnership with home care agencies and

Medicare, resulting in a mandate that certified home care agencies collect outcomes data through the use of OASIS. Other systems such as the American Nurses Association NDNQI, although used by some, has not gained widespread acceptance within nursing. A data set that is used widely is the one the National Committee for Quality Assurance developed: the *Health Plan Employer Data and Information Set* (HEDIS). This data set was developed to provide a standardized system for managed care organizations to use in measuring and reporting quality performance.

Trends in outcomes measurement include the collection of complex, interactive, and multidimensional data across multiple levels. The inputs of health care services include clients, families, providers, organizations or systems, and community environment characteristics. Outcomes occur at multiple levels and may be related to clients, families, providers, organizations or systems, and populations or communities. Multidisciplinary, cross-site investigations provide useful outcome data for improving the health and well-being of communities. Leaders in health care must provide direction in outcome management to ensure detailed descriptions of important outcomes. Nurses must continue to analyze outcome data sensitive to nursing interventions, refine computerized data support for nursing-sensitive outcomes, and facilitate multidisciplinary teams toward comprehensive outcomes management. Outcomes must be evaluated at all levels: individual, organizational, and population or community-related. Jennings and colleagues (1999) presented a framework for classifying outcome indicators across disciplines (medicine, nursing, and health services) to include client-focused (diagnostic and holistically focused), provider-focused (professional provider, family caregiver focused), and organization-focused (access, cost, length of stay, morbidity, mortality, other rate-based measures).

Accurate and timely data are essential to effective leadership in outcomes measurement and management. Managers often evaluate the common cause of variability in order to manage services effectively. Special causes such as sentinel events are easy to identify, but common causes are more subtle and difficult to identify. Tools to organize and visually display data to examine common causes of variation include Pareto charts, run or trend charts, histograms, control charts, scatter diagrams, flow charts, and cause-and-effect diagrams. Nurse leaders have a powerful arsenal using a combination of outcomes thinking, multidisciplinary teamwork, and statistical data tools to manage outcomes in nursing practice. Outcomes measures for quality, service, and cost are important for employers, clients, and managers. There is a trend to design performance

286

management data systems to fit the organizational needs of a nursing service (Gregg, 2002). Report cards and dashboards are final reports generated from performance management data systems. Balanced report cards have four areas for data evaluation: internal business processes, learning and growth, customer, and financial. Dashboards identify the key factors for which nurse managers need to monitor data frequently in order to manage quality and costs. Standardized report cards are being developed and used in health care organizations to improve quality, cost, access, and services. Standardized reports also are being used to compare health care organizations in communities. Nurse leaders also can use systems that describe and classify nursing-sensitive outcomes. Examples of nursing-sensitive systems are the OMAHA system, the Nursing Intervention Classification and the Nursing-Sensitive Outcomes Classification, and the American Nurses Association NDNQI.

LEARNING TOOLS

Assessment: Outcomes

Purpose

To analyze the outcomes measures of an organization to determine whether they are nursing sensitive.

Directions

1. Conduct a short interview with a registered nurse, charge nurse, and nurse manager on the unit to which you are assigned for clinical experiences. Ask each of the individuals the following questions:

Interview Format for Outcome Measures

1. Does the unit use nursing-sensitive outcomes systems to collect and analyze data? (Examples of nursing-sensitive outcomes systems include the OMAHA system, Nursing Intervention Classification Nursing-Sensitive Outcomes Classification, and the American Nurses Association NDNQI.)

   _____

2. What is the process used to collect outcome data for this unit?

   _____

3. How often is outcome data collected on this unit?

   _____

4. Who is responsible for collecting and analyzing the outcome data?_____

5. What are the outcome measures monitored for this unit? _____

6. How is the outcome data reported to the staff of the unit? _____

7. What interventions are implemented based on outcome data? _____

2. List the outcome indicators in two categories as to nursing sensitive or non-nursing sensitive.

Outcomes Measures by Category

Nursing-Sensitive Outcomes

_____

_____

_____

_____

_____

_____

_____

_____

_____

_____

Other (Non–Nursing-Sensitive) Outcomes

_____

_____

_____

_____

_____

_____

_____

_____

_____

287

3. Add the total number of outcomes measures for the clinical unit. Are there more nursing-sensitive outcomes or non-nursing-sensitive outcomes? If there are more non-nursing-sensitive outcomes, what outcomes could be added to measure nursing interventions effectively?

4. Share the findings of the interviews with your colleagues. What did they discover? What are key outcomes for nursing? Why is it important to collect nursing-sensitive outcomes.

CASE STUDY

Jill Jordan, a nurse manager for a midsized primary health care center in Carter, Wisconsin, conducted a clinical outcomes study on all clients diagnosed with diabetes, asthma, and hypertension. The outcomes measures were high for clients who had been diagnosed with hypertension and asthma. Clinical outcomes measures for clients with a diagnosis of diabetes were low. Nurse Jordan was not surprised when the data showed that clients were meeting clinical outcomes when diagnosed with asthma or hypertension. Jon Jones, a primary care physician, had developed a client education system and managed most of the clients who were diagnosed with hypertension. Jen Jergens, a family nurse practitioner, had developed a client education system and managed most of the clients who were diagnosed with asthma.

Case Study Questions

1. What is the problem in Nurse Jordan's office?

2. Whom should Nurse Jordan involve when developing potential strategies to improve client outcomes of those with a diagnosis of diabetes?

3. Is process important in outcomes management? If so, how is process important?

4. What may be useful outcomes measures for those who have a diagnosis of diabetes?

5. How will clients, employers, and the providers in Nurse Jordan's office benefit by improving the outcome scores for those who have a diagnosis of diabetes?

LEARNING RESOURCES

Discussion Questions

1. Should nurses collect indicators that are not exclusively nursing-sensitive indicators? If so, why should they collect these indicators?

2. What is the proper balance between process and outcomes in the provision of health care services?

3. What outcomes measurement systems are there, and what is the purpose of each of these systems?

4. What are the goals of outcomes management? How can outcomes management positively affect the profession of nursing?

5. What are nursing-sensitive indicators? Provide examples.

Study Questions

Matching: Write the letter of the correct response in front of each term.

_____ 1. Outcome

_____ 2. Indicators

_____ 3. Performance measures

_____ 4. Outcomes measurement

_____ 5. Outcomes monitoring

_____ 6. Outcomes management

A. The result of care or end product

B. A valid and reliable measure

C. A quantitative tool

D. A multidisciplinary process that uses process activities for improving outcomes

E. Repeated quantification of outcomes data based on observation of indicators

F. Measuring the results of care

True or False: Circle the correct answer.

T   F   7. The Health Plan Employer Data and Information Set was designed for outcomes measurement in home care agencies.

T   F   8. Outcomes management provides relatively little data for internal use within health care organizations.

T   F   9. The majority of outcomes data collected in health care organizations is nursing sensitive.

T   F   10. The lack of documentation of effectiveness of client services and the variations in practice have triggered the demand for outcomes measurement.

T   F   11. Pareto charts, histograms, and scatter diagrams are tools designed to organize and visually display data to examine common causes of variation.

T   F   12. Outcomes are complex, interactive, and only occur in a single level such as that of client or provider.

T F 13. The Visiting Nurse Association developed the Omaha System to improve its client record system.

T F 14. The goal of outcomes management is to educate health care providers on holistic health care.

T F 15. There is significant variation in medical treatment based on geographical area.

REFERENCES

Agency for Healthcare Research and Quality. (2004). *Outcomes research fact sheet.* Washington, DC: Author. Retrieved January 11, 2005, from *www.ahrq.gov/clinic/outfact.htm*

American Nurses Association (ANA). (2004). *National database of nursing quality indications.* Silver Spring, MD: ANA.

Aydelotte, M. (1962). The use of patient welfare as a criterion measure. *Nursing Research, 11*(1), 10-14.

Daubert, E. (1979). Patient classification system and outcome criteria. *Nursing Outlook, 27,* 450-454.

Gregg, A. C. (2002). Performance management data systems for nursing service organizations. *Journal of Nursing Administration, 32*(2), 71-78.

Horn, B. J., & Swain, M. A. (1978). *Criterion measures of nursing care quality* (DHEW Pub. No. PHS78-3187). Hyattsville, MD: National Center for Health Services Research.

Hover, J., & Zimmer, M (1978). Nursing quality assurance: The Wisconsin system. *Nursing Outlook, 26,* 242-248.

Huber, D., & Oermann, M. (1998). Do outcomes equal quality? *Outcomes Management for Nursing Practice, 3*(1), 1-3.

Jennings, B. M., Staggers, N., & Brosch, L. R. (1999). A classification scheme for outcome indicators. *Image: Journal of Nursing Scholarship, 31*(4), 381-388.

Joint Commission on Accreditation of Healthcare Organizations. (2004a). *Glossary of terms for performance measurement.* Oakbrook Terrace, IL: Author. Retrieved December 13, 2004, from *www.jcaho.org/accredited+organizations/long+term+care/oryx/glossary+of+terms/glossary.htm*

Joint Commission on Accreditation of Healthcare Organizations. (2004b). *Performance measurement in health care.* Oakbrook Terrace, IL: Author. Retrieved July 21, 2004, from *www.jcaho.org/pms/index.htm*

SUPPLEMENTAL READINGS

Bryant, L. L., Floersch, F., Richard, A. A., & Schlenker, R. (2004). Measuring healthcare outcomes to improve quality of care across post-acute care provider settings. *Journal of Nursing Care Quality, 19*(4), 368-376.

Deaton, C., & Grady, K. L. (2004). State of the science for cardiovascular nursing outcomes. *The Journal of Cardiovascular Nursing, 19*(5), 329-338.

Donabedian, A. (1985). *The methods and findings of quality assessment and monitoring: An illustrated analysis* (Vol. 3). Ann Arbor, MI: Health Administration Press.

Goodman, G. R. (2003). Outcomes measurement in pain management: Issues of disease complexity and uncertain outcomes. *Journal of Nursing Care Quality, 18*(2), 105-113.

Lageson, C. (2004). Quality focus of the first line nurse manager and relationship to unit outcomes. *Journal of Nursing Care Quality, 19*(4), 336-342.

Martin, V. (2001). Managing outcomes. *Nursing Management, 8*(1), 33-37.

Chapter 40: Measuring and Managing Outcomes (pp. 869-884)

1. Are outcomes more important than processes? Why or why not?

The outcomes of care provision have always been a focus for nurses. Although outcomes are an important measure of quality service and client care, delivery processes cannot be ignored or discounted. The path or mechanism used to achieve desired outcomes may reveal insightful or disturbing revelations regarding the attainment of outcome goals. By examining processes, nurses can make modifications and adjustments to the current system to make it more efficient, effective, and client-focused while actualizing desired outcomes.

2. Do outcomes equal quality? Discuss the rationale for why or why not.

Although related, outcomes and quality are two separate entities. Outcomes in health care are the result of providing care, whereas quality is a measurement of how well care was given. However, quality is a difficult phenomenon to measure because it holds different meaning for different groups. For example, clients, health care professionals, organizations, and regulatory agencies may view the concept of quality from different perspectives. Organizations and insurance companies may view quality from a resource management or cost-effectiveness perspective, whereas clients and families may evaluate quality by degrees of satisfaction. Health care professionals may assess quality by the amount of time and staff available for the delivery of personalized care.

3. What are the key indicators and outcomes for nursing?

Traditionally, morbidity and mortality rates were used to measure the outcome of nursing care. In addition to death and disease, other outcomes included assessment of disability, dissatisfaction, and discomfort. More recently, outcomes measures have expanded to include psychological, physiological, functional, behavioral, knowledge, home functioning, family strain, safety, symptom control, quality of life, goal attainment, client satisfaction, cost and resource allocation, and resolution of diagnosis. Examples of nursing quality indicators include incidence of client injury, occurrence of nosocomial infections, presence of pressure ulcers, and the frequency of medication errors.

4. Why are outcomes measures not defined consistently across organizations?

Several governmental and accrediting agencies have created outcomes measures that are used across organizations. Databases have been developed to evaluate outcomes for Medicare and Medicaid recipients, the quality of care provided by large health care organizations, and the effectiveness of nursing care. To identify trends and initiate changes that will improve the quality of care delivered and reduce risk, it is imperative that outcomes measures be compared by organizational location, size, and clientele. Differences in clients' health status and the presence of comorbid conditions, as well as staffing ratios and personnel mix, may explain variations in outcomes measures between organizations.

5. How do you know whether an outcome is sensitive to nursing?

Efforts to develop outcomes that are sensitive to nursing were initiated in the past 2 decades. Nursing's initial efforts to quantify its contribution to the health care system included the development of standardized nomenclature necessary to obtain comparative nursing-sensitive data. A nursing-sensitive outcome is one that focuses on the care recipients and their perceptions, conditions, and behaviors in response to nursing interventions.

6. Should nurses ignore outcomes not sensitive to nursing?

Nursing must be cognizant of outcomes that affect the gamut of health care delivery. Moreover, nurses need to examine organizationally sensitive outcomes that may mask the positive impact of nursing care. As nurses make astute clinical decisions that maximize client outcomes while reducing health care expenditures, the ability to discern the cost savings for the institution would provide data that were nursing sensitive.

7. How do nurses determine nursing-sensitive indicators?

Nursing-sensitive indicators can be developed as a result of process improvement initiatives, or nurses can use standardized health care performance indicator data sets from regulating bodies or related health care quality assessment organizations such as the American Nurses Association. The American Nurses Association has the National Database of Nursing Quality Indicators based on its Nursing Quality Indicator initiative (American Nurses Association, 1996, 2004). Nurses also can survey clients and families to determine what factors are considered important client and family satisfiers.

Chapter **40 Measuring and Managing Outcomes**

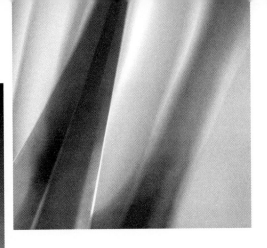

Answer Key

CHAPTER 1: LEADERSHIP PRINCIPLES

Fill in the Blank

1. Autocratic: Direct leadership is needed.
2. Democratic: Direction is needed through facilitation and coordination.
3. Democratic or laissez-faire approach: Direction is provided, but group leadership is allowed and team work is facilitated

True or False

4. T
5. F
6. F
7. T
8. T
9. F
10. F
11. T
12. F
13. T

Matching

14. B
15. H
16. F
17. C
18. G
19. A
20. D
21. E

CHAPTER 2: MANAGEMENT PRINCIPLES

True or False

1. F
2. F
3. T
4. T
5. F
6. T
7. F
8. T
9. F
10. T

CHAPTER 3: PROFESSIONAL PRACTICE AND CAREER DEVELOPMENT

Matching

1. G
2. A
3. F
4. H
5. B
6. E
7. C
8. D

True or False

9. T
10. T
11. F
12. T
13. F
14. T
15. F
16. F
17. T
18. F
19. T
20. T
21. T
22. F

CHAPTER 4: MANAGING TIME AND STRESS

True or False

1. T
2. F
3. F
4. F

Matching

5. J
6. I
7. G
8. F
9. C
10. D
11. H
12. B
13. A
14. E

CHAPTER 5: HEALTH POLICY, HEALTH, AND NURSING

True or False

1. T
2. F
3. F
4. T
5. F
6. F
7. F
8. T
9. T
10. F
11. F
12. F
13. T

CHAPTER 6: CRITICAL THINKING SKILLS

True or False

1. F
2. T
3. F
4. T
5. F
6. F
7. T
8. T
9. F
10. F
11. T
12. F

Matching

13. G
14. C
15. E
16. F
17. D
18. B
19. A
20. H
21. I

CHAPTER 7: DECISION-MAKING SKILLS

True or False

1. F
2. T
3. T
4. F
5. T
6. T
7. F
8. F
9. F
10. F

Matching

11. E
12. D
13. G
14. H
15. F
16. C
17. A
18. B
19. I
20. J

CHAPTER 8: THE HEALTH CARE SYSTEM

Matching

1. D
2. E
3. B
4. C
5. F
6. A
7. G

True or False

8. T
9. F
10. T
11. F
12. T

CHAPTER 9: ORGANIZATIONAL CLIMATE AND CULTURE

True or False

1. T
2. T
3. F
4. F
5. T
6. F
7. F
8. T
9. T
10. T

Multiple Choice

11. B
12. A

CHAPTER 10: MISSION STATEMENTS, POLICIES, AND PROCEDURES

True or False

1. T
2. F
3. F
4. T
5. F
6. F
7. F
8. T
9. T
10. T

Matching

11. B
12. D
13. A
14. C
15. E
16. F

CHAPTER 11: ORGANIZATIONAL STRUCTURE

Matching

1. I
2. C
3. D
4. E
5. F
6. A
7. B
8. J
9. G
10. H
11. S
12. R
13. T
14. Q
15. P
16. O
17. N
18. M
19. L
20. K

True or False

21. F
22. T
23. T
24. F
25. T

CHAPTER 12: DECENTRALIZATION AND SHARED GOVERNANCE

True or False

1. F
2. F
3. T
4. F
5. F
6. T
7. T
8. T
9. F
10. F
11. F
12. T

CHAPTER 13: DATA MANAGEMENT AND INFORMATICS

Matching

1. E
2. C
3. A
4. B
5. D
6. F
7. J
8. G
9. H
10. I

True or False

11. T
12. T
13. F
14. T

CHAPTER 14: STRATEGIC MANAGEMENT

True or False

1. T
2. T
3. T
4. F
5. F
6. F
7. T
8. T
9. T
10. F

CHAPTER 15: MARKETING

Matching

1. D
2. I
3. H
4. A
5. F
6. B
7. G
8. E
9. C

True or False

10. T
11. F
12. T
13. T
14. T
15. F

CHAPTER 16: MODELS OF CARE DELIVERY

True or False

1. F
2. T

Matching

3. J
4. I
5. E
6. D
7. B
8. C
9. F
10. A
11. G
12. H

CHAPTER 17: CASE MANAGEMENT

Matching

1. D
2. E
3. B
4. C
5. A

True or False

6. T
7. F
8. T
9. T
10. T
11. T
12. F
13. T
14. F
15. F
16. T
17. T
18. F
19. T
20. T
21. T
22. T
23. T

CHAPTER 18: DISEASE MANAGEMENT

Matching

1. C
2. J
3. D
4. B
5. H
6. F
7. I
8. G
9. E
10. A

CHAPTER 19: PATIENT AND FAMILY CULTURAL VALUES

True or False

1. T
2. T
3. F
4. F
5. T
6. T
7. F
8. F
9. T

Matching

10. D
11. A
12. C
13. B
14. E

CHAPTER 20: COMMUNICATION, PERSUASION, AND NEGOTIATION

True or False

1. F
2. F
3. F
4. F
5. F
6. F
7. F
8. T
9. T
10. T
11. T
12. T
13. F

Matching

14. I
15. J
16. F
17. E
18. H
19. A
20. B
21. G
22. C
23. D

CHAPTER 21: ALL-HAZARDS DISASTER PREPAREDNESS

True or False

1. T
2. T
3. T
4. F
5. F
6. F
7. T
8. T
9. F
10. F
11. T
12. T
13. T
14. T

CHAPTER 22: EVIDENCE-BASED PRACTICE: STRATEGIES FOR NURSING LEADERS

Matching

1. B
2. A
3. D
4. J
5. C
6. H
7. E
8. G
9. L
10. I
11. F
12. K

CHAPTER 23: MOTIVATION

Matching

1. D
2. E
3. F
4. A
5. G
6. C
7. B

True or False

8. T
9. F
10. F
11. T
12. F

CHAPTER 24: POWER AND CONFLICT

Matching

1. D
2. C
3. J
4. H
5. I
6. A
7. B
8. E
9. G
10. F

True or False

11. F
12. T
13. F
14. F
15. T
16. T
17. T
18. F
19. T
20. F
21. T
22. F

CHAPTER 25: DELEGATION

Matching

1. J
2. I
3. H
4. G
5. F
6. B
7. D
8. E
9. C
10. A

True or False

11. T
12. F
13. T
14. F
15. T

CHAPTER 26: TEAM BUILDING AND WORKING WITH EFFECTIVE GROUPS

True or False

1. T
2. F
3. F
4. F
5. T
6. F
7. T
8. F
9. T
10. F
11. F
12. T
13. F
14. T

Matching

15. C
16. A
17. B

CHAPTER 27: CONFRONTING THE NURSING SHORTAGE

True or False

1. F
2. F
3. T
4. T
5. T
6. F
7. F
8. F
9. T
10. T

CHAPTER 28: CULTURAL AND GENERATIONAL WORKFORCE DIVERSITY

True or False

1. T
2. T
3. T
4. F
5. F
6. T
7. F
8. F

Matching

9. D
10. A
11. C
12. B

CHAPTER 29: STAFF RECRUITMENT AND RETENTION

Matching

1. C
2. E
3. H
4. G
5. B
6. K
7. A
8. J
9. I
10. D
11. F

CHAPTER 30: PERFORMANCE APPRAISAL

Matching

1. E
2. F
3. I
4. J
5. G
6. H
7. A
8. B
9. D
10. C

CHAPTER 31: PREVENTION OF WORKPLACE VIOLENCE

True or False

1. T
2. F
3. F
4. T
5. T
6. T
7. F
8. T
9. T
10. T

CHAPTER 32: COLLECTIVE BARGAINING

Matching

1. G
2. E
3. F
4. H
5. D
6. I
7. J
8. A
9. C
10. B

True or False

11. T
12. F
13. T
14. T
15. F

CHAPTER 33: STAFFING AND SCHEDULING

True or False

1. F
2. F
3. T
4. T
5. F
6. F
7. T
8. F
9. F
10. T

CHAPTER 34: LEGAL AND ETHICAL ISSUES

True or False

1. F
2. T
3. F
4. F
5. T
6. F

Matching

7. B
8. E
9. C
10. A
11. D
12. F

CHAPTER 35: FINANCIAL MANAGEMENT

Matching

1. D
2. C
3. B
4. F
5. E
6. H
7. A
8. G
9. J
10. I

True or False

11. T
12. T
13. F
14. T

CHAPTER 36: BUDGETING

Matching

1. E
2. F
3. G
4. D
5. H
6. I
7. J
8. C
9. B
10. A

True or False

11. F
12. T

CHAPTER 37: PRODUCTIVITY AND COSTING OUT NURSING

True or False

1. F
2. F
3. F
4. T
5. F
6. F
7. F
8. F
9. T
10. F
11. T
12. F
13. T
14. T
15. F

CHAPTER 38: CHANGE AND INNOVATION

True or False

1. T
2. T
3. F
4. F
5. F
6. T
7. T
8. T
9. F
10. T

CHAPTER 39: QUALITY IMPROVEMENT AND HEALTH CARE SAFETY

True or False

1. F
2. F
3. F
4. F
5. F
6. T
7. T
8. T
9. T
10. F
11. F

CHAPTER 40: MEASURING AND MANAGING OUTCOMES

Matching

1. A
2. B
3. C
4. F
5. E
6. D

True or False

7. F
8. F
9. F
10. F
11. T
12. F
13. T
14. F
15. T